An Introduction to
Removable Denture Prosthetics

An Introduction to Removable Denture Prosthetics

Alan A. Grant MSc DDSc FRACDS

Professor of Prosthetic Dentistry, University of
Manchester; Consultant in Restorative Dentistry,
Central Manchester Health Authority; External
Examiner to the Universities of Dublin and Dundee
and the Manchester Polytechnic; Former Examiner
to dental students in the Universities of Baghdad,
Cardiff, Leeds, Liverpool, London, Malaya,
Melbourne and Singapore; Formerly Visiting
Associate Professor of Dental Materials,
Northwestern University, Chicago.

Wesley Johnson BSc MSc LDS

Senior Lecturer in Prosthetic Dentistry, University
of Manchester; Consultant in Restorative Dentistry,
Central Manchester Health Authority; Examiner and
Assessor to the City and Guilds of London Institute
for the Dental Technician's Certificate; Formerly
Visiting Associate Professor of Dental Materials,
Northwestern University, Chicago.

CHURCHILL LIVINGSTONE
EDINBURGH LONDON MELBOURNE AND NEW YORK 1983

CHURCHILL LIVINGSTONE
Medical Division of Longman Group Limited

Distributed in the United States of America by Churchill
Livingstone Inc., 1560 Broadway, New York, N.Y. 10036, and
by associated companies, branches and representatives
throughout the world.

First published 1983
  Reprinted 1986

ISBN 0-443-02377-8

British Library Cataloguing in Publication Data
Grant, A.A.
    An introduction to removable denture prosthetics.
    1. Dentures   2. Dentistry — Laboratory manuals.
    I. Title   II. Johnson, W.
    617.6'92'028   RK656

Library of Congress Cataloging in Publication Data
Grant, A.A.
    An introduction to removable denture prosthetics.
    Bibliography: p.
    Includes index.
    1. Complete dentures. 2. Partial dentures,
Removable. I. Johnson, W. (Wesley) II. Title [DNLM: 1.
Denture, Complete. 2 Denture, Partial, Removable. 3. Dental
prosthesis. WU 530 G76li]
RK656.G67 1983   617.6'92   82-17806

Produced by Longman Singapore Publishers Pte Ltd
Printed in Singapore

Preface

This book has been prepared principally for the undergraduate student who is about to undertake the study of clinical prosthetic dentistry. The text has been kept to a minimum in the interests of simplicity. No laboratory procedures have been included as it is common practice in most undergraduate dental courses for the student to acquire a background in dental technology prior to the commencement of the clinical course.

In common with other clinical disciplines, prosthetic treatment cannot be learned by rote and then applied as a series of procedures which will be equally appropriate to all patients. The physiological differences and psychological individuality of human beings as well as their physical form, health status, social circumstances and other innumerable factors which make up the individual must all be considered. They point to the impossibility of a single approach being successfully applied to all patients. The main thrust of this work has therefore concentrated on principles. Detailed description has been included only where existing works differ in some respect from a suggested approach. Further reading lists have been included in the hope that they will be consulted for three main reasons. First, as a means of expanding the content of the relevant chapter. Second, to introduce the student gently to some of the controversies that exist in the clinical field. Third, to initiate or strengthen the habit of consulting the literature, for it is here that the quality of professional life is nurtured.

Given the introductory nature of this book, which is directed towards undergraduate dental students, it is hoped that it may also be of value to the various dental auxiliary groups where it may contribute to their understanding more readily than do more advanced texts.

Manchester 1983
                                                    A.A.G.
                                                    W.J.

Acknowledgements

All the illustrations have been produced by Anne-marie Grant to whom we are deeply indebted for her skills and forbearance. The bulk of the typing was carried out by Mrs O'Neill, assisted by Mrs T. Quinn and our gratitude for their patience through the tedious drafting procedures and in producing the manuscript is gratefully recorded. Proof reading has been greatly assisted by Mrs O'Neill and Mrs Quinn.

Finally, we acknowledge the support of Heather and Anne over the period of development of the book. We apologise for our lack of attention to domestic matters over the time concerned and record our deep appreciation for the support they have given.

Contents

Part I — Basic aspects

1. Essential anatomy and physiology of
   the masticatory system   3
2. Denture retention   18
3. Principles related to denture design   24
4. Psychological aspects   29
5. Examination   32
6. Diagnosis and treatment planning   45
7. Preparation of the mouth for
   prosthetic treatment   51
8. Principles of impression procedures   56
9. Principles of registering jaw
   relationships   61
10. Dental articulators and their selection   68
11. Principles of tooth selection   75

**Part II — Special aspects relating to partial
denture treatment**

12. Introductory considerations   87
13. Component elements   92
14. Designing partial dentures   116
15. The impression stage of treatment   127
16. The jaw registration stage of treatment   136
17. The principles of tooth arrangement   142
18. The trial denture stage of treatment   145
19. The insertion stage of treatment   151
20. The review stage of treatment   154
21. The free-end saddle partial denture   159

**Part III — Special aspects relating to complete
denture treatment**

22. The impression stage of treatment   169
23. The jaw registration stage of treatment   179
24. The principles of tooth arrangement   191
25. The trial denture stage of treatment   200
26. The insertion stage of treatment   207
27. The review stage of treatment   213
28. The overdenture   223
Further reading   226
Index   227

PART I

Basic Aspects

1

Essential anatomy and physiology of the masticatory system

INTRODUCTION

A knowledge of the anatomy and physiology of the masticatory system is essential to the treatment of patients requiring prosthetic service. It must be appreciated that the provision of removable dentures represents an attempt to replace lost vital tissues, and to this end harmony of the appliance with the biological environment in which it is placed is of fundamental importance. This can only be achieved where the structure, function and functional interdependence of the related tissues is appreciated.

In this chapter it is intended to consider only those aspects of the anatomy and physiology of oral structures which are of direct importance in removable denture treatment. Further details of related tissues and their functions may be obtained from the current literature.

ANATOMY

The anatomical features relevant to the provision of a removable denture service may be considered as follows:-
1. Extra-oral surface anatomy.
2. Intra-oral surface anatomy.
3. Structures influencing the periphery of dentures.
4. Deeper anatomy.

Extra-oral surface anatomy

Figure 1.1 illustrates those structures which will be referred to in the descriptions of clinical procedures in later chapters.

Fig. 1.1 Important landmarks on the face: A, Outer canthus; B, Tragus; C, Ala; D, Columella; E, Naso-labial groove; F, Philtrum; G, Angle of mouth; H, Labio-mental groove.

It has been observed that the naso-labial angle, i.e. the angle formed between the columella and the upper lip in the sagittal plane is, on the average, approximately 90°. Where the teeth are retroclined, the angle tends to be obtuse, and proclination of the upper anterior teeth is often accompanied by an acute naso-labial angle (Fig. 1.2).

As with all generalisations relating to human anatomy the above may be considered useful guidelines only. The value of observations of this nature in the restoration of lost natural tissue is inestimable.

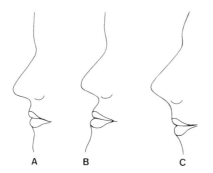

Fig. 1.2 The naso-labial angle in the sagittal plane. A, Right angle; B, Acute angle; C, Obtuse angle.

Intra-oral surface anatomy

Figure 1.3 is a diagrammatic representation of the surface features of the dentate mouth and the edentulous mouth.

With the loss of natural teeth, the alveolar ridge resorbs and becomes the residual alveolar ridge. Resorption is initially rapid following tooth loss and then continues, sometimes intermittently, through the lifetime of the patient. The height of the residual alveolar ridge is reduced in both the maxilla and mandible, but in other aspects the pattern of bone loss in the upper and lower jaws differs.

Resorption of the maxillary ridge occurs mainly labially and buccally (Fig. 1.4A and B). In the anterior region, the incisive papilla appears to become more prominent and situated on the 'crest' of the residual alveolar ridge. When the natural incisors are in situ, the midpoint of the incisive papilla is on the average 10 ± 1 mm posterior to the labial aspect of the contact point of the central incisors (Fig. 1.5).

In the edentulous mouth, a thin fibrous band may sometimes be seen passing from the incisive papilla posteriorly along the crest of the residual alveolar ridge. This represents the collapsed palatal gingival margins following extraction of the teeth, and is called the lingual gingival remnant.

Resorption of the lower residual alveolar ridge occurs mainly labially and buccally towards the anterior part of the mouth. In the lower molar regions the residual alveolar ridge tends to retain its width, or, because of the form of the bone in the posterior segment may even appear to become wider (Fig. 1.4 C).

The sulci

The alveolar ridges are defined labially and buccally by a trough of soft tissue called the sulcus.

Fig. 1.3 Some surface features of the dentate mouth (left) and the edentulous mouth (right). A, Labial frenum (upper); B, Incisive papilla; C, Rugae; D, Buccal frenum; E, Median raphe; F, Residual alveolar ridge (upper); G, Fovea palatinae; H, Tuberosity; I, Palatoglossal arch; J, Retromolar pad; K, Residual alveolar ridge (lower); L, Buccal frenum; M, Gingivae; N, Vestibule; O, Labial frenum (lower).

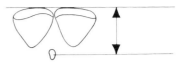

Fig. 1.5 Relation between the incisive papilla and the mid incisal point. The average distance as indicated is 10 ± 1 mm.

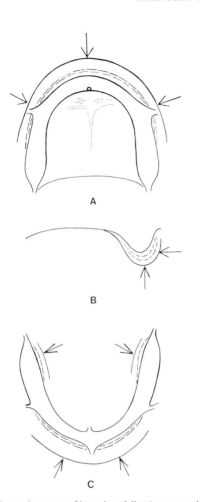

Fig. 1.4 General pattern of bone loss following extractions for the upper and lower arches. A, Upper residual ridge and palate in plan view. Rapid resorption of the residual alveolar ridge occurs in the regions indicated by the arrows. B, Sagittal section of the upper residual alveolar ridge. C, Lower residual ridge. Greatest change in the form of the residual alveolar ridge occurs in the regions indicated by the arrows.

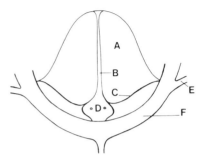

Fig. 1.6 Diagram of some structures visible with the tongue elevated. A, Tongue; B, Lingual frenum; C, Sublingual fold; D, Sublingual papillae; E, Buccal frenum; F, Residual alveolar ridge.

lower buccal sulci in the premolar regions. A lingual frenum is present in the midline of the lower lingual sulcus formed by the reflection of the mucosa from the lingual aspect of the midline to the underside of the tongue.

Under the ventral surface of the tongue on both sides of the lingual frenum is a fold of tissue in which many ducts from the sublingual salivary glands are situated. At the frenal end of each sublingual fold is an elevation called the sublingual papilla (Fig. 1.6). The openings of the ducts from all the submandibular, and some of the sublingual, salivary glands occurs via the sublingual papillae.

The palate

The palate consists anteriorly of the hard palate and posteriorly, the soft palate. Anatomically, the division between hard and soft palates is at the posterior margins of the palatal processes of the palatine bones.

The functional division between hard and soft palates is of more significance in removable denture construction, and this may not coincide with the anatomical division. The functional division is often called the vibrating line and is that imaginary palatal line of tissue which just fails to vibrate

The sulcus is formed by the reflection of the mucosa attached to the tissue overlying the bony ridges into the lips and cheeks. The depth of the sulcus varies in different parts of the mouth.

The lower alveolar ridge also possesses a lingual sulcus formed by the reflection of the mucosa into the tissues of the floor of the mouth.

Within the sulci are seen frenal attachments (or frenula) which are bands of mucous membrane. A labial frenum occurs in the midline of both the upper and lower jaws. Buccal frenal attachments are present usually one on each side of both upper and when the patients says 'aah'. The form of the vibrating line is generally that of a bow, concave posteriorly, whereas the anatomical division between hard and soft palates is that of a double bow, concave posteriorly.

Anteriorly the palate shows a number of transverse ridges of soft tissue known as the palatal rugae. Their functions is obscure, but may be associated with stabilisation of food during mastication.

In many patients two small depressions occur on either side of the midline in the region of the functional division between hard and soft palates. These are the fovea palatinae and it is thought that they represent the common ductal openings of some of the palatal salivary glands.

A torus palatinus may be present in the midline of the hard palate. This is a mound of bone usually covered by a layer of thin mucosa. It is a benign structure of variable size and form.

More rarely, the mandible may show the torus mandibularis. This is a benign mound of bone which occurs bilaterally in the lingual aspects of the mandible in the premolar region.

The retromolar pad

The mandibular alveolar ridge terminates distally in an elevated pad of soft tissue called the retromolar pad. This represents the tissue covering the lower anterior part of the ascending ramus of the mandible. Where the last molar tooth has been lost, in some cases a pear-shaped pad is seen just anterior to the retromolar pad. This structure represents the collapsed papilla related to the last molar tooth.

The tissue covering approximately the anterior third of the retromolar pad is fixed, and beyond this the tissue moves during functional movements of the mouth due to the presence of muscle tissue.

The mucous membrane

The mucous membrane of the mouth is of the stratified squamous type.

A classification of the oral mucous membrane is as follows:
1. Masticatory — covering the hard palate and most regions of the gingivae.
2. Lining — covering the oral surfaces of the cheeks and lips, the labial and buccal sulci, the floor of the mouth, ventral surface of the tongue and the soft palate.
3. Specialised — covering the dorsal surface of the tongue.

The masticatory mucosa covers immobile tissue and is keratinised, whereas lining mucosa covers mobile tissues and is usually non-keratinised. Specialised mucosa is a mixture of both keratinised and non-keratinised types.

The mucous membrane and submucous tissues which cover the palate and alveolar ridges is of varying thickness and consistency. This tissue may be several millimetres thick and resilient in character, or thin with minimal sub-epithelial tissue, and wide variation may exist in a single patient.

The mucosa covering the dorsal surface of the tongue is highly specialised, with the anterior two-thirds covered with filiform and fungiform papillae and deliniated from the posterior third by the circumvallate papillae.

Smooth mucous membrane covers the lateral borders of the tongue anteriorly. Posteriorly, several parallel vertical folds of tissue called foliate papillae occur and these may be prominent in some patients.

The ventral surface of the tongue is covered with smooth mucosa through which blood vessels may be seen. Some elderly people show a nodular enlargement of the superficial veins of the ventral surface of the tongue and these lingual varicosities, when prominent, are readily visible.

The functions of the oral mucosa are both protective to the underlying structures, and sensory — providing temperature, pressure, taste, and possibly proprioceptive functions.

Structures influencing the periphery of dentures

The periodontal tissues

The periodontium consists of the investing and supporting tissues of the teeth and includes the gingivae, the periodontal ligament, the cementum and the alveolar bone. The periodontium supports the tooth, provides proprioceptive sensory function and has also a metabolic function.

The most readily observable of these tissues is

the gingival tissue which is that portion of the oral mucous membrane which surrounds the neck of the tooth and covers the alveolar bone crest. The gingival tissues may be divided into three portions:

1. *The free (marginal) gingivae.* This is the most peripheral portion and comprises a narrow smooth rim which follows the cervical contours of the tooth. It terminates at the gingival margin on the tooth side and apically at the gingival groove which demarcates the free and attached gingivae.

2. *The attached gingivae.* Apically, the attached gingivae merges into the alveolar mucosa at the mucogingival junction, except palatally where no mucogingival junction exists. The attached gingiva is characterised by a stippled appearance which results from interconnection of the epithelium — connective tissue interface.

3. *The interdental gingivae.* This is the tissue located at and within the interproximal space of adjacent teeth. Between posterior teeth which are in contact, the interdental gingiva consists of two elevated portions — the vestibular and lingual papillae — having an apically curved col between them.

Cementum provides a means for attachment of the periodontal fibres. It may become exposed to the mouth as a result of age or periodontal disease. The other periodontal tissues are not visible on examination of the mouth. However, a detailed appreciation of all the periodontal tissues is an essential part of the knowledge required by the prosthetist, and to this end a reference text should be consulted. In particular, note should be made of the structure of the periodontal ligament and the arrangement of the fibres, which appear to permit best resistance to forces directed down the long axis of the tooth.

Figure 1.7 is a diagram of a mesiodistal section through the gingival tissues, showing their relationship to other periodontal tissues.

The remainder of this section will be considered in respect of complete denture bases in order that all the peripheral structures are dealt with.

The maxillary denture periphery (Fig. 1.8)

The most anterior part of the periphery of the denture base is grooved by the labial frenum. Further distally, in the region of the lateral incisor, the fibres of the incisivus labii superioris arise from the alveolar border of the maxilla and arch laterally to become part of the muscle tissue comprising part of the orbicularis oris muscle. The tissue overlying this muscle limits the denture periphery in the region of the lateral incisor.

In the region of the canine fossa and inferior to the infra-orbital foramen is the origin of the levator anguli oris muscle. This muscle is also inserted into the muscular tissue forming the orbicularis oris muscle.

The buccal frenum limits denture base extension in the premolar region. Distal to this the

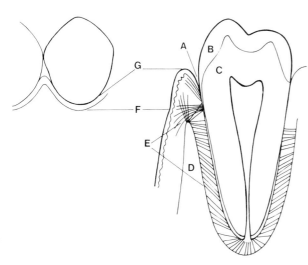

Fig. 1.7 The gingival tissues, showing their relationship to other periodontal tissues. A, Gingival crevice; B, Enamel; C, Dentine; D, Bone; E, Fibres of the periodontal ligament; F, Gingival groove; G, Free (marginal) gingivae.

Fig. 1.8 Lateral view of an upper denture showing structures which influence the peripheral form. A, Labial frenum; B, Incisivus labii superioris muscle; C, Levator anguli oris muscle; D, Buccal frenum; E, Zygomatic process of maxilla; F, Buccinator muscle; G, Pterygomandibular raphe.

Fig. 1.10 Lateral aspect of a lower denture showing the structures which influence the peripheral form. A, Mentalis muscle; B, Incisivus labii inferioris muscle; C, Depressor labii inferioris muscle; D, Depressor anguli oris muscle; E, Mental foramen; F, Buccinator muscle.

Fig. 1.9 Structures related to the left tuberosity region in plan view (left) and lateral view (right). A, Tuberosity; B, Hamular notch; C, I ateral pterygoid plate; D, Medial pterygoid plate; E, Pterygoid hamulus.

zygomatic process of the maxilla — sometimes known as the root of the zygomatic arch — limits extension of the denture base.

Further distally, the buccinator muscle arises from the buccal surface of the alveolar process of the maxilla in the region of the upper molar teeth and also from the pterygo-mandibular raphe. The tissue overlying both these structures influences the denture base extension.

Between the tuberosity of the maxilla and the upper end of the pterygomandibular raphe a delicate tendinous band bridges the gap between the maxilla and the hamulus of the pterygoid bone. A few fibres of the buccinator muscle arise from this band and form a concavity in the overlying mucous membrane which is known as the hamular notch (Fig. 1.9).

After passing from the buccal sulcus around the maxillary tuberosity, the hamular notch is the limiting structure to denture base extension.

The vibrating line lies between the hamular notches and represents the functional division between fixed and movable palatal tissue. It is commonly, but not invariably, just anterior to the fovea palatinae and defines the posterior anatomical extension of the fully extended maxillary denture base.

The mandibular denture periphery (Fig. 1.10)

The most anterior part of the labial denture base periphery is usually grooved by the labial frenum.

Lateral to the labial frenum and arising from the incisive fossa of the mandible is the mentalis muscle. The fibres of the mentalis muscle descend to their insertion in the skin of the chin. Further laterally, the periphery is influenced by the tissues overlying the incisivus labii inferioris which arises at a similar level to the mentalis muscle. The incisivus labii inferioris is inserted into the orbicularis oris muscle.

More distally, the depressor labii inferioris muscle arises between the symphysis menti and the mental foramen and is inserted into the orbicularis oris muscle. Passing further distally the periphery is influenced by the tissues overlying the depressor anguli oris muscle. It arises from the oblique line of the mandible below and lateral to the depressor labii inferioris muscle and up to the mesial aspect of the first molar tooth. This muscle is also inserted into the orbicularis oris muscle.

A buccal frenum is usually present superior to either the depressor anguli oris or the depressor labii superioris muscles, and this structure limits the peripheral denture extension in this region.

Lateral to the first molar teeth the tissue overlying the buccinator muscle delineates the buccal sulcus. This muscle is attached to the external oblique ridge of the mandible and the pterygo-mandibular raphe, and mingles with the superior fibres arising from the maxilla.

Distally, the denture base covers the anterior third of the retromolar pad only, as buccinator fibres are inserted into the posterior two-thirds and this latter position therefore moves when buccinator activity occurs.

As the outline of the lower denture proceeds lingually, the attachment of the buccinator muscle

Fig. 1.11 Lingual aspect of a lower complete denture showing structures which influence the peripheral form. A, Genioglossus muscle; B, Geniohyoid muscle; C, Sublingual gland; D, Mylohyoid muscle; E, Superior pharyngeal constrictor; F, Palatoglossal arch; G, Buccinator muscle.

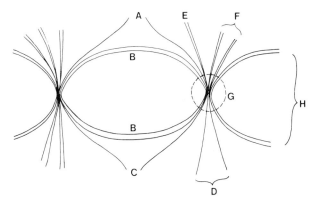

Fig. 1.12 Illustration of the circumoral musculature. A, Incisivus labii superioris muscles; B, Orbicularis oris muscle; C, Incisivus labii inferioris muscles; D, Depressor anguli oris and caninus muscles; E, Levator anguli oris muscles; F, Zygomaticus muscle; G, Modiolus; H, Buccinator muscle.

to the pterygo-mandibular ligament and also the superior constrictor muscle of the pharynx limits possible denture base extension. The forward movement of the palatoglossal arch during actions such as swallowing defines the posterior lingual extension of the denture base (Fig. 1.11).

The lingual extension of the complete lower denture base is mainly influenced by the tissues overlying the mylohyoid muscle which has as its origin the whole length of the mylohyoid line. It inserts via a midline fibrous raphe to fibres from the opposite side, also to the anterior aspect of the body of the hyoid bone at its inferior border.

More anteriorly, the sublingual salivary gland lies superior to the mylohyoid muscle. In the midline, the tissue overlying the genioglossus muscle at its attachment to the superior genial tubercles deliniates the extension of the denture base.

Deeper anatomy

A number of the deeper anatomical structures of the head also influence the shape of removable dentures, especially the surface aspects of the appliance.

Anteriorly, the oral sphincter and the associated obicularis oris muscle have a strong influence.

Near the angle of the mouth the decussation of the fibres of muscles associated with the orbicularis oris, together with those of the buccinator form the modiolus (Fig. 1.12). A number of the muscles of facial expression are also inserted into the modiolus. The modiolus is a region of intensive muscular activity and may have a strong influence on denture design in the premolar region. This is further considered in Chapter 3.

The relationship of the muscle tissue about the periphery of a lower denture when shown in a plan view gives an indication of its importance in denture base design (Fig. 1.13).

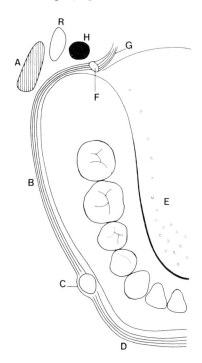

Fig. 1.13 Relationship of musclar tissue to the periphery of the right half of a lower denture in plan view. A, Masseter muscle; B, Buccinator muscle; C, Modiolus; D, Orbicularis oris muscle; E, Tongue; F, Pterygomandibular raphe; G, Superior constrictor muscle; H, Medial pterygoid muscle; R, Ramus of mandible.

The temporomandibular joint

The temporomandibular joint is the joint between the cranium and the mandible. The bony elements involved are the articular eminence, glenoid tubercle of the temporal bone and the condyle of the mandible.

The joint is paired and the right and left joints are not independent of each other as the cranial and mandibular elements are, in effect, single bones.

The glenoid fossa is lined with a thin layer of fibrous tissue which is much thicker anteriorly, covering the articular eminence. The slope of the articular eminence varies widely between individuals and may be subject to change during life.

The mandibular condyle is roughly elliptical in form with the long axis being directed medio-laterally and the short axis antero-posteriorly. The articular surface is covered with a layer of fibrous tissue which is thickest over the convexity of the condyle.

Interposed between the cranial and mandibular elements of the joint is the articular disc or meniscus. The disc is not uniformly thick having a thin central area and thickened anterior and posterior portions.

Posteriorly, the disc is composed of two layers. The upper lamina of the disc attaches to the squamo-tympanic fissure and the lower lamina to the posterior surface of the neck of the condyle. The upper lamina contains loose white fibroelastic tissue. Anteriorly, the disc is attached to the anterior edge of the articular eminence and the articular margin of the condyle (Fig. 1.14).

The capsule of the joint is thin anteriorly and posteriorly, but is strengthened medially and laterally by the capsular ligaments.

The structure of the disc and its attachments are such that a considerable range of movements of the condyle relative to the temporal bone can occur. Movement of the disc relative to the roof of the glenoid fossa can take place and also a limited amount of movement between the disc and the condyle.

The lateral poles of the condyles are approximately 1 cm beneath the skin and can be placed in the region of a point some 12 mm anterior to the tragus of the ear on a line extending to the outer canthus of the eye.

A detailed knowledge of the components and relations of the joint is essential to an understanding of the temporomandibular articulation, and reference to the literature should be made. The above description is intended to serve as a basis for considering the complex and variable nature of possible movements within the joints.

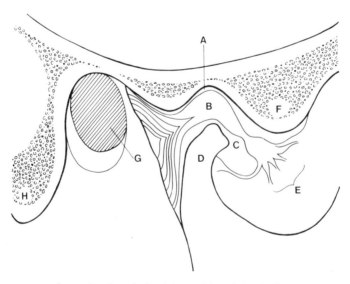

Fig. 1.14 Diagram of an anteroposterior section through the right condyle and glenoid fossa. A, Upper joint compartment; B, Disc; C, Lower joint compartment; D, Head of condyle; E, Lateral pterygoid muscle; F, Articular eminence; G, External auditory meatus; H, Mastoid process.

MANDIBULAR MOVEMENTS

In addition to the movements which may occur in the joints themselves, a knowledge of the movements of the mandible is of fundamental importance to an understanding of functional occlusion of the teeth and dentures.

Mandibular movements are generally represented as the excursions of the mid-incisal point of the mandible.

In order to understand some of the points referred to in considering relations between the jaws, it is necessary first to consider the basic terms used in this field.

Jaw positions and related terminology

There are many positions which the mandible may occupy relative to the maxilla, and also different positions in which the teeth may contact. In order to avoid confusion in description of jaw and teeth positions which are used throughout this text, it is important that a standard form of terminology be adopted.

The position of the mandible is usually described relative to the maxilla and is termed a jaw relation, which may be defined as 'the positional relationship which the mandible bears to the maxilla', and is usually considered in a vertical or horizontal plane.

When referring to tooth contact, the term occlusion is used and may be defined as 'the contact relationship of the masticatory surfaces of the teeth or their equivalent'.

The rest jaw relation

The rest jaw relation of a person is the relationship of the mandible to the maxilla when the person is seated at ease in an upright position with the Frankfort plane horizontal and the muscles controlling the mandible in equilibrium. In rest relation the opposing teeth are not in occlusion and the amount by which they are separated is known as the interocclusal distance or freeway space.

The rest jaw relation is dependent on a balance of muscular forces between the muscles attached to the mandible. The resting posture of the mandible is subject to variations both in short and long term periods. Since muscular forces are involved, a change in the posture of the patient will produce a change in the interocclusal distance. For a patient with the trunk erect, if the head is tilted forward, the interocclusal distance becomes smaller and the mandible moves anteriorly. Tilting the head backwards causes the mandible to move postero-inferiorly.

Other factors which affect the rest jaw relation include emotion, physical health, age, proprioception from the teeth, muscles and oral mucosa, and the pattern of tooth loss. Because of the clinical significance of the rest jaw relation it is important that the student familiarise himself with the current literature on this topic.

Measurement of interocclusal distance

The interocclusal distance between individual teeth is rarely measured directly and a convenient clinical method for assessing its magnitude can be obtained from reference points chosen on the midline of the face.

With a patient seated upright as described above, the interocclusal distance has been estimated to average between 2 and 4 mm.

The presence of an adequate interocclusal distance is essential to the success of removable denture treatment. Over- or under-estimation of the interocclusal distance may result in the clinical effects described in Chapter 9.

Horizontal relations

Horizontal relations between the jaws and teeth may be considered to exist anteroposteriorly in the sagittal plane and laterally in the coronal plane.

Retruded jaw relation (centric jaw relation). Retruded jaw relation is the unstrained, most retruded relation of the mandible to the maxilla at the established vertical dimension of occlusion. It should be noted that although this is essentially a horizontal jaw relation, reference is made also to the position of the mandible in the vertical plane. When the retruded jaw relation is recorded the clinician establishes the vertical dimension of the occlusion either by accepting contact of the patient's natural teeth, or by reference to the rest vertical dimension, so that an adequate interocclusal distance will result.

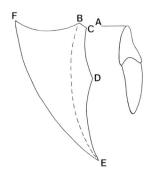

Fig. 1.15 Illustration of various condyle positions. A, Anterior part of fossa; B, Condyle; C, Maximal intercuspal position; D, Retruded jaw relation; E, Muscular stimulation.

Fig. 1.16 Border movements of the mandible in the sagittal plane. A, Represents a pointer attached to the mid-incisal point of the lower incisors; B, Teeth in maximal intercuspal position; C, Teeth in retruded jaw relation; D, Extent of hinge movement of the mandible; E, Maximum opening; F, Maximum protrusion. Line EB represents the path of habitual closure from the position of maximum opening.

Maximal intercuspal position. This is the relation of opposing occlusal surfaces at which the cusps of the maxillary and mandibular teeth contact with maximum intercuspation. It is dependent upon the presence of tooth contact, whether natural or artificial, in the molar and/or premolar regions of both maxilla and mandible.

A further position to which reference may be made is the muscular position which is the horizontal contact relation of the teeth determined by the habitual muscle pattern.

In many dentulous subjects, retruded jaw relation and the maximal intercuspal position do not correspond (Fig. 1.15).

In the treatment of edentulous subjects, however, the teeth are arranged in the maximal intercuspal position and must contact in this position in the mouth when the mandible is in the retruded jaw relation.

Border movements of the mandible

Border movements are the maximum excursive movements of the mandible which can be achieved. These movements are rarely, if ever, performed during normal functional activity such as occurs during mastication and speech. Consequently, most functional movements are intra-border movements.

Recording of border movements in the sagittal plane produces the form of excursion illustrated in Figure 1.16.

Hinge movement (or terminal hinge movement) is considered to be a purely rotational movement of the mandible about an intercondylar axis and occurs over a short distance at the commencement of opening between closure and approximately the rest position of the mandible.

In the coronal plane the border movement appears as in Figure 1.17.

In the horizontal plane, the border excursions appear as shown in Figure 1.18.

The form of excursion in the horizontal plane from the retruded jaw relation to the extremity of lateral movements produces a pattern which has been styled a gothic arch (Fig. 1.19) and has been adapted to a clinical technique. This is considered in Chapter 23.

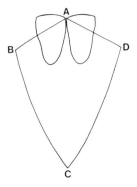

Fig. 1.17 Border movements of the mandible in the coronal plane. A, Teeth in retruded jaw relation; B, Right lateral excursion of the mandible; C, Maximum protrusion; D, Left lateral excursion of the mandible;

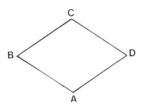

Fig. 1.18 Border movements of the mandible in the horizontal plane. A, Teeth in retruded jaw relation; B, Right lateral excursion of the mandible; C, Maximum protrusion; D, Left lateral excursion of the mandible.

Fig. 1.19 The gothic arch form. A, Retruded jaw relation; B, Right lateral excursion of the mandible; C, Left lateral excursion of the mandible;

Bennett movement

A further detail of movements of the mandible which occurs during lateral excursions should be appreciated, especially in relation to restoration of the natural dentition. This is known as the Bennett movement and consists of a bodily lateral translation of the mandible to the side towards which the mandible is moving and is illustrated in Figure 1.20. The condylar movement which

Fig. 1.20 Plan view of the mandible. The position of the mandible following a right lateral excursion is shown by the dotted outline. Bennett movement is shown by the lateral movement of right condyle.

occurs on the side towards which the mandible moves is of the order of 1–2 mm.

The muscles producing mandibular movement

Primary movements of the mandible result from the contraction of muscles attached to the mandible. The principal muscles involved are designated the muscles of mastication and they are the:
1. Masseter
2. Medial pterygoid
3. Lateral pterygoid and
4. Temporalis muscles

The digastic, geniohyoid, mylohyoid and platysma muscles are also associated with depression of the mandible.

From a functional point of view the muscles of mastication may be divided into 4 groups as illustrated in Figure 1.21.

In considering the movements of the mandible, it is important to appreciate that various combinations of muscle groups are always involved and that contraction of similar muscles of the right and left sides do not necessarily occur simultaneously and equally. The nature of the muscle activity which takes place is that of co-ordinated and reciprocal actions of the elevator and depressor muscles. In addition, reflex actions are known to occur during mandibular functional activities.

Saliva

Saliva is secreted from three large pairs of glands — the parotid, submandibular and sublingual salivary glands — and many others situated in the lips, tongue and palate. Salivary secretion is controlled by the autonomic nervous system.

Many functions have been ascribed to saliva including:

1. Moistening and lubrication of soft tissues, keeping them pliable and preventing drying.

2. Solvent action — dissolving solids and thus aiding in appreciation of food and taste bud stimulation.

3. Preparation of food for swallowing — altering the consistency and forming a lubricated plastic mass of food.

4. Digestive function — the presence of, for ex-

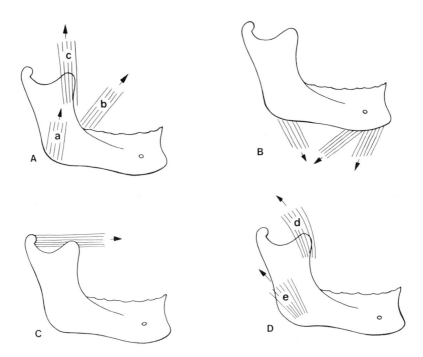

Fig. 1.21 Illustration of the activity of the mandible resulting from contraction of the major muscle groups. A, Elevators. a. Superficial and medial layers of masseter muscle; b. Medial pterygoid muscle; c. Vertical fibres of temporalis muscle. B, Depressors, including digastric, geniohyoid, platysma and posterior vertical fibres of mylohyoid muscle. C, Protractors. Lateral pterygoid muscles. D, Retractors. d. Horizontal fibres of temporalis muscle; e. Deep layers of masseter muscle.

ample, amylase, may help to dissolve starchy food substances.

5. Regulation of water balance — drying of mucous membranes results in a sensation of thirst.

6. Excretory function — many drugs and electrolytes are excreted in saliva.

7. Buffering function — saliva buffers acid in the diet and also acts as a temperature buffer against hot and cold foods.

8. Peripheral seal — saliva acts to form a peripheral seal necessary for the retention of some removable dentures and also an oral seal during the suckling process.

From the prosthetic viewpoint the formation of a peripheral seal for a denture is an important function. A further effect related to saliva is that of oral galvanism — i.e., the development of an electrical potential difference between dissimilar metals in saliva, which is a good electrolyte.

The amount of saliva secreted each day varies from individual to individual. In addition, saliva is not an homogeneous fluid but is probably best considered as a suspension of bacteria, food particles, cellular elements and other particulate elements. The composition and physical properties of saliva from an individual may vary widely throughout the day.

The property of viscosity is one which has received considerable attention in considering the retention of dentures, and in general it has been shown that there is a relationship between viscosity and adhesive capacity. In this respect the secretions of the palatine mucous glands have been

Fig. 1.22 The hatched areas indicate the approximate distribution of the palatine mucous glands.

shown to be important in the retention of a complete upper denture (Fig. 1.22).

The role of saliva in denture retention is further considered in Chapter 2.

Variations in flow

The quantity of saliva secreted may be:
1. Diminished (Xerostomia)
2. Increased (Sialorrhoea)

A temporary decrease in salivary flow may result from an emotional reaction such as fear. A large number of systemic conditions can also cause Xerostomia and it may also result as an ageing effect as the glands atrophy and may be a side effect of drug therapy.

Xerostomia may result in a 'burning' sensation of the oral tissues and tongue and cracking of lips. The oral mucosa becomes dry, smooth and translucent and denture retention is frequently severely diminished. Mucous membranes become susceptible to frictional effects from dentures and are much more friable and readily traumatised.

It is important that an abnormally reduced salivary flow be detected at the examination stage of denture construction in order that steps may be taken to redress the situation. A possible xerostomia which was previously undetected by a patient may become obvious when a new appliance is provided, with the result that the patient may 'blame' the condition on the treatment provided.

Sialorrhoea or profuse salivary secretion is commonly caused by local irritation such as sharp teeth, pathology — e.g. ulcers — or a new denture. It may also result from some diseases of the nervous system. When caused by a 'foreign body' such as a new prosthesis, the effect will be temporary and the rate of flow will return to normal within a few days.

Oral galvanism

Oral galvanism may result in corrosion of metallic restorations in the mouth, and pain resulting from the electrical potentials developed between dissimilar metals in the mouth has been reported. The presence of metallic and non-metallic ions in the saliva create good conditions for the fluid to act as an electrolyte.

Speech

Because of the importance of the oral cavity in the production of intelligible speech it is necessary to have an understanding of phonetics before attempting to design prostheses for insertion into the mouth.

The sounds of speech are all created by obstructing or shaping the stream of the breath. The shaping and the interruption of the expired air produces sounds known as vowels and consonants.

The organs involved in varying the contours of the air stream are the lips, the tongue, the teeth, the alveolar ridges and hard and soft palate and the vocal folds.

Vowel sounds are made by the free and unobstructed passage of air through the various cavity resonators: the larynx, the pharynx, the nasal cavity and the oral cavity. Varying the lip, jaw and tongue positions changes the vowel sounds and makes them different from one another.

To form consonants the air passage is either closed or narrowed, thus preventing the air passing freely from the mouth. The interruption of the air stream creates the sound. Sounds made when the narrowing or closure of the air passage is created by contact between the teeth, alveolar ridges and palate and another of the organs of speech, are particularly susceptible to possible difficulties following the loss of teeth on the insertion of a denture.

The tongue is a remarkably adaptable organ and usually requires only a relatively short period of readjustment to changes occurring in the mouth following tooth extraction or prosthetic treatment. In respect of the insertion of dentures into the mouth, this statement assumes that the appliance is carefully designed, being well retained and providing adequate tongue space.

Dentures and speech

Vowel sounds. The tip of the tongue lies on the floor of the mouth during the production of the vowel sounds and either contacts, or is very close to, the lingual surfaces of the lower anterior teeth. Any denture having a component to be placed in this part of the mouth should not encroach on the space required to accommodate the tongue.

Consonant sounds. As the consonant sounds require contact between various anatomical elements, it is convenient to consider a classification in terms of the parts concerned:

1. Labials — sounds requiring contact between the lips. e.g. 'b', 'p' and 'm'. These sounds may be altered if changes in the occlusal vertical height or forward positioning of teeth make lip contact difficult.

2. Labiodentals — sounds requiring contact between the lips and teeth, e.g. 'f', 'ph', 'v'. A change in the level of the incisal edge of the upper incisor teeth may affect these sounds.

3. Linguodentals — sounds requiring contact between the tongue tip and the upper incisors, e.g. 'th'. This sound may be affected when the horizontal overlap between the upper and lower incisors is excessive or when an excessive occlusal vertical height has been provided.

4. Linguopalatals — sounds requiring contact between the tongue and the palate. These may be considered as subgroups according to whether the anterior, and/or lateral, portions of the hard palate or the soft palate are involved.

a. Sounds requiring contact between the tongue and hard palate, e.g. 'd', 't', 'l', 'ch', 'j'. A change in palatal contour such as may be created by reducing the inter premolar width may produce cramping of the tongue causing particular problems with sounds requiring the lateral margins of the tongue to contact the lingual surfaces of the upper posterior teeth.

b. Sounds requiring contact between the tongue and soft palate, e.g. 'h', 'g', 'ng'. The thickness and positioning of the posterior border of a denture or a palatal bar may cause it to be contacted by the dorsal surface of the tongue in making these sounds and can result in a feeling of nausea and possibly impair speech.

5. Nasal — Where air cannot escape via the mouth, sounds may emerge via the nose, e.g. lip contact in the production of 'm'. The occlusal vertical height and also the inter arch width of a denture may be implicated where difficulties with the nasal sounds occur.

Apart from the immediate post-insertion period, speech difficulties arising from removable dentures are not common where the appliance has been carefully designed, provides maximum stability in the mouth, and replaces lost tissue with the minimum of encroachment on tongue activity.

FURTHER READING

Afonsky D 1961 Saliva and its Relation to Oral Health. University of Alabama Press, Alabama

Atkinson P J and Woodhead C 1968 Changes in human mandibular structure with age. Arch Oral Biol 13: 1453

Atwood D A 1971 The reduction of residual ridges. A major oral disease entity. J Prosthet Dent 26: 266

Ballard C F 1955 A consideration of the physiological background of mandibular posture and movement. Dent Pract Dent Rec 6: 80

Barker B C W 1971 Dissection of regions of interest to the dentist from a medial approach. Austral Dent J 16: 163

Barrett S G and Haines R W 1962 Structure of the mouth in the mandibular molar region and its relation to the denture. J Prosthet Dent 12: 835

Bates J F, Stafford G D and Harrison A 1975 Masticatory function — a review of the literature. Part 1. The form of the masticatory cycle. J Oral Rehab 2: 281

Brill N, Lammie G A, Osborne J and Berry H T 1959 Mandibular position and mandibular movements. Brit Dent J 106: 391

Chierici G and Lawson L 1973 Clinical speech considerations in prosthodontics: perspectives of the prosthodontist and speech pathologist. J Prosthet Dent 29: 29

Christensen F G 1969 Some anatomical concepts associated with the temporomandibular joint. Parts I and II. Anals Austral Coll Dent Surg 2: 39

Jackson R A and Ralph W J 1980 Continuing changes in the contour of the maxillary residual alveolar ridge. J Oral Rehab 7: 245

Martone A L and Edwards L F 1962 Anatomy of the mouth and related structures. Part III. J Prosthet Dent 12: 206

Matthews E, McIntyre H, Wain E A and Bates J F 1961 The full denture problem. Brit Dent J 111: 401

Myer J, Alvares D F and Gerson S J 1976 The structure and function of the oral mucosa. In: Scientific Foundations of Dentistry. B Cohen and I R H Kramer Eds Heinemann London

Nairn R I 1975 The circumoral musculature: structure and function. Brit Dent J 138: 49

Preiskel H W 1972 Lateral translatory movements of the mandible: critical review of investigations. J Prosthet Dent 28: 46

Posselt U 1968 Physiology of Occlusion and Rehabilitation. 2nd Edn. Blackwell, Oxford

Rees L A 1954 The structure and function of the mandibular joint. Brit Dent J 96: 125

Schroeder H E 1976 Gingival tissue. In: Scientific Foundations of Dentistry. B Cohen and I R H Kramer, Eds., Heinemann, London

Scott J H and Dixon A D 1978 Anatomy for Students of Dentistry. 4th Edn. Churchill Livingstone, Edinburgh.

Tanaka H 1973 Speech patterns of edentulous patients and morphology of the palate in relation to phonetics. J Prosthet Dent 29: 16

Thompson J R 1946 The rest position of the mandible and its significance in dental science. J Amer Dent Assoc 33: 151

2

Denture retention

INTRODUCTION

It is fundamental to the success of prosthetic treatment that appliances placed in the mouth should maintain their planned relationship to the tissues which they contact. In the absence of adequate retention, dentures are unlikely to be functionally effective or physiologically acceptable.

The retention of a denture may be defined as the resistance it possesses to withdrawal from its planned position in the mouth.

Another descriptive term often coupled with that of retention is stability. Stability is a measure of the ability of a denture to remain firm, steady and constant in position when forces are applied to it.

The difference between retention and stability may be illustrated by reference to a simple clinical test applied to dentures to assess qualitatively these properties. Retention is generally tested by attempting to remove a denture by means of a force applied in the opposite direction to that in which the appliance was seated in position. Stability may be assessed by observing any movement which occurs by the application of a force in the same direction as that by which the denture was seated in position. A denture may remain in close contact with the underlying tissues (i.e. have good retention) but by virtue of the displaceability of those tissues demonstrates appreciable movement when subjected to occlusally directed forces (i.e. it may demonstrate poor stability). Methods of overcoming clinical situations which may lead to instability of a denture are considered in the appropriate sections relating to impression procedures, jaw relationships and tooth arrangements.

FACTORS AFFECTING DENTURE RETENTION

The factors affecting denture retention can be divided into:
1. Physical
2. Mechanical and
3. Physiological forces.

Physical factors

Forces associated with the salivary film

The physical properties of cohesion, surface tension, adhesion and viscosity, all play a part in denture retention.

Cohesion. Cohesion refers to the forces of attraction between like molecules. The cohesive forces in a fluid (such as saliva) will act to maintain the integrity of the fluid whether the fluid is moving or at rest.

Surface tension. The intermolecular forces responsible for cohesion in a fluid act equally on all molecules within the bulk of the fluid. At the surface, one component of these forces is missing, thus resulting in a net attractive force towards the interior of the liquid (Fig. 2.1). This directional

Fig. 2.1 Intermolecular forces within the bulk of a fluid act equally in all directions. At the surface, the net force is directional towards the interior.

Fig. 2.2 A, Very small contact angle in a spreading system e.g. alcohol and clean glass; B, θ is just less than 90° e.g. water and acrylic resin; C, High contact angle in a non-wetting system e.g. water and wax.

energy gives rise to the phenomenon of surface tension which counteracts forces tending to break the surface of the liquid and also tends to give the fluid the smallest possible surface area.

Solids also possess surface tension.

Adhesion. Adhesion refers to the forces of attraction between unlike molecules. For adhesion to be accomplished between a solid and a fluid, wetting of the solid by the fluid must take place, and the degree to which this occurs will depend on their relative surface tensions. The wetting characteristics of a fluid may be described in terms of the contact angle formed with the solid surface on which it is placed — a high contact angle indicates poor wetting (Fig. 2.2).

In considering the role of cohesion, wetting characteristics and adhesion in denture retention, the adhesive forces between the saliva and oral mucous membrane present no problems in (physiologically) normal circumstances. This is because saliva effectively wets oral mucous membrane.

The wetting characteristics between saliva and the denture base material will determine the effectiveness of the adhesion of saliva to the denture. Most commonly used non-metallic denture base materials are effectively wet by saliva.

The cohesive forces within the saliva will complete the mucous membrane–saliva–denture system, and with good adhesion between the saliva and the oral mucous membrane and the denture, these forces will make a significant contribution to denture retention.

Early workers attempted to relate the above factors regarding the relationship between the denture and the underlying tissue as similar to that of two flat parallel plates as follows:

$$F = \frac{2\gamma A}{H}$$

where F is the force required to separate the plates, γ is the surface tension constant of the interposing fluid film, A is the surface area of the plates and H is the distance separating the plates.

It is now appreciated that the above relationship represents an oversimplified account of the problem.

In the clinical situation there is considerable variation between patients in respect of, for example, the area covered by the denture base and the direction and magnitude of the displacing forces applied. It also takes no account of the role played by the viscosity of the saliva.

Viscosity. Viscosity is the resistance to flow of a fluid resulting from intermolecular forces acting within the fluid.

When a fluid is set in motion, the cohesive forces within the fluid act as a form of intermolecular friction to oppose the movement. If a fluid tends to move between parallel plates, the molecules nearest the plates move only slowly because of the adhesive forces acting, while the central molecules move the fastest. The closer the two plates are together the closer the flow of fluid comes to the speed of the fluid nearest the plates, so that a thin film of fluid resists flow more readily than a thicker film (Fig. 2.3). In addition, fluids having a high viscosity resist flow more effectively than those of lower viscosity.

Experimental work which has been carried out in respect of denture retention and viscosity of saliva has shown that the retention between glass plates increases with increase in viscosity of an interposed film of saliva. It has also been shown that for a given viscosity value, high retention values result when a denture is subjected to high forces of short duration, and conversely that small forces acting over an extended period may dislodge a denture. This is because there is little time for

Fig. 2.3 Fluid near the walls of the plates moves slowly while that in the centre moves more rapidly.

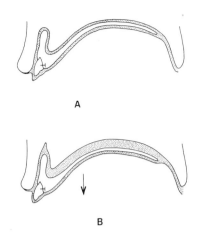

Fig. 2.4 A downward displacing force causes additional saliva to be drawn under the denture. A, Denture at rest; B, Denture subjected to a downward displacing force.

flow of saliva to occur when a force is applied suddenly.

When in position in the mouth the denture is covered over all surfaces by a continuous film of saliva. Should the denture be subject to a force tending to displace it, a reduced pressure will result in the salivary film under the denture relative to that in the oral cavity. This will cause additional saliva to be drawn under the denture (Fig. 2.4).

The additional saliva will result in loss of retention of the denture because of the resultant increase in distance between the denture and the mucosa. It is therefore essential that the relationship between the periphery of the denture and the surrounding tissue is such that the closest possible adaptation exists. Close adaptation

Fig. 2.5 The two diagrams on the left illustrate wide openings and consequent easy displacement of the plate and denture. On the right side the plate and denture fit closely against the sides and upward displacement is more difficult because more time is required for fluid to pass through the restricted opening.

about the periphery will have the effect of delaying the rate of influx of saliva under the denture base (Fig. 2.5). This aspect of close adaptation of the denture base to the tissues is usually referred to as peripheral seal, and is referred to again in the section on physiological forces.

Clearly the viscosity of the saliva will have a significant effect in the above description, and it should be appreciated that the viscosity of saliva varies markedly between patients and even in a single patient under varying circumstances.

An analysis of factors involved in the separation of two plates in an analogous situation to that of a denture completely surrounded by saliva has produced the following relationship:

$$F = \frac{3\eta A^2}{2h^3} \cdot \frac{dh}{dt}$$

where F is the force required to separate the two plates of surface area A, η is the viscosity of the fluid in which the plates are immersed, h is the distance between the plates and dh/dt represents the rate of separation of the plates.

The above formula indicates that increasing the viscosity will increase the force required for separation of the plates and that the greater the area covered, the higher will be the separation force required since this factor is raised to the second power. Low values of h, i.e. the distance between the plates, are very significant as this factor is cubed. The period of time over which the force producing separation occurs is also taken into account.

As indicated above, the forces derived from cohesion, adhesion and wetting characteristics contribute to denture retention. Thus, in order to obtain the maximum possible benefit for denture retention from the physical forces related to the salivary film, the denture base should:

1. Cover the maximum usable area,
2. Provide for the closest possible adaptation between the denture base and the oral mucous membrane,
3. Provide for accurate peripheral seal.

Gravity

A further force which should be considered in relation to denture retention relates to the weight of the appliance. In the upper jaw, light weight is advantageous as lower gravitational forces will be acting on it. In the lower jaw, however, additional weight may help to keep the denture in place. Care must be exercised in this latter case to ensure that the mass of any appliance is kept within the physiological limits of tolerance for the patient, so that neither muscular fatigue nor accelerated bone resorption occur.

Magnetic forces

Magnetic forces of repulsion have occasionally been used in an attempt to stabilise dentures. The like poles of permanent magnets are contained in opposing dentures, so that the forces of repulsion act to seat the dentures firmly when the dentures are at or near contact. This has not been shown to be effective. More promising is the use of the force of attraction in the overlay denture where one element of the magnetic system is attached to the remaining root face of the patient, and the other to the denture which fits over the root face.

Vacuum devices

This type of device aims at the production of a reduced pressure in a circumscribed area of the denture base — usually in an upper complete denture. The dangers of older devices such as rubber suction discs — a sucker-like attachment to the tissue side of the palate of an upper denture — are well documented. Their use is now condemned.

Relief areas are sometimes used in upper dentures in order to compensate for unequal displaceability of the tissues contacted by an overlying denture and so improve stability. Such areas have the effect of increasing the distance between the denture and the tissue over the area relieved, and as a result cause a reduction in the retentive forces derived from close contact between the denture and the tissues.

Relief areas may be supplemented by valves which are designed to enable the patient to evacuate the relief area by sucking on the valve. There is no evidence of continuing effectiveness of these valves as the relief area is quickly filled by saliva and tissue, which proliferates into the area.

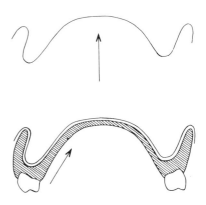

Fig. 2.6 Attempts to insert the denture vertically will fail because of the undercuts present. Inserting the denture from the side allows it to contact the residual ridge and will provide for mechanical resistance to a direct downwards force.

Mechanical factors

Engagement of undercuts

The use of undercut areas in edentulous regions of the mouth may be possible. This is illustrated in Figure 2.6.

Springs

Mechanical devices such as springs are used only rarely to assist the retention of complete dentures in such circumstances as post surgical rehabilitation, and are considered to be outside the scope of this text.

Most removable partial dentures depend for their retention on friction or direct mechanical interlocking.

Friction

Friction may be utilised by virtue of contact between parts of a partial denture and the remaining teeth which may be modified in order to provide for more effective retention. Either naturally present contact points such as are used in the Every design denture, or tooth and restoration surfaces modified to produce guiding planes are examples.

In the majority of circumstances where partial dentures are to be provided, additional retention in the form of

1. direct or
2. indirect retainers
will be required.

Direct retention is obtained by means of clasps, or by the use of preformed (precision) attachments.

Clasps

Clasps provide resistance to a displacing force because they are so designed that the terminal end rests on an undercut surface. For the denture to be displaced, it is necessary for the clasp arm to be moved over the most bulbous portion of the tooth. Provided that the force tending to dislodge the denture is less than that required for the clasp arm to be displaced from the undercut, the denture will be retained in position (Fig. 2.7).

Fig. 2.7 The tip of the clasp arm must deform to allow its withdrawal over the tooth. A, Clasp arm; B, Survey line (maximum convexity of the tooth with respect to the direction of surveying).

Preformed (precision) attachments

These comprise a male component which is usually attached to the saddle (q.v.) of the denture, and a female part which is fabricated into an inlay or crown of an abutment tooth. When assembled in the mouth a dovetailed, ball and socket, or hinged joint is formed which provides for mechanical retention. (Fig. 2.8).

These two types of direct retainer will be considered in more detail in respect of their place in partial denture treatment.

Physiological forces

These relate to the musculature of the oral cavity. In this respect the buccinator, orbicularis oris and the musculature of the tongue may be regarded as the most important.

Active muscular fixation of dentures may be obtained by careful attention to the form of those surfaces which contact their environmental tissues. The tongue on the lingual surface and the peripherally placed muscles of the lips and cheeks may be considered to act as antagonists, so that in the event of careful, clinically developed denture form, the simultaneous contraction of the two muscle groups may stabilise the denture and retain it against its foundation (Fig. 2.9).

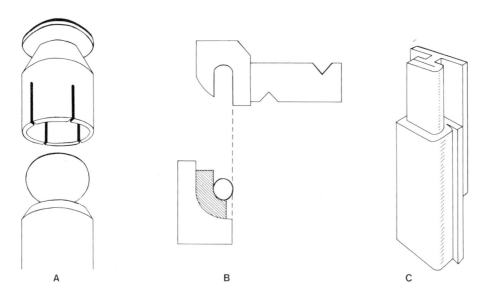

Fig. 2.8 Some types of precision attachment: A, Ball and socket; B, Hinge; C, Dovetailed slot.

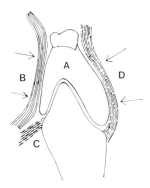

Fig. 2.9 Opposing muscle groups acting to stabilise a lower denture. A, Denture; B, Tongue; C, Mylohyoid muscle; D, Buccinator muscle.

The accurate approximation of the tongue, cheeks and lips to a denture also acts to impede the flow of saliva about the denture, thus increasing the effective area for retention. When a small displacing force is applied to a denture, the reduced pressure which develops in the salivary film under the denture will cause the soft tissues about the periphery of the denture to move inwards, thus reducing the potential flow of saliva under the denture. Inaccurate extension of a denture may allow increased saliva and even air to enter under a denture and cause loss of retention. Because of the small surface area covered by a complete lower denture relative to the length of border, the potential for saliva and air leaks is high. For the upper denture, there is little or no moveable tissue available at the posterior palatal border, so that the breakdown of the film of saliva in this region may occur on only slight displacement. Consequently a specially formed addition to the denture is provided to assist in retention in this region. This addition is called the posterior palatal seal or post-dam, and is considered in Chapter 25.

It may be helpful to think in terms of retention derived by accurate denture base extension and approximation to the adjacent tissues as resulting from interfacial seal.

Careful development of the form of the 'polished' surfaces of dentures can be a powerful aid to denture retention. This is well illustrated by the common clinical experience whereby the dentures worn by a patient for many years can be shown to be poorly adapted to the foundation tissues and yet are regarded by the patient as being a good 'fit'.

In such a situation, muscular fixation has compensated for the loss of retention via physical factors which pertained at the initial insertion of the denture.

Provision for musclar fixation is required in the design of both complete and partial dentures.

FURTHER READING

Avant W E 1971 Factors that influence the retention of removable partial dentures. J Prosthet Dent 25: 265

Barbenel J C 1971 Physical retention of complete dentures. J Prosthet Dent 26: 592

Bates J F 1980 Retention of partial dentures. Brit Dent J 149: 171

Brill N 1967 Factors in the mechanism of full denture retention — a discussion of selected papers. Dent Pract 18: 9

Caldwell R C 1956 A method of measuring the adhesion of foodstuffs to tooth surfaces. J Dent Res 38: 188

Clayton J A and Jaslow C 1971 A measurement of clasp forces on teeth. J Prosthet Dent 25: 21

Laird W R E, Grant A A and Smith G A 1981 The use of magnetic forces in prosthetic dentistry. J Dent 9: 328.

O'Brien W J 1980 Base retention. Dent Clin North Amer 24: 123

3

Principles related to denture design

INTRODUCTION

The functions to which the oral tissues contribute depend on sensory processes for their control. In the context of removable dentures, the functions related to mastication and speech are of particular interest. In addition, the large number of transient tooth contacts made throughout the day such as, for instance, in swallowing saliva, must also be considered.

It will be helpful to consider briefly some functional aspects of normal occlusion of the natural teeth at this stage.

FUNCTIONAL OCCLUSION

In Chapter 1 the term occlusion was used to define the contact relationship between opposing teeth. During function, the upper and lower dentitions move relative to each other. The dynamic relationships which exist during sliding of the opposing teeth while they are in contact is called articulation.

Balanced occlusion refers to an arrangement of the teeth so that in any occlusal relationship as many teeth as possible are in occlusion. When changing from one occlusal relationship to another and a smooth, sliding contact is maintained free from cuspal interference balanced articulation is said to exist. The features of a functionally optimum occlusion include:

1. The teeth should receive occlusal stresses consistent with the physiological requirements of the supporting structures. It has been shown that a tooth must be stimulated to maintain the support provided by the periodontal ligament. Too much

or too little stimulation may lead to damage or atrophy of the ligament. The arrangement of the tooth in its socket is such that the periodontium is capable of resisting axial forces better than those directed laterally.

2. The effects of occlusal forces are minimised by firm interproximal tooth contacts and simultaneous occlusal contacts.

3. Closure into the maximal intercuspal position must be even and without premature contacts and cuspal interference.

4. An acceptable amount of freeway space is an essential part of the functional occlusion.

5. During mandibular movements such as in chewing, when occlusal contacts are made other than in the maximal intercuspal position, the teeth usually slide back to that contact relationship before another masticatory cycle commences. Ideally, balanced articulation should exist, but this is rarely achieved with the natural dentition.

The functional occlusion is controlled by a complex neuromuscular mechanism in which various sensory elements play a part.

RESTORATION OF THE DISRUPTED OCCLUSION

The loss of parts of the dental tissues is accompanied by the loss of some of the exteroceptive and proprioceptive apparatus. This will have a direct effect on the ability of the remaining oral components to function normally. In addition, when attempts to replace the lost tissue by means of a prosthesis have been made, the nervous mechanisms about the mouth may suffer further interference.

On the basis of a knowledge of the functional anatomy and normal occlusion, a number of principles of design for removable prostheses may be defined. These are as follows:

1. The restoration must not interfere with normal physiological processes.
2. The restoration must not prejudice the health of the remaining hard and soft tissues.
3. The restoration must be tolerated in the mouth.

These factors are interdependent, but they will be considered separately. It should, however, be appreciated that there is considerable overlap between them.

Interference with normal physiological processes

The nervous pathways controlling mandibular movements include voluntary and reflex mechanisms. Only the sensory component of the neuromuscular control mechanism will be considered here because of its direct relationship to tooth loss.

The sensory nerve endings provide exteroceptive and proprioceptive sense. Exteroceptive sense is that of pressure, temperature, etc., and proprioception is the awareness of position in space.

Proprioceptive elements are located in the tendons, muscles, ligaments (including the periodontal ligaments) and joints of the jaws. Exteroceptive innervation lies in the periodontal ligaments, the epithelial surfaces of the oral cavity, tongue muscles, muscles of mastication and the temporomandibular joints.

Some examples of the way in which removable prostheses may influence sensory mechanisms about the mouth follow and are intended to illustrate the severe interference to normal function which may result.

Premature contact between opposing teeth

In the context of removable dentures this is a situation which might occur where uneven contact between a natural tooth and part of a denture in the opposing jaw takes place. The proprioceptive nerve endings of the periodontal ligament serve an important function. When a tooth is contacted prematurely, these receptors send impulses through a reflex arc to the muscles of mastication,

which contract in a manner which attempts to avoid the premature contact. As pointed out above, the ideal situation exists when the teeth contact simultaneously without interference. This produces simultaneous firing of the periodontal receptors and reinforces the habitual path of closure. If the premature contact cannot be avoided several consequences may follow:

1. The neuromuscular system attains asynchronous contraction patterns which causes increased muscle tonus and may act as a trigger for bruxism (grinding or forceful clamping together of the teeth and jaws).
2. Pain may develop in the periodontal membrane.
3. Pain may develop in the temporomandibular joint due to eccentric closure of the jaws in attempting to avoid the pain of premature contact.
4. A general effect on the nervous system may occur when continual attempts to avoid pain must be made.

Errors in jaw relations

Temporomandibular joint proprioception is thought to play a key role in identifying mandibular position and in control of muscular activities about the jaws. Errors in securing jaw relations in respect of either the vertical or horizontal component might therefore be expected to interfere severely with oral function. This type of error is more likely to be associated with patients who have lost several teeth from one or both jaws.

Clasps

As already pointed out, natural teeth can withstand forces directed along the long axis of the tooth much more effectively than laterally directed forces. Some laterally directed forces are generated during normal mastication and, in addition, where a removable partial denture is present a clasped tooth will receive stimuli from forces applied to the opposite side of the denture through the denture. Lateral stresses to a tooth contacted by a denture may therefore build up to physiologically unacceptable levels.

In addition, the presence of an inaccurately constructed clasp about a tooth can cause a stream of nervous signals to be produced which may cause interference with the normal controlling mechanism of the masticatory system. This aspect is further considered in the section on surveying, as it is fundamentally important that clasps be accurately constructed, and that any appliance contacting the natural teeth is passive when not in function.

Prejudice to the health of the hard and soft tissues

It is clear that the above examples of possible interference with physiological processes could also be considered in this section. It is, however, intended to consider here two further aspects:
1. Trauma
2. Plaque control

Trauma

Mention has been made of the effects on the nervous control mechanism of the masticatory apparatus by an inaccurately clasped tooth. Inaccuracy may also result in direct traumatic injury to the periodontal membrane. Similarly, any part of partial or complete dentures which contacts any part of the oral mucous membrane inaccurately may cause traumatic injury. Margins or flanges of dentures which extend excessively onto moveable tissues are included in this category, and the trauma produced may result in mild inflammation at one end of the scale, to ulceration of the epithelium and subepithelial tissues or even hyperplasia of the soft tissues where persistent, severe and prolonged damage has occurred.

Dentures which contact the tissues accurately but where the teeth occlude inaccurately, may also result in trauma to the underlying tissues as a result of the transmission of unplanned forces through the denture. In this context the diminished sensitivity of the oral mucous membrane on which a denture is placed after tooth extraction, relative to that of the natural tooth, should be borne in mind. The sensitive receptors in the periodontal membrane of the natural tooth provide much better protection to possible tissue overload that does the mucous membrane.

Surfaces of dentures which are not adequately smooth or polished may cause trauma to the cheeks, tongue or mucoperiosteum covering the residual alveolar ridges or palate. In addition, where artificial teeth are not accurately placed in relation to the opposing teeth, trauma in the form of cheek, lip, or tongue biting may result.

Plaque control

The presence of a removable denture in the mouth provides an increase in the surface area to which plaque may be retained.

A discussion of plaque formation and the damaging effects of plaque accumulation is beyond the scope of this text. It is, however, important to bear in mind that the presence of plaque accumulations can result in dental caries and periodontal disease. The very fact of a patient seeking removable denture treatment is often an indication that natural teeth have been lost as a result of tooth decay or periodontal disease. Such a patient might be regarded as being particularly at risk in this respect, and particular attention will need to be given to his education in oral hygiene measures.

The design of an appliance to be placed in the mouth must be carried out with an appreciation of the need to minimise plaque retention, coupled with the importance of educating the patient in oral and denture hygiene measures.

A removable partial denture often involves many natural teeth and gingival margins, and covers a large area of the other oral tissues; it is very demanding of good plaque control or periodontal disease and caries may occur.

Similarly, complete dentures present large areas for the retention of plaque. In this case, however, no natural teeth or gingival margins are present and the effects of plaque accumulation will be on the soft tissues covered by the denture and may encourage candidal infection of the mucous membrane.

Details of methods by which the effects of plaque accumulations on removable dentures may be minimised are considered in Chapters 19 and 26.

Tolerance in the mouth

The great majority of patients become accustomed to the wearing of a prosthesis following tooth loss.

This may include even those patients who express strong doubts as to whether they will ever 'get used to' an appliance.

The only somatic mechanism by which a patient can become accustomed to a foreign appliance in the mouth is through readjustment to the changed nervous responses about the oral cavity which result from tooth loss, and the subsequent placement in the mouth of a denture. This requires a carefully designed appliance to facilitate reeducation of the tissues which comprise the denture environment. The space available for removable appliances to be placed in the mouth is a major consideration in this respect, and is discussed below.

Psychological factors can be very powerful in respect of dental treatment, and there are a number of dental conditions which are thought to have psychological involvement. The conditions are best described as psychosomatic processes. The literature includes the following as amongst those in which a psychosomatic component may be present: gagging, temporomandibular joint dysfunction, bad taste, periodontal disease and maxillo-facial pain.

Consideration of psychological factors is regarded as an advanced aspect of prosthetic treatment, and the student is referred to the current literature for details, beyond those presented in Chapter 4.

The space available for removable dentures

The space available is dependent on the nervous mechanisms discussed above and also the functional activity of the environmental musculature.

The term used to describe the space which a removable denture may occupy in the mouth is the 'denture space', and may be described as that space limited by the tongue, cheeks, lips, residual alveolar ridges and any remaining teeth.

A simplified version of the denture space in the edentulous mouth is shown in Figure 3.1 and is based on the concept:
1. That the force developed by the cheek is exactly balanced by that of the tongue and
2. That such a balance of forces is likely to occur at, or near, the crest of the residual alveolar ridge.

While it is possible that this situation may occur

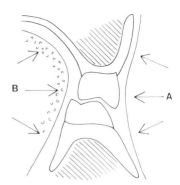

Fig. 3.1 Diagram to illustrate the concept that the force developed by the cheek (A) may balance that developed by the tongue (B).

during rest, it is unlikely that such a balance of forces would exist except, perhaps, momentarily during functional activity.

The terms 'neutral zone' and 'zone of equilibrium' have been applied to the concept that equilibrium may exist at any given site in the mouth between the buccally and lingually directed forces generated by muscular activity during rest and in some functions. It is known that this equilibrium does not exist in the natural dentition, and because of the individuality of the teeth in the natural state such a balance of forces may have no significance in terms of the stability of the dentition.

If one considers the extreme example of a complete denture, the placement of a denture in a zone of equilibrium would have clear advantages in respect of its retention and stability. The results of the application of a force to an artificial tooth affects the whole denture base to which the tooth is attached. However, a disturbance of equilibrium at one site on a denture does not preclude the possibility that muscular activity in another site might resist displacement of the denture.

In this context several clinical techniques have been devised in an attempt to define a zone of equilibrium for an individual patient. Such treatment forms are costly in time and resources, and as a consequence the great majority of removable dentures conform to an 'average' approach to denture design in terms of bucco-lingual tooth placement. Where only a few natural teeth are missing, a clear guide to tooth placement might be obtained from a study of the position of the remaining teeth.

For complete dentures the 'average' is based, in general, on the assumptions of Figure 3.1 — having due regard to the known patterns of resorption of the residual alveolar bone following tooth loss. The assumptions include:

1. That the pressures of the cheeks and tongue tend to be balanced in repose, and
2. That the polished surfaces of the dentures should be a series of inclines so that forces generated from the muscular environment will help to retain the denture in position.

THE SURVEYOR IN RELATION TO DESIGN PRINCIPLES

Mention has already been made of the biological necessity for ensuring that any part of a removable denture in contact with a natural tooth be passive when not in function.

It is similarly essential from the biological point of view that no part of an appliance meant for insertion and removal from the mouth without modification should be fashioned in such a manner as to have rigid portions which enter undercut regions of the mouth.

To avoid the damage which will inevitably result if the above criteria are not met, an instrument called the cast surveyor is used. The cast surveyor is a precision instrument which enables the position of maximum contour of individual teeth and alveolar ridges to be located as one of its functions.

A detailed description of the cast surveyor and its use is included in Chapter 5. Because of its importance in denture design for placement of retaining elements for removable dentures, it is often thought of as having a purely mechanical function. It is important to appreciate the fundamental biological necessity for the use of the surveyor.

FURTHER READING

Bergman B, Hugoson A and Olsson C O 1977 Caries and periodontal status in patients fitted with removable partial dentures. J Clin Periodont 4: 134

Brill N, Tryde G and Schubeler S 1959 The role of exteroceptors in denture retention. J Prosthet Dent 9: 761

Crum R J and Loiselle R J 1972 Oral perception and proprioception. A review of the literature and its significance in prosthodontics. J Prosthet Dent 28: 215

Fish S F 1967 Adaptation and habituation to full dentures. Brit Dent J 129: 19

Heath R M 1971 A study of the morphology of the denture space. Dent Pract Dent Rec 21: 109

Ramfjord S P and Ash M M 1971 Occlusion. 2nd Edn. Saunders, Philadelphia

Stipho H D K, Murphy W M and Adams D 1978 Effect of oral prostheses on plaque accumulation. Brit Dent J 145: 47

The Academy of Denture Prosthetics 1977 Principles, concepts and practices in prosthodontics, 1976. J Prosthet Dent 37: 204

4

Psychological aspects

INTRODUCTION

In the provision of a removable denture service, the need for an appreciation of the patient from the psychological viewpoint is essential to the success of treatment.

Indeed, the emotional characteristics of both the dentist and the patient, and the relationships which develop between them, may affect the diagnosis and treatment plan adopted by the dentist and also acceptance by the patient of the treatment provided.

Inability to establish empathy with the patient may lead to failure regardless of the excellence of the treatment provided. Mutual respect and understanding must be developed between the dentist and patient at the earliest moment and be maintained throughout treatment.

Within the practice environment the state of mind of the patient will depend on many factors. These include the ability and reputation of the dentist, the health of the patient and the atmosphere of confidence, trust and security created by the dentist and his surroundings.

MENTAL ATTITUDE

While it has long been appreciated that people cannot be classified into 'types', it can be helpful to recognise the attitudes of patients seeking removable dentures as an aid to approaching their treatment. Four groups based on those suggested by House may be considered. It must be emphasised that these groupings are suitable largely as an aid to the comparison of patients' attitudes.

Philosophic

Patients having a philosophic attitude trust the dentist and will generally accept without question the advice and treatment plan provided. Even where the conditions in the mouth of the patient present difficulties, these patients are content in the knowledge that the dentist will exercise to the maximum his skill and judgement in their treatment.

Exacting or critical

Patients having a critical attitude often doubt the ability of the dentist to provide satisfactory treatment. They tend to be highly critical of previous dental treatment and are always ready to provide advice and instruction to the dentist on the way in which treatment should proceed.

It is essential that this attitude be recognised before the commencement of any treatment, and attempts at re-education of the patient be commenced immediately. A careful and sympathetic attitude in dealing with the critical patient is needed in order that accuracy may be achieved in diagnosis and treatment planning. It must be borne in mind that ill-health may be a factor involved in their outlook.

Hysterical or sceptical

This attitude may have been fostered by previous failures of treatment resulting in a conviction on the part of the patient that they are a 'hopeless' case and that no form of treatment can ever be successful for them. These patients may make impossible demands in respect of efficiency and appearance of their dentures. An unfortunate social background (such as a bereavement) may be present, and poor health is often a contributing factor.

For this group the development of confidence in the dentist by the patient is paramount, and must commence as early as possible in the first appointment.

Indifferent

These patients appear unconcerned about their appearance or the need for replacement of lost natural teeth. Treatment is often sought because of the insistence of relatives and if early problems with dentures are encountered, they generally do not bother to seek adjustments but prefer simply to discard the appliances.

APPLICATION OF PSYCHOLOGY TO THE DENTURE PATIENT

The classification of attitude suggested by House may be considered a useful starting point in patient assessment, but it must be appreciated that there are many factors which influence the individual under treatment. These may be considered as:
1. Intrapersonal factors
2. Interpersonal factors

The intrapersonal feelings of the patient influence strongly the interpersonal relationships between the dentist and the patient.

Intrapersonal factors

The most important of these are body image and fear and anxiety.

Body image

Body image refers to the unconscious representation possessed by each individual of the image and appearance of the body and associated organs. The retention of this representation of the mental image of the body is important in maintaining a sense of security, and the prospect of change may be interpreted as a threatening action. The adjustment to change takes time and this has important implications in connection with prosthetic dentistry because of the important part played by the mouth in body image.

Silverman found that body image was important in denture acceptance, especially for the older patient.

Fear and anxiety

Many people experience some kind of anxiety in the dental surgery, and the reaction which results is highly individual. The role of the dentist in this respect should be an educational one, directed towards helping the patient to manage his anxiety and adjust it to a tolerable level in each situation.

Interpersonal factors

A knowledge of the individual needs of the patient is of basic importance to the success of treatment. By the careful development of his powers of observation and listening ability the dentist can go a long way towards getting to 'know' the patient before the commencement of treatment.

The dress and posture of the patient, the way he copes with or dramatises symptoms, his handshake, any speech defects, the number of previous dentures and his expectations, are all part of the many factors which contribute to the evaluation of the patient.

Good communication is one of the factors of such importance that it cannot be over-emphasised in respect of its contribution to a satisfactory dentist–patient relationship. The ability to present information to the patient in respect of the treatment to be undertaken, and interpreting the thoughts of the patient are abilities which must be acquired and developed.

DEVELOPING RAPPORT WITH THE PATIENT

The relationship between the dentist and patient is directly related to the degree to which the patient feels satisfied with each appointment.

Patient satisfaction may be increased by the application of the factors considered above which give rise to the following practice of dealing with the denture patient:

1. Determine the expectations of the patient in respect of dentures, and if it is unlikely that they can be met, explain why.

2. Determine the causes of concern of the patient and do not simply confine the diagnostic visit to gathering objective information about the oral conditions and medical background.

3. Provide full information to the patient concerning the diagnosis and treatment plan.

4. Adopt a friendly attitude rather than a purely business-like one.

5. Spend some time in conversation of a non-dental type. This helps to make it clear to the patient that you have an interest in him as an individual.

Increased satisfaction of the patient with each appointment will result in increased co-operation. The key to increased satisfaction is good communication.

FURTHER READING

Miller A A 1970 Psychological considerations in dentistry. J Amer Dent Assoc 81: 941

Silverman S, Silverman S I, Silverman B and Garfinkel L 1976 Self-image and its relation to denture acceptance. J Prosthet Dent 35: 131

Smit G L 1978 Psychological considerations in dentistry: a survey of the literature. J Dent Assoc Sth Africa 33: 375

Winkler S, Davidoff A and Lee M H M 1972 Dentistry for the Special Patient: The Aged, Chronically Ill and Handicapped. Saunders, Philadelphia

5

Examination

INTRODUCTION

In the preceding chapters some of the factors relating to the provision of prosthetic treatment have been referred to. Generalisations concerning anatomical and physiological factors have been considered, but it must be appreciated that there is substantial individual variation between patients in respect of these factors and the way in which they may affect treatment.

Some reference has also been made to psychological factors related to treatment, but no mention has been made of the many other individual and personal factors which affect the approach to, or the outcome of, treatment.

Before treatment is commenced, the operator must undertake a thorough assessment of the patient, who can then be advised on the most appropriate form of treatment. In addition, a careful examination will allow for any possible difficulties to be anticipated, together with the degree of success likely to be achieved.

To do this effectively an understanding of conditions which might have an effect on the jaws or their movement is required. Skill in recognising general conditions and those disease states confined to the oral cavity is also required. In addition, the effects of drug therapy on denture retention and tolerance must be appreciated.

It is proposed in this chapter to outline an approach to gathering all the information necessary to form a detailed diagnosis and treatment plan for the patient seeking prosthetic treatment. The information obtained will also enable an assessment of the likely degree of success or outcome of treatment to be made, i.e. a prognosis can be formed.

The procedure by which information gathering is carried out is known as history taking and examination of the patient.

HISTORY TAKING

History taking consists of communicating with the patient in order to obtain essential personal details, including health information.

When properly conducted, the history taking phase of treatment can, in addition to the essential information obtained, provide an opportunity to initiate the development of rapport between the dentist and the patient. Any doubts or fears the patient may have in respect of dental treatment should be elicited as early as possible as a sympathetic consideration of these may suggest the need to vary the routine approach to information gathering and treatment.

Details which will be required may be considered under the following headings:
1. Personal details
2. Social details
3. Reason for attendance
4. Dental history
5. Medical and surgical history

Personal details

The name, address and telephone number of the patient must be recorded so that positive identification may be made and the patient can be contacted as required.

The age of the patient should be determined. For an adult this is usually best obtained by asking for the date of birth. In general, older patients may have more difficulty in adapting to removable dentures than younger patients. Chronological age of itself is not always a good guide in this context, and an estimation of the physiological age of the patient may be helpful. A 'young' sixty-five year-old can be much more adaptable to change than an 'old' fifty year-old. Some pathological conditions, e.g. carcinoma, are known to be age related.

The name and address of the patient's physician should also be recorded in case it may be necessary to obtain details of any aspect of the health status of the patient.

Where a patient has been referred by a professional colleague, details of this should also be recorded.

Social details

Occupation can provide an indication of the socio-economic class of the patient and may indicate possible difficulties with regular attendance for appointments, e.g. if the patient is a shift worker. Special treatment needs might also be indicated by the patient's occupation, e.g. wind instrument players who may have special needs in respect of the formation of an embrochure; singers may have special needs concerning retention of an appliance and the placement of teeth.

Social conditions relating to the patient's personal life may also be significant, e.g. severe emotional disturbance following the death of a spouse or other stress-inducing circumstances can result in apparently excessive reactions to minor trauma, or clenching or grinding of the teeth, or an inability to cope with what would normally be a non-stressful situation.

Reason for attendance

Determining the exact reason for the patient's attendance should be carried out at an early stage in the interview. The patient may never have worn a removable denture before and the reason for presenting might be the absence of some or all of the teeth and a desire for their replacement. If a denture has been worn or an attempt has been made to wear a denture and a replacement is sought, the reasons for requesting a new denture must be determined so that treatment planning will include overcoming the present difficulties. If a replacement denture is sought because of fracture of an existing appliance, it is important to determine whether the denture broke during normal use or if it was dropped and fracture occurred outside the mouth.

Whether or not a denture is present, the attitude and expectations of the patient to removable denture treatment must be determined. The attitude of the patient is often conditioned by knowledge of a third party who has been treated regardless of whether or not the same type of treatment was required. An enquiry as to why the patient has sought treatment at this particular dental practice may therefore be useful in this context.

In questioning patients about difficulties they have experienced with dentures, it must be appreciated that they use their own terminology which must be interpreted by the interviewer. It should also be borne in mind that the length of time a previous denture has been worn will be of significance in relation to the criticism offered, e.g. a complaint of looseness of a denture only a few weeks old may have a different basis to that of a denture which is considered to be loose after many years of use.

If the appearance of the denture is said to be unsatisfactory, it is important to know if the patient has initiated the complaint or, as is common with more elderly patients, another member of the family has done so. An exact description of the nature of the complaint should be obtained.

Where looseness is the complaint it will be important to know the circumstances in which the dentures feel loose. During mastication a feeling of looseness may be related to faults in tooth positioning or occlusion or the stability or extension of the bases. During speech a feeling of looseness could result from tongue interference.

If pain is complained of, it will be necessary to determine the character of the pain, whether it is local or general about the mouth or jaws, and if it is present all the time or relieved by removal of the dentures.

Clicking noises during speech or eating could result from looseness or incorrect vertical height estimation.

Retching may result, for example, from stimulation of the soft palate by overextension of an upper denture or placement of the upper posterior teeth lingually so that they contact the dorsal surface of the tongue. It is important to know whether it is a chronic problem or has just developed.

The above are examples only and do not represent the whole range of reasons for replacement of dentures or of all the possible bases for the complaints.

At this stage information in the patient's own words is sought and this phase of history taking merges into the next phase.

Dental history

Where dentures are being worn, questions should be asked concerning their age, how many dentures have been made following the loss of the natural teeth, how long each lasted and why they were replaced. This will give valuable information concerning the tolerance of the patient to dentures and may give an indication of the rate at which resorption of the residual alveolar ridges has occurred. Comments on the appearance of the dentures should be encouraged.

If the missing teeth were not extracted by the dental surgeon who is conducting the interview with the patient, information regarding the extractions should be sought. The order in which the teeth were extracted may be significant in that uncommon masticatory habits may have developed. Where a history of difficult extractions is elicited, the possibility of retained roots in apparently edentulous regions of the jaws should be borne in mind.

Where natural teeth are present in the mouth it is essential that the oral hygiene habits of the patient are fully explored and also the regularity of attendance for dental treatment. It is known that the success of removable partial denture treatment is strongly dependent on good oral hygiene and the importance of early motivation of the patient to this end cannot be overemphasised. The denture hygiene habits of the patient must also be determined.

If dentures have never been worn before, it is important to understand exactly what the patient expects and if it is clear that such expectation cannot be met by removable denture treatment, a careful explanation of the limitations of this type of treatment must be given.

Medical and surgical history

The health status of the patient may have a direct bearing on the approach to, or the outcome of, treatment either as a direct result of a disease process or of any medication.

A convenient starting point for this part of history taking is to ask whether the patient has ever suffered from a serious illness or been subjected to a period of hospitalisation. Any current treatment being undertaken should be elicited.

A direct question should be asked concerning any medicine, tablets, capsules or other form of medication being taken. It is possible that a patient may have been consuming tablets as a matter of routine for a prolonged period and come to accept these as part of a daily routine rather that considering themselves as taking a drug.

It has been shown that this part of history-taking can be assisted considerably by allowing the patient to read a list of relevant conditions before history-taking commences. An example of a suitable list is shown in Figure 5.1. This is not an exhaustive list of conditions known to influence dental treatment, but it does include many which have direct relevance and it has been shown to act as an effective memory promoter for patients about to undergo dental treatment.

There are many general conditions which have a direct bearing on the treatment of patients seeking removable denture service.

General disorders of the neuro-muscular system such as may occur with Parkinson's disease can result in poor control of the muscles about the jaws together with excessive salivation. The ability to manage removable dentures in these circumstances is severely diminished. In the diabetic patient the timing of appointments in relation to dietary control of the condition may be important, and in addition, healing of lesions in the mouth is likely to be slow and the periodontal tissues will require special care where natural teeth are present. The patient suffering from nutritional disturbances or blood dyscrasias may show an abnormal response of the oral mucous membrane to denture trauma.

A history of allergy will alert the operator to possible abnormal reactions to materials or drugs which may be used in treatment. The existence of epilepsy in a patient will introduce design con-

Before being examined and treated, the following questions should be read carefully.
Your answers are *important* in your own interests.
If you have any disease, condition or complaint not listed below that you think should be taken note of, please inform the person attending to you.
Any matters arising from this questionnaire will be dealt with more fully by the person attending to you, but will in any case be treated in confidence.

HEALTH
1. Are you in good health?
2. Are you under the care of a doctor at the present time?
3. Have you ever had any serious illness or operation at any time?
4. Have you ever been in Hospital, especially within the past year?

ILLNESS
Do you suffer from, or have you had, any of the following:-

RHEUMATIC FEVER
RHEUMATIC HEART DISEASE
CHOREA (St. Vitus Dance)
CONGENITAL HEART DISEASE (Blue baby)
HEART MURMUR or VALVULAR DISEASE OF THE HEART
ANAEMIA
HEART TROUBLE, HEART ATTACK
STROKE, PARALYSIS or THROMBOSIS
TUBERCULOSIS, BRONCHITIS, CHEST PAINS
PERSISTENT COUGH or SHORTNESS OF BREATH

FAINTNG SPELLS, BLACKOUTS, FITS
EPILEPSY or LOW BLOOD PRESSURE
ASTHMA, HAY FEVER (Summer colds)
BLOCKED NOSE, ECZEMA or HIVES
  (Urticaria)
DIABETES
JAUNDICE (Yellowing of the skin)
  especially after operation
ARTHRITIS (Rheumatism)
KIDNEY TROUBLE

MEDICINES
1. Are you taking, or have you taken, any of the following medicines, tablets or drugs during the past year?
  (a) Antibiotics (Penicillin, etc.) (b) Tablets for high blood pressure (c) Nerve tablets for depression (d) Insulin or others for Diabetes (e) Anticoagulants (to thin the blood) (f) Cortisone (Steroids) (g) Tranquillisers (sedatives) (h) Digitalis, etc. for the heart.
2. Do you habitually take alcohol?

BAD REACTIONS
1. Are you, or have you been, allergic, sensitive or hypersensitive to any drug, medicine or anything else such as:-
  (a) Local Anaesthetic (b) Penicillin or other antibiotic (c) Sleeping Pills (d) Aspirin or similar pain killing drugs (e) Sticking Plaster (f) Iodine (g) Any other drug (h) Any type of food (i) Ointments.

DENTAL COMPLICATIONS
1. Have you been to the dentist during the past six months?
2. Have you needed treatment for bleeding following dental extractions, operation or injury?
3. Do you bruise easily?
4. Are you employed in any situation which regularly exposes you to X-rays or other ionising radiation?
5. Have you had any bad reactions to any form of dental treatment?
6. Have you or your relatives had any bad reactions to a general anaesthetic (going to sleep for an operation)?

FOR WOMEN
Are you pregnant or taking the contraceptive pill?
FOR PATIENTS OF AFRICAN OR MEDITERRANEAN DESCENT
1. Have you or members of your close family suffered with Sickle Cell Anaemia or Cooley's Anaemia?
2. Have you had a blood test for these diseases?

Fig. 5.1 List of relevant conditions to be read by patient before history-taking commences.

siderations so that any appliance provided will not present an additional hazard to the patient. Where an infective condition is suspected, proper protection will need to be provided to the operator and other members of the dental team — nursing staff, receptionists, and technicians — as well as to other patients attending the practice.

These few examples are intended to underline the need to obtain a full and accurate medical history, and where any doubt may exist the patient's own physician should be contacted.

An additional aspect of the patient's health which is important in removable denture treatment relates to drug therapy, which may be either prescribed by a doctor or represent self-medication by the patient. In either case drugs being taken must be accurately identified.

Some examples of drug therapy relevant to denture treatment include undue dryness of the oral mucosa with a resultant predisposition to damage from minor trauma and potential problems with denture retention. This can occur with the use of tricyclic antidepressant drugs and also with anti-hypertension drugs. Diuretic drugs can cause rapid fluid loss from the tissues resulting in an apparently altered 'fit' of a soft tissue supported denture causing looseness and local trauma. The prolonged use of phenothiazines or similar psychotropic drugs can produce abnormal and unpredictable movements of the oral musculature. The use of non-soluble forms of aspirin can cause ulceration which may simulate other lesions in the mouth.

CLINICAL EXAMINATION

This will be considered as a series of stages which should be followed as a routine so that no aspect is overlooked. It is all too easy to examine only that feature of which a patient may complain and in so doing overlook another condition which might be present.

The clinical examination requires the following to be carried out:
1. Extra-oral examination
2. Intra-oral examination
3. Examination of existing dentures both intra- and extra-orally
4. Special tests where indicated

In addition, the production of study casts will be required for all dentate and some edentulous patients before a final diagnosis can be made.

Extra-oral examination

The overall appearance of the patient should be noted as this may provide a guide to the importance the patient places on aesthetic values. The symmetry of the face should also be noted, and any abnormal movements about the jaws during speech. It may also be possible to detect abnormal clenching or grinding habits.

The general development of the facial musculature should be observed, as a well developed musculature may indicate that heavy forces are generated during mastication.

The lips should be observed for their general characteristics such as length, relationship to the teeth, mobility during speech and whether they appear tense and might therefore exert strong lingually directed forces against the anterior teeth. Any deep creasing, inflammation or scarring at the angles of the mouth should also be noted, as this might indicate possible vertical dimension loss of the facial height, or the presence of an active or healed angular cheilitis.

The apparent skeletal base relationship should be noted following observation of the profile, as this information will be useful in assisting the development of correct tooth positions. The naso-labial angle may also be determined by profile observation of the patient.

Temporomandibular joint activity should be observed and any asymmetry of action during opening and lateral movements of the jaws noted. The presence of any clicking or crepitus or any present or past pain in the region of the joints should be recorded.

Any palpable or tender lymph nodes about the face, jaws or neck should be noted and their cause determined, as these may have a direct relationship to the patient's dental condition and treatment.

The amount of freeway space should be measured and noted on the record card as this will have a direct influence on decisions relating to the vertical dimension provided during the subsequent treatment procedures.

Intra-oral examination of existing dentures

Any dentures should be examined while in position in the mouth and the extension, retention and stability noted. Methods for testing these properties have been referred to in Chapter 2, and in addition careful note should be made of the relationship between the periphery of the denture and the adjacent soft tissues during their manipulation. Where clasped partial dentures are present, the position of clasps and rests and their relationships to tooth surfaces and soft tissues should be noted. Any observable soft or hard tissue lesion related to the *in situ* dentures should be recorded.

Where no natural teeth are present, the horizontal relationship of the anterior teeth to the lips should be noted, and also the tooth arrangement and their colour. The same procedure should be followed where natural teeth are present, and, additionally, the relationship, form and colour of the artificial teeth and natural teeth should be noted.

The occlusion in the retruded jaw relationship is next observed and whether balance exists in eccentric contact relationships between the teeth and/or dentures.

Observations made during the above procedures often relate to the difficulties to which the patient may have referred during the history taking stage.

Extra-oral examination of existing dentures

At this stage, the existing dentures are removed from the mouth and carefully examined. Note should be made of the type of base material used, any relief area, and any other elements present. The material and form of the denture teeth should be noted also. Any evidence of chipping of denture teeth may indicate lack of balanced occlusion. Loss of substance from the teeth should be looked at in terms of the length of time the denture has been in use and also the method used for cleaning the appliance. This is necessary in order to decide whether wear has been excessive, in which case the use of a more abrasion resistant material may be indicated.

The state of hygiene of the denture will give an indication of the attitude of the patient to oral hygiene, and the degree of care likely to be exercised to the remaining teeth or a replacement denture. Similarly, broken flanges, distorted clasps, etc. may point to lack of adequate education of the patient by previous dentists, or a careless patient.

Where any palatal relief has been provided this should be noted. The general arch form and arch width of the dentures should be recorded so that a reduction in tongue space or tissue support may be avoided in a new denture.

Intra-oral examination

This phase of the clinical examination requires a knowledge of disease states affecting or involving the hard and soft tissues of the mouth.

The mucous membranes

The mucous membranes covering the lips, cheeks, floor of the mouth, tongue, hard and soft palate, tonsillar areas, the jaws and residual alveolar ridges should be carefully examined in turn. Any areas of inflammation or other pathology should be noted and the cause identified wherever possible. This may involve special tests or referral for diagnosis to a specialist. It will be necessary to institute treatment of any lesions found before undertaking removable denture treatment.

Where natural teeth are present the gingival condition must be carefully assessed. The standard of oral hygiene must be noted, and by means of a Plaque or Debris Index and a Gingival Index the periodontal state should be recorded. This will also necessitate recording the mobility of the teeth and a careful radiographic assessment (see later). The condition at the time of examination must be recorded to provide a base line so that the effects of treatment can be determined objectively.

The teeth

The teeth present in the mouth must be charted and the form of the occlusal surfaces noted. Any caries and restorations, and the materials of which they are made should be noted. The length of the clinical crowns of the teeth and the amount of abrasion present should be noted. Wear facets on the teeth should be observed in relation to the age of the patient, and the number of teeth present. Apparently excessive wear might point to the possibility of parafunctional jaw activity as a cause. Vitality tests may be indicated. The occlusion should be examined with special reference to the numbers of teeth in contact on closure of the jaws. Disturbances of normal closure from the rest position to tooth contact should be noted, together with any lack of balance in mandibular excursions. Any mobility of each tooth should be assessed and noted.

The upper jaw

The overall size and form of the maxillary alveolar ridge and residual ridge should be noted. The forward movement of the coronoid processes lateral to the tuberosities should be observed in case there is limited space available for a denture flange which may be required in this region. The form of the hard palate may provide a possible clue to the retention which might be expected for a denture which does not involve the use of tooth-borne retainers. A flat, horizontal palatal form with well formed ridges and covered by evenly displaceable mucoperiosteum will give most favourable conditions where soft tissue support is required. The nature of the mucoperiosteum — whether firm or displaceable — will influence the support and stability which might be expected.

Note should be made of the presence and prominence of the frenae as these will influence the peripheral form and possibly the positioning of clasps.

The presence of a torus palatinus and/or undercut regions will affect treatment, and note should be made of the position and form of such features.

The mandible

The overall size and form of the mandibular alveolar ridge and residual ridge should be noted. The presence and size of frenae should be noted as these will have an influence on denture base design, and possibly on clasp placement. In edentulous patients particularly the prominence of the mylohyoid ridge and the genial tubercles should be noted. The displaceability of the covering mucoperiosteum and its evenness or otherwise, and also the presence of undercuts, should be noted. The presence of a torus mandibularis will influence denture design and should be noted and described.

The tongue

The tongue will have a strong influence on denture design, especially for a lower denture, and note should be made of its size and mobility. Where posterior teeth have been missing for many years, the tongue may tend to spread laterally because of the lack of restriction postero-laterally, and may result in difficulty in the patient adjusting to a denture replacing the missing teeth. A large tongue may also suffer mechanical irritation resulting from friction with a denture.

Saliva

It has been pointed out that the presence of saliva is essential for denture retention, particularly for complete denture wearers, and is also important to the comfort of the patient wearing removeable dentures.

Lack of saliva may result in frictional effects, general oral discomfort and trauma. Excessive saliva may tend to cause drooling, and good support of the corners of the mouth will be required. Both of these conditions will require care in the choice of impression materials and the design of any appliance provided.

SPECIAL TESTS

Radiographic examination

In order to assess further patients presenting for removable denture treatment, a radiographic examination may be required. Where partial denture treatment is being considered, all the teeth which may be directly associated with the denture must be radiographed. In some instances this will involve radiographs of all standing teeth. The amount of bony support available, interproximal caries and any pulpal or periapical pathology, may all be disclosed using radiographs.

In edentulous areas, the presence of unerupted teeth, retained roots or other pathological entities may be disclosed. The nature of the residual alveolar bone may provide a valuable indication of possible reactions to denture treatment. Where a sound layer of dense cortical bone is present with a clearly defined pattern of trabeculae in the cancellous bone, good support for a denture might be anticipated. The recommended X-rays for suitable examination of the teeth and jaws include an orthopantomographic type scan of the jaws, supplemented by intra-oral views of any area which is specifically indicated.

Other special tests

The soft tissue condition in the oral cavity may require bacteriological examination. Biopsy may be indicated in the presence of suspected neoplasia. Blood tests may be indicated where anaemia or other deficiency conditions are thought to exist.

Where suspicion is aroused regarding possible allergy to dental materials, skin sensitivity tests may be indicated.

STUDY CASTS FOR DENTATE MOUTHS

Because of the difficulties involved in close examination of parts of the mouth and in assessing tooth relationships and their contours accurately, study casts are required to provide additional information to assist in planning the treatment to be undertaken.

Study casts are an accurate representation of the teeth, jaws and sulci. They should be fabricated of a durable material such as dental stone. The casts must be mounted on an adjustable articulator. Mounting of the upper cast is accomplished using a face-bow record in order to ensure its correct relationship to the condylar mechanism of the articulator. An accurate record of retruded jaw relation is obtained for attachment of the lower cast to the articulator in its correct relationship to the upper.

Functions of study casts

1. They reveal the surface morphology of the tissues about the jaws unencumbered by surrounding tissues and the presence of saliva.

2. A detailed study of the occlusion, including the lingual aspects in retruded jaw relation, can be made.

3. The occlusion and its balance in retruded jaw relation and eccentric positions can be examined. A decision to adjust the occlusal surfaces by, for example, judicious grinding or crown modification using restorative procedures may be reached in order to:

a. Improve tooth contact in retruded jaw relation, or provide freedom of movement and more favourable distribution of occlusal loads in lateral movements.

b. Adjust the level of the occlusal plane of the remaining natural teeth.

4. The need for further extractions might be indicated following examination of the study casts and in the light of the information obtained in the clinical examination. A third molar, for example, could be malpositioned and mitigate against successful denture design, either by virtue of being in contact with the opposing residual alveolar ridge, or by interference with occlusal balance, or perhaps because of a nearly horizontal inclination. Tooth extraction or crown modification will therefore be required.

5. The casts can be surveyed and the pathway by which the denture may be seated into position in the mouth determined. Surveying the casts enables many other decisions relating to partial dentures to be reached. These are considered below.

6. They provide an excellent visual aid for discussion of treatment with the patient.

7. They can be used in the production of special impression trays for subsequent impression procedures and for the production of temporary splints where a change in the patient's vertical dimension of occlusion is contemplated.

8. They are an essential guide to the technician for subsequent laboratory stages.

SURVEYING

The next step in diagnosis and treatment planning is to survey the study casts. Surveying consists of locating the maximum contour of individual teeth and of the alveolar ridges and residual ridges. The maximum contour is located by means of a vertical plane, which is brought into contact with the cast. If a carbon marker is substituted for the vertical plane, a mark which is called a survey line can be produced on the cast. All parts of the surveyed

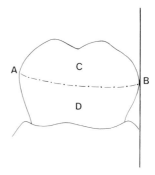

Fig. 5.2 Undercut and non-undercut areas. A, Survey line; B, Plane of survey; C, Non-undercut area; D, Undercut area.

cast above the survey line are non-undercut areas and all parts below are called undercut areas with respect to the direction in which the survey was carried out (Fig. 5.2)

The objects of surveying

1. To determine the path of insertion of a denture. The path of insertion of a denture is the path or direction followed by the denture in being seated into position in the mouth. The procedure for selecting the path of insertion is outlined below.

2. To ensure that no rigid portion of a partial denture lies in an undercut relative to the path of insertion (and of removal) of the denture.

3. Undercuts useful for retention of a denture can be located.

4. The amount of horizontal undercut of the teeth selected for clasping can be determined. A corollary to this object is that where no undercut is present on a tooth otherwise suitable for clasping, modification of the tooth surface to form an undercut may be considered.

The cast surveyor

A large number of cast surveyors (also called model surveyors or dental surveyors) are available, and they all have the same basic property of providing a means whereby a vertical plane can be bought into contact with a cast.

In brief, the cast surveyor consists of a horizontal platform or base from which a rigid vertical post projects. Attached to the vertical post is a horizontal arm which supports another vertical post which is adjustable upwards and downwards. The adjustable vertical post is designed in such a manner that the lower end carries a mandrel which can hold the various tools used in surveying, clasp positioning and cast modification. For mounting the cast, a cast table is provided. This consists of a heavy metal base which, by means of a universal joint, carries an adjustable top capable of being locked in any position to provide the chosen amount of tilt. Provision for firm attachment of the cast to the top of the cast table is required. A diagram of one type of cast surveyor is shown in Figure 5.3.

Fig. 5.3 Diagram of a cast surveyor. A, Base; B, Vertical rod; C, Hinged horizontal arm; D, Vertical spindle; E, Chuck for surveying tools; F, A surveying tool; G, Cast retainer; H, Table of surveyor.

The tools used in the surveyor include:
1. Analysing rod   (Fig. 5.4 A)
2. Carbon marker   (Fig. 5.4 B)
3. Undercut gauges   (Fig. 5.4 C)
4. Chisels or trimmers   (Fig. 5.4 D)

The analysing rod is a smooth metal rod used for diagnostic purposes (analysis) in selecting a path of insertion and thus the desired tilt of the cast table, and in determining the presence of undercuts.

The carbon marker is similar in form to the analysing rod and is used for marking the survey line

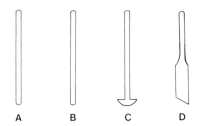

Fig. 5.4 Tools used in the surveyor. A, Analysing rod; B, Carbon marker; C, Undercut gauge; D, Chisel or trimmer.

Fig. 5.5 Use of the undercut gauge. A, Undercut gauge; B, Survey line; C, Undercut dimension.

on the cast once the direction in which surveying is to be carried out has been determined.

Undercut gauges are used to measure the amount of horizontal undercut on a tooth. These guages are available in three sizes (0.25 mm, 0.50 mm and 0.75 mm) and the method of use is shown in Figure 5.5. The use of these gauges is essential to decisions regarding the position in which clasp arms may be placed, the material of which they may be constructed, and their dimensions.

The chisels or trimmers are used in the elimination of unwanted undercuts. Where a cast is to be used in the production of a partial denture it is essential that unwanted undercuts are eliminated in the same axis as that chosen for insertion and removal of the denture. If the denture is to be produced on a duplicate cast, e.g. such as that used for a cast partial denture base, the undercuts are eliminated using wax prior to the construction of the duplicate cast. Where the denture is to be produced directly on the master cast, unwanted undercuts are eliminated using plaster of Paris. Elimination of unwanted undercuts is essential to ensure that no rigid part of a partial denture can enter an undercut area relative to the paths of insertion and removal. In addition to undercuts about the teeth, the elimination of undercuts related to soft tissues may be required in order to prevent injury to the superficial tissues when such areas are to be included within the denture outline.

Selecting the path of insertion

The selection of the path of insertion for a removable partial denture is fundamental to further detailed planning of the appliance.

Two basic schools of thought may be said to exist in relation to selection of the path of insertion.

1. A vertical path of insertion, where the occlusal plane is horizontal during surveying, should be used. The forces which tend to dislodge a denture during mastication and which are generated by the adhesion of foodstuffs to opposing occlusal surfaces are at a maximum at the moment of first separation of the jaws. These forces act at right angles to the occlusal plane and retention for the denture should be provided to resist these displacing forces. Such an approach would provide for a single vertical path of insertion and withdrawal for the denture so that the patient would not have any complicated manoeuvres to learn. Where complex insertion and removal procedures are involved, the possibility of inducing excessive stresses in the periodontium exists.

2. If a vertical path of insertion is used, displacement of the denture is resisted only by clasps. Where the path of insertion is not at right angles to the occlusal plane, rigid portions of the denture will resist displacement in the vertical plane during mastication. Thus the cast should not be surveyed with the occlusal plane horizontal (Fig. 5.6).

The choice between these two approaches is not always so clear cut as would appear from the above, and there are several other factors which may appear to be in conflict in any given clinical situation:

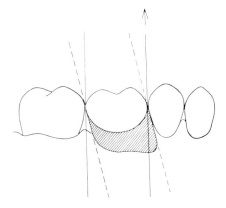

Fig. 5.6 By tilting the cast, rigid portions of the denture can engage undercuts relative to the vertical path of displacement. The solid line represents a vertical direction of survey, and the broken line that of a survey with the cast tilted.

Fig. 5.7 Guiding planes are indicated by the broken lines

1. *Guiding planes.* These are parallel surfaces of teeth and residual ridges which form a clear pathway along which the denture may be guided to its planned position in the mouth (Fig. 5.7).

Where effective guiding planes are present, part of the retention of the denture may be affected by friction between the denture and the guiding plane, thus reducing the need for reliance on clasps. Where no guiding planes exist, limited modification of tooth substance may be undertaken in order to produce them. Guiding planes are also significant in considering effective reciprocation for individual clasps (Fig. 5.8).

2. *Retention undercuts.* Ideally, undercuts utilised for retention should be equally distributed over the teeth to be clasped.

3. *Undercut areas enclosed by the denture.* These

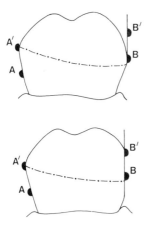

Fig. 5.8 The presence of a guiding plane on a tooth enables the reciprocating arm (B) of the clasp to oppose the action of the retentive arm (A) in all positions of contact of the retentive arm with the tooth. Note how the absence of a guiding plane in the upper diagram results in loss of contact of the reciprocating arm while the retentive arm still engages an undercut region of the tooth.

are in effect dead spaces and should be minimised either by averaging them out in selecting the path of insertion, or by adjusting the form of the abutment teeth.

4. *Appearance.* When clasps are required about the anterior parts of the mouth, a minimal display of metal must be aimed at.

5. *Saddles.* Several may be present, each having different characteristics.

Procedure for surveying

The cast to be surveyed is removed from the articulator and firmly attached to the cast table which is placed on the base of the surveyor.

The occlusal plane of the cast is then orientated with respect to the base of the surveyor, i.e. a degree of tilt is applied to the cast. In the first instance zero tilt, i.e. with the occlusal plane horizontal, should be adopted. The analysing rod is placed in the surveyor and gently brought into contact with the cast. Guiding planes may be present on the lingual aspect of the remaining teeth; undercuts in regions where retention by means of clasps will be sought should be checked. It may be found necessary to modify the tilt of the cast in order to even out undercuts and dead spaces. Areas where minor modification of a tooth surface to produce suitable guiding planes are required should be noted. When the final degree of tilt has been decided upon, the analysing rod should be substituted by the carbon marker. All undercut areas should then be recorded including that part of the cast representing soft tissue.

Where moderate to severe abutment tooth inclination exists the method of averaging abutment inclination offers a good starting method for tilting the cast. In this approach the abutment tooth inclinations in the lateral plane are marked on the cast and the average of these taken to provide the degree of lateral tilt for the cast. The anteroposterior tilt is similarly averaged from the mesiodistal inclination of the abutment teeth. The vertical movable post of the surveyor is then made parallel to this average of inclinations of the abutment teeth.

Whatever approach is used, compromises often need to be made to allow for simplicity of insertion consistent with the availability of suitable under-

Fig. 5.9 Downwards tilting of the anterior part of the cast enables the distal aspect of |4 to be used as a guiding plane.

cuts and diminishing dead spaces which are potential areas for stagnation of food debris.

In general, surveying the cast with the occlusal plane horizontal is preferred because:

1. A single path of insertion and removal is obtained where this is possible.

2. Clasps may be designed to provide maximum retention in the plane where displacement is most likely to occur.

The main exceptions to this generalisation where model tilting is required are:

1. To tilt the anterior aspect of the cast downwards where a free-end saddle exists so that the distal surface of the abutment tooth can be used as a guide plane (Fig. 5.9).

2. To try to bring parallel oblique abutments into a vertical alignment and so eliminate the need for blocking out undercuts.

SUBSEQUENT PROCEDURES

Following surveying of the cast, the final design of the denture can be considered, including particular types of clasp most suitable to the survey lines produced. These aspects are further considered in Chapters 13 and 14. The position of the retentive tips of clasp arms relative to the survey lines will require the use of the undercut gauges described above. In general more flexible materials can engage deeper undercuts, e.g. a long wrought gold alloy clasp arm can engage an undercut of up to 0.75 mm without exerting damaging forces on the clasped tooth during withdrawal of the denture. On the other hand, a cast cobalt chromium clasp must not engage an undercut in excess of 0.25 mm.

Finally, in association with a knowledge of the occlusion between opposing teeth, a decision regarding the need for, and the position of, any rest seat preparation and other forms of tooth modification should be made and carried out. It is, of course, essential that all preparation of the mouth be completed before attempting to obtain an impression to produce the working cast on which the denture will be constructed.

STUDY CASTS FOR EDENTULOUS MOUTHS

Apart from the function of providing a means for producing special trays in order to obtain a working impression, there are two further principal reasons why study casts for edentulous mouths may be required.

1. Where lack of space appears to be a possible problem, study casts should be mounted on an adjustable articulator using a record of the retruded jaw relationship. This type of problem is most frequently seen in the posterior part of the mouth, and an adjustable articulator will give an opportunity to assess the tissue proximity during mandibular excursions. A knowledge of the health status of the patient, X-rays of the region concerned and, following discussions with the patient, a decision to adopt a surgical approach prior to denture construction might be made. Alternatively, a modified denture base might be considered — possibly by not including the region concerned in the denture outline.

2. Where unyielding undercuts are present, especially when bilateral. A common site for this to occur is in the tuberosity region of the upper denture bearing area. By using the surveyor the extent of the undercuts will be revealed. Where these are minimal, it may be decided to eliminate the undercut on one or both sides by means of plaster of Paris applied to the cast, and subsequently using a chisel or trimmer on the surveyor in order to minimise the area of the denture base which will be affected.

For deeper undercuts, surgery may need to be considered and/or modification of the denture base outline. Alternatively, where surgery is contra-indicated and the use of an undercut is required for adequate retention, the flange of the denture may be constructed using a soft lining material.

FURTHER READING

Atkinson H F 1953 Partial denture problems. Designing about a path of withdrawal. Austral J Dent 57: 187

Bremner V A and Grant A A 1971 A radiographic survey of edentulous mouths. Austral J Dent 16: 17

Boitel R H 1971 Problems of old age in dental prosthetics and restorative procedures. J Prosthet Dent 26: 350

Coy R E and Arnold P D 1974 Survey and design of diagnostic casts for removable partial dentures. J Prosthet Dent 32: 103

Ettinger R L 1981 Xerostomia — a complication of ageing. Austral Dent J 26: 365

Franks A S T and Hedegard B 1973 Geriatric Dentistry. Blackwell, Oxford

House M M 1958 The relationship of oral examination to dental diagnosis. J Prosthet Dent 8: 208

Katulski E A and Appleyard W N 1959 Biological concepts of the use of a mechanical cast surveyor. J Prosthet Dent 9: 629

Langer A 1979 Prosthodontic failures in patients with systemic disorders. J Oral Rehab 6: 13

Levine E M 1960 Gagging — a problem in prosthodontics. J Canad Dent Assoc 26: 70

Mack A O 1964 Complete dentures: functional difficulties. Brit Dent J 117: 92

Neill D J and Walter J D 1977 Partial Denture Prosthetics. Blackwell, Oxford.

Rothwell P S and Wragg K A 1972 Assessment of the medical status of patients in general dental practice. Brit Dent J 133: 252

Schole M C 1959 Management of the gagging patient. J Prosthet Dent 9: 578

Szymaitis D W 1977 Considerations in treatment of alcoholics. J Amer Dent Assoc 95: 592

Woods R G 1978 Drug therapy and denture patient (Letter). Austral Dent J 23: 431

6

Diagnosis and treatment planning

INTRODUCTION

In principle, diagnosis and treatment planning for dentate and edentulous patients seeking prosthetic treatment are similar.

Following the history taking and examination procedures, the basic reason for the patient seeking treatment will become apparent. Indeed, where natural teeth are missing, the patient will often ask for a specific type of treatment, e.g. for partial or complete dentures, and may be unaware that such treatment may be inappropriate or that other treatment may be required before their requirements can satisfactorily be met. Thus, having obtained all the relevant information regarding the dental condition of the patient, consideration is next given to the possible alternative forms of treatment available. Any preliminary treatment required to bring the mouth to an optimal state of health is then carried out.

Details of the prosthetic treatment can then be planned, including any necessary modifications of the hard or soft tissues of the mouth.

Diagnosis is the identification of a disease state by its signs and symptoms. For prosthetic treatment the term diagnosis must take into account any conditions which might necessitate preliminary treatment such as the presence of any pathology, and also modifications of any hard or soft tissue which might mitigate against effective treatment. (The consideration of alternative forms of treatment which might be available to a patient might be regarded as a differential diagnosis.)

Treatment planning refers to the order in which the proposed treatment is to be carried out and includes an outline of the clinical techniques to be used in the various stages of treatment.

While the principles are similar, there are considerable differences in detail between dentate and edentulous mouths in respect of diagnosis and treatment planning and they will be considered separately.

Plaque control

Wherever natural teeth are present, the damaging effects of plaque must be borne in mind and also that the capacity for the retention of plaque by removable dentures is well established. The risks of the effects of this on the remaining dentition and supporting tissues may outweigh any possible benefits of the denture. It is therefore basic to the success of removable denture therapy that the establishment of plaque control and instruction in appropriate oral hygiene procedures are given at the outset of treatment. Plaque control must be established for all patients as an integral part of removable denture treatment.

Poor plaque control in the dentate patient may result in periodontal breakdown with the ultimate loss of the natural teeth. The edentulous patient wearing complete dentures must also be aware of the need for plaque control in order to avoid soft tissue lesions such as those resulting from trauma caused by the build up of plaque on the fitting surface of dentures, and candidal infection.

WHERE NATURAL TEETH ARE PRESENT

The treatment alternatives for the patient who has lost some natural teeth are:
1. No prosthetic treatment.
2. The provision of fixed appliances.
3. Removable partial denture treatment.
4. Extraction of some or all of the remaining teeth

and the provision of complete dentures. A common means by which the conversion of a dentate patient to a complete denture wearer is achieved is by the provision of immediate dentures. This topic is considered to be outside the scope of this text and the reader should refer to the literature for details of the procedures available.

No prosthetic treatment

Health

In some circumstances it might be considered to be in the best interests of the health of the patient not to replace missing teeth by means of a removable partial denture. Where a patient is known to be severely epileptic, for example, the presence of a removable denture in the mouth might represent a danger to the patient. Similarly, where a functional but incomplete dentition exists in a patient who, by virtue of physical or mental handicap, is incapable of inserting or removing a denture from the mouth, it might be considered better not to provide prosthetic treatment by means of a removable appliance.

The number and position of the missing teeth

Both must be considered. In a mouth from which only the third molars are missing it is unlikely that a denture would be required. Where the second and third molars have been lost from one side only of the upper or lower arch, in the absence of over-eruption of the opposing teeth it might be considered preferable not to replace the missing teeth using a removable denture.

Age

The age of the patient may also be a factor to be considered. An elderly patient having several teeth missing and an adequate number of opposing teeth to provide for effective mastication may find adjustment to a denture difficult. In addition, the extra care of the mouth and the appliance required might represent too difficult a task to be undertaken on a regular basis. Chronological age is not of itself the criterion on which to base decisions of this nature. It is the biological age of the patient which is important in this context.

Plaque control

This important factor has already been considered above. It is repeated here to remind the reader that where there is a lack of appreciation of the need for good oral hygiene the provision of a removable partial denture may have a harmful rather than a beneficial effect on the dental status of the patient.

The provision of fixed appliances

A bridge which is permanently cemented into the mouth is in every way a more acceptable form of treatment than that using removable partial dentures. Bridges occupy a similar amount of space in the mouth to the teeth they replace and this is rarely true of a removable denture. Being entirely tooth borne they may withstand greater masticatory force than a mucosa borne denture. A further advantage is that the patient is never conscious of movement of a bridge, whereas some patients may detect partial denture movement during function. Where anterior teeth are involved, and excessive loss of residual alveolar bone has not occurred, the aesthetic result achievable with fixed bridgework may be superior to that obtained using removable partial dentures.

Bridgework is the method of choice in the treatment of handicapped patients where suitable oral conditions exist, e.g. the physically handicapped patient who is unable to manipulate a removable partial denture; or in severe epilepsy where a denture may become dislodged.

Fixed bridgework, however, is only recommended for use over relatively short spans depending on the suitability of the abutment teeth to which the bridge is cemented. It is always necessary to prepare the abutment teeth for crowns to provide retention, and where such teeth are free of any lesion, the loss of tooth substance from a healthy tooth may not be acceptable.

Where fixed bridgework is contemplated, it must be borne in mind that adaptation of the appliance to further tooth loss is often impossible. Thus, where the life expectancy for other teeth is limited, this can be an important consideration.

In addition to being somewhat less versatile in that partial dentures are usable over a wider variety of clinical conditions, the clinical time required for the preparation of the abutment teeth involved tends to make bridges more expensive than dentures, so that an economic factor may also need to be considered.

Removable partial denture treatment

Where the dentition is incomplete, its restoration by removable partial denture treatment may be contemplated. There are a number of clinical circumstances in which removable partial denture treatment may be indicated:

1. Where fixed bridgework is contraindicated, e.g. if the span of the edentulous ridge is too long for the available abutments; or where periodontally involved teeth remaining would benefit from cross-arch bracing; or where the contemplated abutment teeth are unblemished.

2. Where excessive loss of residual bone has followed tooth loss, e.g. in the anterior region, the aesthetic requirements in such cases cannot be met by bridgework.

3. Where there is need for replacement of posterior teeth having an abutment tooth at one end of the edentulous ridge only.

4. In children and adolescents where growth of the jaws or tooth roots might still be taking place.

5. Where it is required to attach an obturator, e.g. for a cleft palate patient, to the denture.

6. Where there is a short life expectancy for other remaining teeth.

7. As a transitional prosthesis, e.g. where total tooth loss is anticipated and it is desired to accustom the patient to denture management before the provision of complete dentures; where alteration to the vertical dimension is indicated and the decision as to the permanent form of restoration is to be guided by the reaction of the patient to a temporary appliance.

Extraction of some, or all, of the remaining teeth and the provision of complete dentures

The removal of the remaining teeth of a patient from one or both jaws is an irreversible procedure having very serious implications. It must never be undertaken lightly and should only be carried out where alternative forms of treatment are inappropriate.

The principle reasons for the loss of several teeth are trauma, advanced caries, and loss of bony support for the teeth. The condition of the mouth of a patient on examination will also have been subject to many other factors. For example, the attitude of the patient to dental treatment and home dental care will have been factors of long term influence, as will the nature and quality of the dental care provided for the patient.

The age of the patient may also be a factor of some significance, where the long term prognosis for the retention of the natural teeth is poor. In such circumstances it is important to remember that the older patient requires, in general, a longer period for adaptation to dentures than a younger one.

In some cases an older patient may be beyond the point where control of dentures can be learned, and consequently all patients beyond the middle 50's should be carefully assessed with this in mind. It may be more desirable from a long term point of view to convert these patients to complete denture wearing while they can learn new muscular activities. No such problem exists where the prognosis for retention of the remaining natural teeth is good.

Where only a few pairs of opposing natural teeth can be retained, they may provide the basis for better masticatory effectiveness than complete dentures.

Caution should be exercised in considering a complete denture in one jaw opposed to natural teeth in the other. The prognosis for a complete upper denture opposed by natural teeth can be fair provided that there is a minimum of potential displacing contacts between the teeth and the denture. Modification of the natural tooth surfaces may be required to achieve this. The situation in which natural upper teeth oppose a lower complete denture should be avoided as the small surface area covered by the denture does not allow for protection of the underlying mucosa from the high masticatory forces developed.

One of the common problems presented by a patient with only a few teeth remaining is the very long clinical crowns of the teeth resulting from bone resorption in the edentulous regions. Such teeth may be susceptible to tilting forces because of their length, and may be mobile. This does not necessarily mean that the teeth must be extracted, as by endodontic treatment where necessary, and reduction of the length of the tooth crown, the tooth may be rendered suitable for use in the support of an overdenture. Similarly a tooth with advanced damage of the crown by caries can be considered for retention as an abutment for support of an overdenture. This form of treatment is considered in more detail in Chapter 28.

TREATMENT PLANNING WHERE NATURAL TEETH ARE PRESENT AND A REMOVABLE PARTIAL DENTURE IS TO BE PROVIDED

Following the history taking and examination procedure, and having reached a decision concerning the overall treatment to be undertaken, a detailed treatment plan can be drawn up.

This will consist of:

1. Immediate measures for the relief of pain or any acute condition present.

2. Details of the treatment to be undertaken in respect of the provision of removable partial dentures.

3. The details of the proposed treatment which must be noted include:

a. Treatment of any oral lesions such as denture stomatitis, ulceration, candidal infections, etc.

b. Treatment of the periodontal condition and instruction and motivation to effective oral hygiene.

c. Any surgical and conservative treatment necessary to prepare the mouth for removable partial dentures. This will include any necessary extractions and restorations. The provision of any rest seats, modifications to guiding planes or additional retentive regions will have been decided upon with the examination of the study casts. Any conservative treatment must be carried out with reference to that phase of planning.

d. The impression procedure to be used should be planned on the basis of clinical conditions present (Chapter 8).

e. Any special aesthetic requirements must be noted.

f. The type of artificial teeth to be used, in-

cluding the material from which they should be made must be noted (see Chapter 11).

g. The type of articulator required for mounting the working casts and setting the teeth should be recorded (see Chapter 10).

h. The base material of which the denture is to be made — whether metallic or non-metallic, and any requirements for stress breaking using precision attachments or other elements — must be noted.

i. The proposed final design of the removable denture(s) must be recorded on a prescription form in such a manner as to be clearly communicated to the dental technician without possible misinterpretation (see Chapter 15).

WHERE NO TEETH ARE PRESENT

The treatment alternatives where no natural teeth are present are:

1. No prosthetic treatment.
2. The provision of complete dentures.
3. The provision of complete dentures in conjunction with dental implants.

No prosthetic treatment

Where all the teeth have been lost from one or both jaws it is unusual for a patient to be prepared to suffer the deprivation and indignity of edentulousness without seeking denture treatment.

Contraindications to complete denture treatment are rare, and include some advanced neuromuscular disorders and certain mental disorders and other conditions where cooperation of the patient cannot be obtained.

The provision of complete dentures

A detailed treatment plan for the edentulous patient must encompass all treatment necessary to bring the mouth to an optimal condition for the provision of complete dentures.

This will involve:

1. Immediate measures for the relief of pain or any acute conditions present.

2. Treatment for any oral lesions present such as denture stomatitis, candidal infection, ulcer-

ation or any other inflammatory condition. This will include the correction of any condition resulting from ill-fitting dentures and may require the modification, or withholding, of the existing dentures as a preliminary measure prior to undertaking further treatment (see Chapter 7).

3. Any surgical treatment required to prepare the mouth for complete dentures (Chapter 7).

4. Where a single complete denture is opposed by the natural dentition, any tooth modification required to eliminate or reduce occlusal contacts which might tend to displace the denture.

5. The selection of an impression procedure based on the clinical conditions present (Chapter 8).

6. Whether any change in vertical dimension from that provided by an existing denture is required. Where a gross change in vertical dimension is required, it may be necessary to consider incremental changes using the existing dentures with suitable occlusal adjustment over a period of time.

7. Any special aesthetic requirements of the patient should be noted.

8. The type of articulator required for mounting the working cast and setting the teeth should be recorded (Chapter 10).

9. The type of artificial teeth to be used, including the material from which they should be made, must be noted (Chapter 11).

10. The base material from which the dentures will be constructed must be recorded. In some circumstances, a soft lining material may be prescribed.

Soft lining materials

Denture base materials are generally of a rigid nature, being of a rigid polymer or less frequently of metal. Occasionally, the forces transmitted to the underlying mucosa via the denture base are such as to produce pain during functions such as mastication.

The use of a soft material under that part of the denture which contacts the mucosa overlying the residual alveolar ridge may afford relief to the patient. This is considered to occur by virtue of energy absorption of the soft material as it distorts when the masticatory force is applied.

Soft lining materials are most effective where the mucosa is thin and overlies a smooth alveolar crest. They are generally used under complete lower dentures, but may occasionally be used with the upper denture where it is considered essential for the denture base to enter an unyielding undercut.

DENTAL IMPLANTS

A dental implant is an object which is implanted into or onto the surface of the bone of the jaw and which has one or more extensions which project through the mucoperiosteum into the oral cavity with the object of providing anchorage for a denture.

Implants are designated subperiosteal or endosseous, depending on whether they lie beneath the mucoperiosteum and on the surface of the bone (subperiosteal) or actually enter into the body of the bone (endosseous).

They may be used for dentate patients to replace some missing teeth, but are most commonly applied for the edentulous patient having a long history of repeated failure and difficulties with a conventional lower complete denture. In this latter category the subperiosteal implant has been most commonly used. The subperiosteal framework is produced on a model obtained from an impression of the bony ridge at an operation following reflection of the mucoperiosteum. At a subsequent operation the framework is inserted. A denture is fabricated to engage the projecting elements of the framework and so transmit the forces developed during mastication to the bony foundations.

Variable success rates with implant dentures have been reported and the techniques employed are regarded as still being in a developmental stage. For further details the reader is referred to the current literature in this specialised topic.

FURTHER READING

Anderson J N and Storer R 1981 Immediate and Replacement Dentures. 3rd Edn. Blackwell, Oxford

Applegate O C 1957 Conditions which may influence the choice of partial or complete denture service. J Prosthet Dent 7: 182

Beeson P E 1970 The mouth examination for complete dentures: a review. J Prosthet Dent 23: 482

Carlsson G E, Hedegard B and Koivumaa K K 1970 The current place of removable partial dentures in restorative dentistry. Dent Clin North Amer 14: 553

Dawson P E 1974 Evaluation, Diagnosis and Treatment of Occulsal Problems. Mosby, St Louis

Landa J S 1957 Diagnosis of the edentulous mouth and the probable prognosis of its rehabilitation. Dent Clin North Amer 1: 187

Linkow K I and Cherchevre R 1970 Theory and Techniques of Oral Implantology. Mosby, St Louis

Stern N and Brayer L 1975 Collapse of the occlusion — aetiology, symptomatology and treatment. J Oral Rehab 2: 1

Wright P S 1976 Soft lining materials: their status and prospects. J Dent 4: 247

7

Preparation of the mouth for prosthetic treatment

INTRODUCTION

Only when the mouth is in a healthy state should prosthetic treatment be undertaken. Even when the oral tissues have been brought to as healthy a condition as possible, it is often necessary for further treatment to be undertaken to facilitate and maximise the benefits of prosthetic treatment for the patient.

There are many conditions of a general nature having oral manifestations. The operator must be able to recognise general disease states having oral signs and symptoms. Reference should be made to the relevant literature on this important topic, which is considered to be outside the scope of this text. Clearly, any such condition must be recognised and treatment instituted before any dental treatment is undertaken.

For descriptive puposes the common conditions which necessitate treatment prior to denture production have been grouped together. It must be appreciated that there may be overlap between these groups as the treatment required may embrace both surgical and non-surgical procedures.

NON-SURGICAL PREPARATION

Soft tissue preparation

Periodontal treatment

Where natural teeth are present in the mouth of a patient seeking denture treatment, periodontal treatment is likely to be required. Any calculus present will need to be removed at the outset of treatment so that an accurate assessment of the gingival tissues can be made. Even where the teeth are to be extracted calculus removal will be required prior to surgery. Treatment of the periodontal condition of denture patients may require scaling and polishing together with oral hygiene instruction and/or reinforcement, or more advanced forms of periodontal therapy might be indicated. A thorough understanding of this topic is essential to successful restoration of the mouth, and reference to the literature should be made for its full consideration.

The potential denture patient should be required to show evidence of adequate plaque control before treatment is proceeded with.

Tissue distortion

Where continuous use of a soft tissue supported denture which has become ill-fitting has occurred, the uneven forces directed to the mucosa via the denture will result in deformation of the tissues from their resting form. Distortion of the form of tissues occurs to the greatest extent where thickened mucoperiosteum is present and usually some signs of inflammation of the tissues may be seen. Return of the tissues to their resting contour is a time dependent phenomenon, and the simplest and most effective method for achieving this is by removal of the denture until the tissues have recovered.

Even where there are no obvious signs of tissue deformation in patients having thickened mucoperiosterum, up to 90 minutes may be required to allow the tissues to achieve stable contours following removal of the existing denture (Fig. 7.1). It is therefore desirable that this interval be allowed to elapse before impressions are taken.

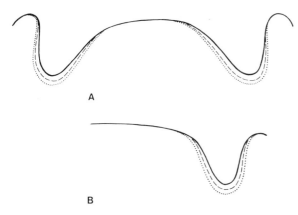

Fig. 7.1 Coronal section through the first molar region (A), and sagittal section through the incisor region (B) for an edentulous patient showing the surface contours at several times following removal of a complete upper denture. Solid line: Immediately following removal; Broken line: 30 minutes following removal; Dotted line: 90 minutes and all subsequent times to 150 minutes following removal.

Denture stomatitis

This is a condition in which chronic irritation of the mucoperiosteum contacted by the denture base has produced an inflammatory response. Denture stomatitis is most commonly seen in association with upper dentures and may appear as a vivid inflammation over an area coincident with that covered by the denture. In less severe cases, small discrete areas of pinpoint inflammation, often associated with the ducts of the palatal mucous glands, may be present. Between these two extremes inflammation of varying extent may be present. A further form of denture stomatitis is described as papillary hyperplasia in which a nodular hyperaemic surface of the mucosa of the denture bearing area is seen. Papillary hyperplasia occurs commonly in the central palatal region and more rarely may extend over the entire denture bearing area.

A large number of causative factors have been implicated in the aetiology of denture stomatitis including:

1. Trauma, usually associated with an existing denture.
2. Endocrine disturbances, e.g. associated with the climacteric; diabetes.
3. Deficiency states (e.g. certain vitamins).
4. During antibiotic therapy.
5. Associated with xerostomia (dry mouth).

The first of these factors is by far the most common, and the trauma induced by a denture may result from occlusal or articulation faults such as premature tooth contacts; roughness of the denture base; poor denture hygiene; faulty adaptation of the denture to the underlying tissues; or incorrect vertical dimension of occlusion. These factors can cause undesirable effects from movement between the mucosa and the denture base, and this trauma produces an inflammatory response in the mucosa. This inflammation is often associated with infection by *Candida albicans* invasion of which appears to be stimulated by trauma to the tissues and also by the nature of the denture base, particularly in the presence of poor oral hygiene.

Treatment is directed towards the elimination of trauma and control of the candidal infection. Denture induced trauma is best eliminated by removal of the denture. Where only relatively minor faults are present in the denture it may be possible for a patient to continue to use the appliance following correction of the faults which are present. The use of a tissue conditioning material may also be required. Details relating to these materials should be obtained from the literature. Control of candidal infections will involve the use of suitable antifungicides on both the oral mucosa and the denture.

Angular cheilitis

This is a condition in which a painful inflammation of the corners of the mouth is present. It commonly occurs as a result of constant wetting of the angles of the mouth by saliva because of lack of lip support following tooth extraction; a poorly designed denture flange lacking the capacity to provide adequate lip support; or loss of occlusal vertical dimension of a denture or a natural dentition lacking opposing posterior teeth. The skin at the angles of the mouth cracks and becomes infected producing painful fissures. Other causes of angular cheilitis include vitamin deficiency and iron deficiency states. Angular cheilitis may be associated with an intra-oral candidal infection.

Angular cheilitis may require antibacterial or antifungal therapy and appropriate medication where a deficiency state exists. It must also be taken into account in planning the design of a new denture.

Denture hyperplasia (denture granuloma)

This condition is characterised by the presence of one or more rolls or flaps of soft tissue, usually associated with the border of a denture flange. It generally results from resorption of the residual alveolar ridge so that the flanges of the denture become overextended with respect to the functional sulcus and the hyperplasia follows the resultant severe tissue irritation.

The treatment of this condition involves removal of the source of irritation, i.e. removal of part or the whole of the denture flange in the region concerned, or removal of the denture, when resolution may occur over a period of weeks. Should resolution fail to take place, surgery may have to be considered.

Other soft tissue conditions

Other soft tissue conditions which will require investigation and treatment prior to denture treatment include:
Hyperkeratosis
Aphthous ulceration
Pseudomembranous candidosis ('thrush')
Chronic hyperplastic candidosis
Leukoplakia
Lichen planus
Tumours
    A suitable text on Oral Medicine should be consulted for details of recognition and management of these conditions.

Tooth preparation

A sound restorative condition of all the teeth is required so that individual restorations throughout the mouth must be of a high standard.

Rest seats, guide planes and undercuts

The exact site for these types of preparation will have been decided during detailed treatment planning and study casts must be available at the chairside when tooth modification is being undertaken. In some instances restorations may exist in teeth in sites where modification to accommodate the planned denture elements is required. In other cases new restorations may be required in positions where rest seats, guiding planes or undercuts are planned and the new restorations must be designed accordingly. It may be necessary to replace existing restorations or, where they are suitable, surface modifications may be adequate to achieve the required feature.

Where a rest seat or guide plane is to be prepared in an unrestored sound tooth, the preparation must remain within the thickness of the enamel. After suitable preparation the abraded surface must be polished and topical fluoride applied. Suitable forms for rest seats are considered in Chapter 13.

If an undercut region is required to assist direct retention a cervical inlay incorporating a dimple may be produced. A ball ended clasp can be constructed to engage the dimple (see Fig. 13.28). A further method for producing an undercut region is to modify the tooth contour by means of a composite restorative material which is attached to the enamel surface following etching of the tooth by a suitable acid. This method has the advantage of leaving the tooth structure intact.

Modification of the occlusion

Because of occlusal relationships which may have developed following the loss of some teeth, it may not be possible to obtain the required occlusal balance between the opposing teeth and removable dentures during treatment. Overeruption of a tooth or teeth, or the presence of a grossly irregular occlusal plane are examples which might suggest the need for occlusal modification. The treatment required might vary from the reduction of the cusps of a tooth, or an increase or reduction in the crown height of a tooth or teeth requiring full coverage crowns. Where the occlusal discrepancy is gross, tooth extraction may need to be considered.

Orthodontic treatment might also be considered as a means of reducing anomalies in tooth relationships prior to denture treatment.

SURGICAL PREPARATION

Treatment of pathological entities

Whenever pathological entities are disclosed during the clinical or radiographic examination of the mouth, their treatment may be indicated. Retained roots and unerupted tooth are possibly the most common problems encountered. Where infection or other pathology is present, treatment is mandatory. Where retained roots and unerupted teeth are in contact with the overlying soft tissues their removal will usually be required. A root or tooth deeply buried in the bone of the jaws and showing no associated pathology will allow a level of election regarding surgery. The basis for a decision concerning treatment will relate to such factors as age, health status and whether their removal will be to the benefit of the patient.

Other conditions such as cysts and soft or hard tissue tumours will require surgical treatment prior to denture treatment.

Modification of the oral tissues

There are a number of surgical procedures which may be useful in providing a better basis for successful dentures than that present in the mouth of the patient on examination.

Soft tissue surgery

Surgical procedures involving only the soft tissues of the mouth and which may facilitate denture treatment include the following:

Frenectomy. Where prominent labial or buccal frenae will interfere with the production of an effective peripheral seal or might predispose a denture to fracture by virtue of the deep notch required to accommodate the tissue, removal or repositioning of the frenae may be undertaken.

Hyperplasia. If hyperplastic tissue associated with a denture fails to resolve on removal of the denture, its surgical removal may be required.

Fibrous enlargement of the tuberosities. Excessive amounts of fibrous tissue can produce problems, e.g. in respect of tooth positioning for a denture by occluding the space required for artificial teeth. The enlargement may also preclude full extension of the denture base. Surgical reduction of the soft tissue may be considered in such cases.

Sulcus extension. Deepening the sulcus at the borders of the denture bearing area on the labial and buccal aspects may be considered as a means of increasing the denture bearing area in edentulous jaws. The method used involves the use of an epithelial inlay formed by lining the surgically opened sulcus with an epithelial graft obtained from a suitable skin surface. The technique has most favourable results where some alveolar bone remains, and the danger of obliteration of the newly formed sulcus as extended healing proceeds is ever present.

Flabby ridges. Where a very mobile ridge is present, such as may occur in the upper anterior region of the edentulous maxilla where a denture has been opposed by natural lower anterior teeth, surgery is occasionally recommended. Surgery is, however, to be avoided in these circumstances where little or no residual alveolar bone remains beneath the mobile tissue.

Hard tissue surgery

Alveoplasty. This is the term applied to altering the form of the residual alveolar ridge by shaping the bony tissue. In its simplest form alveoplasty involves smoothing irregularities of the ridges. The irregularities may take the form of undercut 'knobs' of bone or a very sharp 'knife edge' ridge form which may occur especially in the lower anterior region following the extraction of severely periodontally involved teeth. Lack of intermaxillary space may preclude the provision of denture base coverage and the tuberosity and retromolar pad region are common sites for this problem. It is clearly important to distinguish between large tuberosities present as a result of excess bone from that resulting from fibrous enlargement before attempting treatment for reduction. Occasionally, a general reduction of ridge height is required so that space can be provided for dentures. However, it must be borne in mind that lack of bony support is often productive of difficulties for denture patients later in life, and careful planning with a generally conservative approach is always required.

Exostoses. Torus palatinus or torus mandibularis may require removal when excessively lobulated, or undercut, or so large as to cause a severe reduction in tongue space when covered by a denture base.

Mylohyoid ridge resection. This is really a form of sulcus extension and involves removal of the mylohyoid ridge and the portion of muscle at-tached to it. A sharp, prominent, mylohyoid ridge can be a source of considerable discomfort to a patient. Similarly, the superior genial tubercles may be so prominent, and covered with very thin mucoperiosteum following resorption of the mandibular residual alveolar ridge, that their removal may be indicated.

FURTHER READING

Bowman A J and Green R M 1968 Preprosthetic conservation. Dent Pract Dent Rec 18: 249

Cecconi B T 1974 Effect of rest design on transmission of forces to abutment teeth. J Prosthet Dent 32: 141

Guernsey L H 1971 Preprosthetic surgery. Dent Clin North Amer 15: 455

Hopkins R, Stafford G D and Gregory M C 1980 Preprosthetic surgery of the edentulous mandible. Brit Dent J 148: 183

Klein I and Miglino J 1966 Uses and abuses of tissue treatment materials. J Prosthet Dent 16: 1

Lytle R B 1957 Management of abused oral tissues in complete denture construction. J Prosthet Dent 7: 27

McCracken W L 1956 Mouth preparation for partial dentures. J Prosthet Dent 6: 38

Miller E L 1977 Clinical management of denture induced inflammations. J Prosthet Dent 38: 362

Pawlaak E A and Hoag P M 1980 Essentials of Periodontics. Mosby. St. Louis

Ritchie G M, Fletcher A M, Main D M and Prophet A S P 1969 The aetiology, exfoliative cytology and treatment of denture stomatitis. J Prosthet Dent 22: 185

Walker D M, Stafford G D, Huggett R and Newcombe R G 1981 The treatment of denture induced stomatitis. Brit Dent J 151: 416

Wilkie N D 1975 The role of the prosthodontist in preprosthetic surgery. J Prosthet Dent 33: 386

Winkler S 1979 Essentials of Complete Denture Prosthodontics. Saunders, Philadelphia

8

Principles of impression procedures

INTRODUCTION

In removable denture prosthetics an impression is an accurate negative likeness of the denture supporting tissues associated with the upper or lower jaw.

The impression represents a stage in the prosthetic treatment of a patient and its planning is equally as important and demanding as that of the other stages of denture treatment.

The significance of accuracy of adaptation of the denture base to the dental tissues, and also that of the need for the development of a properly designed border seal has already been considered in Chapter 2. In this chapter a general consideration will be given to principles directed towards the attainment of these objectives.

Just as there is an infinite variety of clinical oral conditions, so there are a large number of impression techniques, as the procedures used are related to the clinical conditions present. Most impression methods, however, fall into relatively few types and it is not intended to consider all possible variations within these groups.

IMPRESSION TRAYS

In order to carry the material used to obtain the impression into intimate contact with the oral tissues in the desired manner, impression trays are used. To obtain the degree of accuracy required to produce the cast on which the denture will be produced, an individually prepared impression tray called a special tray is used. The special tray is made on a cast of the patient's jaw and to produce this it is necessary to use a ready-made impression tray which is known as a stock tray.

Stock trays

These trays can be purchased in a variety of sizes and shapes and may be made of metal or of a plastic material. The metal trays are strong and rigid, and being sterilisable they may be re-used. Plastic trays are disposable and not intended for re-use. Only those plastic trays designed to provide maximum rigidity are considered suitable for use as any distortion of a tray at any stage of the impression procedure will result in distortion of the contained impression.

There are three main types of stock trays:
1. Box trays used to obtain impressions of dentate mouths.
2. Trays for obtaining impressions of the edentulous mouth.
3. Combination trays which are used where only anterior teeth are present in the jaw to be impressed. The anterior section is of a box form and the posterior section is similar to that used for the edentulous mouth.

Trays for the edentulous mouth have a curved form of the body of the tray, whereas those where teeth are present have a square or box section to allow for additional impression material around the teeth. Lower trays differ from upper trays in having space provided to allow the tongue to remain uncovered when taking the impression (Fig. 8.1).

Perforations may be present to provide a measure of mechanical retention which is required to secure some impression materials in the tray. Special adhesives are also required for some impression materials to aid their retention in the tray. It has been shown that perforations alone are not always reliable for this purpose. Any loss of retention of the material in the tray will result in

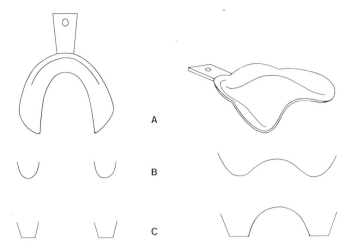

Fig. 8.1 Stock impression trays. A, For edentulous mouths. Lower tray on the left and upper tray on the right; B, Sections through trays for edentulous patients; C, Sections through trays for dentate patients.

distortion of the impression contained therein.

Despite the variety of sizes of stock trays available, they will only very rarely fit the mouth accurately. For example, the trays may have flanges shorter than those required to support the impression material for the clinical conditions present; or the tray may be too large and distort the cheeks and lips, thus altering the form of the functional sulcus.

Perhaps the most common cause for the resultant inaccuracy of fit associated with stock trays is that they do not provide for an even layer of impression material between the tray and the tissues of the mouth. It has been shown that the capacity of impression materials to reproduce accurately the form of the tissues depends on an even and controlled layer being used.

As the preliminary impressions produced using stock trays is required to be as accurate as possible, various methods for modifying the form of the trays are used. Examples of modifications for box type trays appear in Chapter 15.

Special trays

These are constructed on casts produced using the preliminary impressions obtained by means of stock trays, and as the name implies they are specially constructed for the patient being treated.

Special trays may be made of metal; heat or cold cured acrylic resin; baseplate shellac; or impression compound. The materials commonly used for their construction are heat and cold cured acrylic resin and baseplate shellac. Perforations may be required depending on the nature of the impression material to be used. Provision of controlled space is provided for the impression material during the construction of the tray. The space will depend on the material to be used for the impression. Where space is provided, stops or small areas of contact with the tissue to be impressed are fitted. The stops are equal in thickness to the space intended for the impression material. They should be placed in regions of firm tissue which will not be easily displaced during the impression procedure.

The handle provided for the special tray should be centrally placed and must not interfere with lip action. The tray should be rigid, accurately made, and free of undercuts which would interfere with its insertion and withdrawal from the mouth. It should also be finished with smooth surfaces free from any potentially injurious sharp edges and corners.

A guide to some aspects of special trays is presented in Table 8.1.

DISPLACEMENT OF TISSUES

Impressions for dentures are frequently described according to whether they involve pressure, selec-

Table 8.1 Some examples of aspects of special tray design in relation to clinical requirements

Clinical conditions	Secondary impression material	Suitable tray material	Spacer thickness required	Perforations	Adhesive
Edentulous jaw Minimal undercuts Average salivary flow	Plaster of Paris	Shellac	2 mm	No	No
Edentulous jaw Minimal undercuts Average salivary flow	Zinc oxide-eugenol	Acrylic resin	0.5 mm	No	No
Edentulous jaw Deep unyielding undercuts	Alginate	Acrylic resin	3 mm	Yes	Yes
Dentate mouth, average tooth inclination	Alginate	Acrylic resin	3 mm	Yes	Yes
Dentate mouth, severe undercuts	Elastomer	Acrylic resin	1.5 mm	Yes	Yes
Selective pressure impression	Compound/zinc oxide-eugenol	Acrylic resin/compound	As determined by clinical conditions	Provision for escape of material is required	No

tive pressure, or minimal pressure, between the impression material and the soft tissues covering the residual alveolar ridge.

Pressure impressions

Proponents of pressure impressions consider that as the soft tissues contacted by the denture are displaced by the forces transmitted to them via the denture during mastication, the mucosa should be similarly displaced during the impression procedure. In this way the denture made using an impression obtained under pressure will fit the tissues during functional activities. It is, however, considered that non-predictable displacement of the teeth or soft tissues will occur during function since such forces are applied in dynamic and transient circumstances. On the other hand, the forces applied during impression taking under pressure are static and continuous. They are likely, therefore, to produce distortion of the tissues involved. The distorted tissue will always be stressed when a denture produced on such an impression is in the mouth and, therefore, tending to return to its resting state when no forces are acting. Thus a de-

nture prepared using this type of impression may tend to be dislodged under resting conditions.

Pressure techniques may be open mouth techniques or closed mouth procedures, depending whether the pressure is applied by the operator's finger or via the patient's masticatory muscles. Generally, it is considered that closed mouth techniques are fraught with potential difficulties because of the inability of the operator to control the setting impression directly once the tray has been placed in the mouth of the patient. In particular, closed mouth techniques do not permit close control of border moulding procedures.

Selective pressure impressions

In many cases there will be clinical circumstances involving marked differences between the displaceability of the soft tissues covering the various regions of the denture bearing area. This situation can be approached by attempting to control the forces used in obtaining the impression so that the softer areas and those requiring protection from the high forces developed during mastication are stressed least during function. When the denture produced using such an impression is subjected to masticatory and other functional contacts, the aim is to distribute the transmitted forces selectively over the basal tissues to those regions considered best able to withstand them.

Minimal pressure impressions

The objective with impressions obtained using minimal pressure is to obtain an accurate record of the tissues in the resting relationship with each other. In normal circumstances, functions in which high forces are exerted on the denture supporting tissues operate for only a fraction of the time that a denture is in position in the mouth. Proponents of minimal pressure impressions therefore consider that an appliance constructed using such an impression will fit accurately in relationship to the tissues for the greater part of the day. Where differences in tissue displaceability occur over the denture bearing areas, relief areas are provided in the denture base to accommodate these differences. The extent of relief required is carefully judged by palpatation of the denture bearing tissues and relief equal to the difference in displaceability between the harder and softer areas is provided over the clinically determined extent of the hard areas.

INSERTION AND REMOVAL OF
IMPRESSION TRAYS

Impression trays should be inserted into the mouth by a rotational movement about the angle of the mouth. Where the patient is seated upright the lower tray is brought to the region of the mouth with the tray orientated at right angles to the sagittal plane and the junction of the handle and body of the tray by the left angle of the mouth. The operator, standing in front and usually at the right of the patient, uses the left forefinger to retract the right angle of the patient's mouth, and the tray is rotated about the left angle, past the orifice into the mouth.

With the upright patient the upper tray is inserted into the mouth with the operator placed behind the patient. The junction of the handle and body of the tray is placed to the right angle of the mouth and the left forefinger retracts the left angle of the patient's mouth while the tray is rotated into position.

A similar approach may be made with the supine patient. However, if the lower tray is inserted from a cranial direction, with the supine patient and the operator positioned cranially, adequate mandibular support is difficult to achieve.

Once the tray has been inserted into the mouth, it should be held in position and a careful check of the tissue covered by the tray made to ensure inclusion of all the required denture bearing area, and at the same time freedom from interference with the reflected tissue.

SUPPORT FOR THE MANDIBLE

It must constantly be borne in mind that any force applied to the mandible must be adequately reciprocated by support from the operator's fingers or thumbs, as possible damage to the temporomandibular joint may result. Similarly during removal, it is particularly important for all impressions, and especially where high viscosity materials which enter undercuts are used in the mouth, that the patient should be instructed to partially close the mouth before applying the removal force to the lower impression. This will allow the condyle to retract into the glenoid fossa and minimise the possibility of trauma to the temporomandibular joint.

It is also pertinent to note that it is not good practice for the patient to be encouraged to hold the mandible in a forced open position during the lower impression procedure as measurable medial approximation of the lateral segments of this bone will occur under these conditions. Wide opening of the mouth also tends to distort the form of the sulcus and makes the provision of an adequate peripheral seal impossible.

FURTHER READING

Atkinson H F 1966 The physical principles of impression techniques. Austral Dent J 11: 145

Boucher C O 1951 A critical analysis of mid-century impression techniques for full dentures. J Prosthet Dent 1: 472

De Van M M 1952 Basic principles of impression making. J Prosthet Dent 2: 26

Douglas W H, Wilson H J and Bates J F 1965 Pressures involved in taking impressions. Dent Pract Dent Rec 15: 248

Frank, R P 1970 Controlling pressures during complete denture impressions. Dent Clin North Amer 14: 453

Regli C P and Kelly E K 1967 The phenomenon of decreased mandibular arch width in opening movements. J Prosthet Dent 17: 49

Stephens, A P 1969 Special trays for full denture impressions. J Irish Dent Assoc 15:31.

Tucker K M 1971 Personalised impression trays. Dent Dig Part I, 77: 70, Part II, 77: 154

Tuckfield W J 1947 The relative importance of impressions in full denture construction. Austral J Dent 51: 361

9

Principles of registering jaw relationships

INTRODUCTION

As pointed out in Chapter 1, a jaw relationship may be defined as the positional relationship which the mandible bears to the maxilla and is considered in terms of a vertical and horizontal component. These two components are interdependent and one cannot be changed without changing the other. The mandible is capable of adopting an infinite number of positions in both the vertical and horizontal planes and in removable denture production it is essential that the required relationship is established accurately in accordance with the anatomical and physiological needs of the patient.

Once established, the jaw relationship is registered or recorded so that the casts of the patient's jaws can be related in a similar manner to that which pertains in the mouth. The correctly located casts can then be transferred to an articulator. This is an instrument designed to simulate some actions of the jaws and is considered in Chapter 10.

THE VERTICAL COMPONENT OF THE JAW RELATIONSHIP

It has already been pointed out that when the mandible is in the rest jaw relationship the opposing teeth are not in occlusion, being separated by the distance known as the interocclusal distance. When the natural teeth are present in the jaws and in a state of normal occlusion, contact between the opposing teeth determines the vertical dimension of occlusion. Where there is no tooth contact possible because of the absence of teeth, for example, then the vertical dimension must be estimated.

The basis for estimation of the vertical dimension of occlusion is the rest vertical dimension. It is known that the rest jaw relationship which determines the rest vertical dimension may be subject to variation from a number of causes, both short and long term. In general, as the rest jaw relationship is maintained by a balance of the muscle forces acting on the mandible, factors which influence muscle activity will affect the rest jaw relationship.

Short term factors which influence the rest jaw relationship

1. Head posture. As indicated in Chapter 1, tilting the head backwards will increase the rest vertical dimension while inclining the head forwards will result in a decreased value.

2. Stress. This tends to decrease the rest vertical dimension as a result of increased activity of the elevator muscles attached to the mandible.

3. Mouth contents. There is a tendency for the rest vertical dimension to decrease following extraction of the natural teeth, and for a new postural position to develop following the insertion of a lower denture.

4. Pain about or within the mouth or in the muscles supporting the mandible may affect the rest vertical dimension as a protective posture may be assumed.

5. Respiration produces minor variations in the rest jaw relationship.

Long term factors which influence the rest jaw relationship

1. Age and health status. These factors may produce a change in the rest jaw relationship.

With advancing age where natural teeth or dentures have gradually worn down, or a prolonged period of edentulousness has occurred, a decrease in the rest vertical dimension may result. Chronic neuromuscular disorders may also produce a change in the rest jaw position.

2. Bruxism and the developments of habits related to abnormal occlusion are often associated with muscular hypertonicity with a resultant decrease in the rest vertical dimension.

VERTICAL DIMENSION OF OCCLUSION

In the determination of the vertical dimension of occlusion in the absence of natural teeth or of acceptable tooth contacts, the procedure first involves the establishment of the rest vertical dimension. The vertical dimension of occlusion is then obtained by subtracting from the rest vertical dimension an allowance of 2–4 mm to provide for an adequate freeway space or inter-occlusal distance. Thus: Rest vertical dimension – Freeway space = Vertical dimension of occlusion.

ASSESSMENT OF THE VERTICAL DIMENSION

There are many methods in current use which attempt to determine an absolute value for the rest vertical dimension. The variety of methods available is, of itself, an indication of the difficulties involved in assessing this important value. Some of the methods used include:

Swallowing

Niswonger (1934) observed that in swallowing the mandible moves from the rest position to centric jaw relation and returns to the resting position on completion of the act. In adopting this observation to estimation of the vertical dimension, the patient is seated and the head supported with the ala-tragal line parallel to the floor. Two marks are placed on the face in the midline — one on the upper lip and the other on the chin. The patient is instructed to swallow and relax and the distance between the marks measured. This distance represents the rest vertical dimension. The difficulties associated with this approach relate to movement of the marks consequent on movement of the skin, and obtaining adequate relaxation of the patient.

Facial measurements

A number of methods which utilise measurements between various anatomical landmarks have been suggested. Willis considered that the distance from the pupil of the eye to the rima oris was equal to the distance from the base of the nose to the inferior border of the chin at the vertical dimension of occlusion. The Willis Bite Gauge was introduced to assist in measuring the above distances. In other methods it has been suggested that the face can be considered in terms of 'equal thirds' in respect of the forehead, the nose, and the lips and chin.

These and other methods based on facial measurement have been shown to be of little practical value because of the vague nature of the measuring 'points' and also because of individual variation in facial features.

Phonetic methods

Some phonetic methods are based on the 'closest speaking distance' (without tooth contact occurring) which is assumed by the mandibular teeth in relation to the maxillary teeth during the production of sounds such as 's' or 'ch'. It is considered by users of this approach that the near contact position is close enough to be used as a measure of the vertical diversion of occlusion. Obviously the correct relationship between the teeth, lips and tongue would need to be developed for the application of this method and it is considered to be best used as a check on an established vertical dimension at the trial stage of denture production. In another phonetic method, the production of the letter 'm' is used. When this sound is produced, measurement between a mark placed on the upper lip or nose and another on the chin is considered to represent the rest vertical dimension.

Appearance

Some operators simply attempt to judge the rest

vertical dimension on the basis of the appearance of the patient. Such an approach is very subjective.

Biting forces

Boos (1952) considered that the maximum biting force developed at a degree of jaw separation equal to the rest vertical dimension, and he developed an instrument (Bimeter) to enable biting forces to be measured. This method has not been shown to produce reliable results for all operators.

Other methods

These include tactile methods in which a jack-screw can be adjusted vertically between the jaws until the patient considers the degree of jaw separation correct. This is then checked by the operator for reasonableness. A further approach utilises electromyographic recordings on the basis that minimal muscular activity occurs when the mandible is in the resting or postural position.

No reference has been made to pre-extraction records which could be obtained before the loss of the natural vertical dimension 'stop' has occurred, such as would be available for use in the production of immediate dentures. The student is referred to texts on immediate denture service for a description of these as they are considered to be outside the scope of this work.

A method for assessing the vertical dimension

The recommended method consists of a combination of some of the above methods.

Markers should be attached to the midline of the face — one on the nose and the other on the chin. As pointed out above, the action of the muscles of facial expression may produce skin movement, so that the sites chosen for attachment of the markers should be observed carefully and only positions which do not appear to show movement independent of the skeleton should be used. Suitable markers may be of self-adhesive paper or marks produced by a chinagraph pencil. The patient should be seated upright with the head erect. Measurement between the markers is made with the patient in a relaxed and comfortable pos-

Fig. 9.1 Measurement of vertical dimension of the face using the Willis Gauge. A, Markers; B, Willis Gauge.

ition. This can be very difficult to achieve. Requesting the patient to moisten the lips and bring them into light contact may be helpful. Asking the patient to swallow and relax the jaws may be attempted. Observation of the patient's face for signs of muscle activity should be carried out continuously, while suitable encouragement of the patient to be as relaxed as possible should be undertaken. The patient's appearance in a more general sense should be observed also to take into account the general proportions of the face. Verification of the measured dimension by asking the patient to say 'm' may be helpful. Measurements can be conveniently made using a Willis Gauge for example. This instrument carries a scale and can be readily sterilised (Fig. 9.1).

For an edentulous patient a lower denture, if available, should be in the mouth during measurement of the rest vertical dimension to reduce the error resulting from the effect of the absence of teeth from the lower jaw.

The above description provides no indication of the difficulties which may accompany the procedure particularly in respect of achieving, or recognising, the resting posture of the mandible. Considerable experience may be required for successful determination of the rest vertical dimension.

The next step is to estimate the amount of freeway space to be provided as the vertical dimension at which the jaw relationship will be registered is the vertical dimension of occlusion. On the average, the freeway space will be some 2–4 mm in the premolar region. In the absence of suitable guidance, e.g. tooth contacts adequate to establish the vertical dimension of occlusion, dentures which may provide a guide in relation to occlusal wear or show the effects of over- or under-estimation of vertical dimension, it is common practice to provide the average amount of freeway space. At a later stage of removable denture treatment — the trial denture stage — a re-estimation of the adequacy of the freeway space provided is made and, if necessary, re-registration of the jaw relationship at a newly established vertical dimension of occlusion is made. This aspect is further considered in Chapters 18 and 25.

The importance of accurate estimation of the vertical dimension of occlusion cannot be over-emphasised.

Errors in the vertical dimension of occlusion

It is essential that provision for the correct vertical dimension of occlusion be made, as excessive or deficient vertical dimension can produce serious consequences.

Excessive vertical dimension

Excessive vertical dimension will result in deficiency or elimination of the freeway space and the effects may include:

1. Increased risk of trauma to the tissues contacted by the denture. In the absence of freeway space the teeth will be continually clenched. Muscle forces are increased for the first few millimetres of increased vertical height. These two factors may give rise to considerable discomfort. The oral mucosa overlying the denture seating areas may become painful and inflamed and muscle pain, particularly involving the masseter muscle, may also result.

2. It has been postulated that a decreased or absent freeway space may result in accelerated resorption of the residual alveolar bone.

3. The teeth are liable to contact during speech, resulting in an audible clicking sound.

4. Speech defects may arise because of difficulties in bringing the lips together to produce such sounds as 'p', 'b' and 'm'.

5. Poor aesthetics may be apparent. The lips and cheeks are constantly stretched and an open mouth posture may be apparent.

6. Symptoms of temporomandibular joint dysfunction syndrome may develop as a result of increased stress to the tissues related to the joint.

Deficient vertical dimension

A deficient vertical dimension of occlusion is sometimes referred to as 'overclosure' and may result in:

1. Poor aesthetics — lack of proper lip and cheek support together with protrusion of the chin on closure of the jaws may be apparent. This produces a premature aged appearance.

2. Masticatory efficiency is reduced because the muscles which are substantially vertical in their fibre direction are required to operate at a reduced length, thus reducing the forces generated on contraction.

3. Lack of support at the angles of the mouth may result in dribbling of saliva, thus favouring the development of angular cheilitis.

4. The risk of cheek biting because of bunching of that tissue is increased.

5. Symptoms of temporomandibular joint dysfunction syndrome may develop as a result of increased stress to the tissues related to the joint.

HORIZONTAL JAW RELATIONS

Once the correct vertical dimension is determined and allowance for the necessary interocclusal distance or freeway space has been made, the jaw relation in the horizontal plane must be established. This will be considered in two sections, because in the production of removable prostheses, a distinction is made between the horizontal relationships of the jaws depending on the presence or absence of acceptable natural tooth contacts.

Dentate patients where natural tooth contact is accepted

For the patient having natural teeth in sufficient numbers and relative positions to provide a definite intercuspal relationship in the horizontal plane at an acceptable vertical dimension, the maximal intercuspal position is the horizontal relationship to be recorded.

Patients lacking acceptable tooth contact

In all cases where acceptable natural tooth contact is absent, the retruded jaw relationship is that which must be determined and recorded at the vertical dimension of occlusion. These include:

1. All edentulous patients.
2. Dentate patients lacking acceptable tooth contact. Where changes in the normal occlusal relationships have occurred following tooth extraction, e.g. drifting of teeth into edentulous spaces, rotation or overeruption of teeth, the maximal intercuspal contact presented may be achieved by deflection from the normal path of closure following premature contact between opposing teeth. In situations such as these occlusal modification will be required as part of the planned treatment for removable partial dentures.
3. Dentate patients requiring a change in the vertical dimension of occlusion from that provided by natural tooth contact. As a result of tooth loss there may be no occlusal contact between teeth in opposing jaws, or because of gross attrition or abrasion of opposing teeth, contact may only be achieved at an inadequate vertical dimension of occlusion.

While the absolute value of the difference between the maximal intercuspal position where natural teeth are present, and the retruded jaw relationship is relatively small (approximately 1 mm) it is considered by many authorities to be significant in clinical terms where normal occlusal contacts are absent or cannot be maintained.

Reasons for acceptance of the retruded jaw relationship

1. The retruded jaw relationship is reproducable. Only when opposing tooth surfaces in substan-tially normal positions are present in the mouth is the position of maximal intercuspation reproducable.
2. The apparatus used for reproducing some jaw movements and setting the teeth basically operate from the retruded position. Commonly used articulators are incapable of reproducing a retrusive mandibular action.
3. Denture instability will result from abnormal contact between dentures or dentures and natural teeth when set up with the casts in other than the retruded jaw relationship. The non-reproducibility of positions other than the retruded position makes the achievement of balanced occlusion and articulation unlikely.
4. The vertical dimension of occlusion may be altered during function when the teeth are set with casts of the jaws in other than the retruded jaw relationship.
5. Abnormal temporomandibular joint activity related to attempts by the patient to modify chewing action to accommodate incorrect occlusal relationships may result in joint dysfunction.

RECORDING AND TRANSFER OF JAW RELATIONSHIPS

Having established the vertical and horizontal components of the jaw relationship it is essential that the recording of this relationship (the registration) and the subsequent transfer of the jaw relationship record to the articulator is carried out without error.

Clearly, any errors introduced at this stage will be retained in the subsequent stages of denture production and appear as occlusal errors in the completed appliance. It is known that inaccurate occlusal relationships constitute the most common cause of denture failure and tissue damage.

The clinical techniques adopted for recording the above jaw relationships will be considered in Chapters 16 and 23 together with the precautions which should be taken to ensure accuracy.

OTHER JAW RELATIONSHIPS

Protrusive and lateral jaw relationships may also be recorded. These relationships are used primarily to assist in the adjustment of the condylar guidance mechanism of the articulator.

A protrusive jaw relationship pertains when the mandible is postured forward of the accepted retruded jaw relationship. Lateral jaw relationships occur when the mandible is postured towards the right or left side. In each of these movements, one or both condyles is caused to travel downwards and forwards from the retruded position in the glenoid fossa, and in addition lateral movements include a total lateral shift of the condyles.

The form of the bony elements of the temporomandibular joint do not of themselves govern the path taken by the condyles. Most articulators have a straight path which the equivalent of the condyle follows in its movement and this differs from the path taken by the mandibular condyle in its movements. This situation arises because records obtained for adjusting the mechanism of the articulator utilise two static records and the assumption is made that the pathway between these positions is straight. Thus the protrusive movements of the simple adjustable articulator are not identical to those of the mandible. Such records do, however, offer refinements in the development of occlusion between artificial teeth, and artificial and natural teeth, and also provide opportunity for the study of the occlusion of natural teeth.

Protrusive relationships are more commonly used for condylar mechanism adjustment although some clinicians use both protrusive and lateral records while others use left and right lateral records only.

The method of adjustment of the condylar mechanisms of an articulator using the protrusive record utilises the phenomenon observed by Christensen at about the turn of the century. Christensen noted the development of a gap in the molar region of patients having natural teeth, during protrusion of the mandible while contact between the anterior teeth was maintained. This wedge shaped space between the opposing occlusal planes of the upper and lower teeth results from the downward movement of the condyle (Fig. 9.2) and is used as a means of determining the gross downward and forwards movement of the condyle during protrusion.

In practice, an interocclusal record between the upper and lower teeth, or their equivalent, is

Fig. 9.2 Christensen's phenomenon in protrusive jaw relationship. The arrow indicates the downwards and forwards excursion of the condyle. The wedge-shaped gap between the opposing occlusal planes which develops on protrusion of the mandible is shown as a hatched area.

obtained in wax or other suitable medium. This record (protrusive registration) is then transferred to the articulator in which casts of the jaws have been mounted in the appropriate retruded jaw relationship. The condylar mechanism of the articulator is then adjusted to permit the reproduction of the protrusive record between the casts of the patient's jaws. Following adjustment of the horizontal condylar inclination of the articulator, with some articulators adjustment for Bennett Movement may be made in accordance with Hanau's equation (Chapter 10):

$$L = \frac{H}{8} + 12$$

where L = the lateral condylar inclination and H = the horizontal condylar inclination.

Thus, when the horizontal condylar inclination is found to be 24°, the lateral condylar inclination would be 15°. The articulator pillars supporting

Fig. 9.3 Plan view to illustrate adjustment of the condyle mechanism of an articulator for Bennett movement.

the condyle mechanism would therefore be rotated 15° and this would influence the extent of the provision for Bennett Movement by the articulator (Fig. 9.3). As this adjustment is also of a mechanical type dependent on the geometry of the instrument in use, it will be seen that both condylar guidance and Bennett adjustment represent approximations to the patient's mandibular movements.

To date, no mechanism has been devised which can accurately imitate the complex movements which can occur in the temporomandibular joints.

FURTHER READING

Brill N, Schubeler S and Tryde G 1962 Aspects of occlusal sense in natural and artificial teeth. J Prosthet Dent 12: 123

Dyer E H 1973 Importance of a stable maxillomandibular relation. J Prosthet Dent 30: 241

Granger E R 1948 Biologic factors in partial denture design. Austral J Dent 52: 119

Hickey J C, Williams B H and Woelfel J B 1961 Stability of mandibular rest position. J Prosthet Dent 11: 566

Lawson W A 1959 An analysis of the commonest causes of full denture failure. Dent Pract Dent Rec 10: 61

Osborne J and Lammie G A 1974 Partial Dentures. 4th Edn. Blackwell, Oxford

Shanahan T E J and Leff A 1960 Interocclusal records. J Prosthet Dent 10: 842

Swerdlow H 1965 Vertical dimension literature review. J Prosthet Dent 15: 241

10

Dental articulators and their selection

INTRODUCTION

A dental articulator is an instrument in which casts of the upper and lower dentate or edentulous jaws can be attached for reproducing jaw relations and movements of the lower jaw relative to the upper.

The simplest form of articulator consists of two arms or bows united by a hinge. This type of instrument enables an accurate record of a single static relationship between the jaws to be maintained, and the only movement which can be made is an opening and closing one about the hinge. It is known as a simple hinge or plane-line articulator. More complex articulators are able to assume relationships other than a single static one, and instruments capable of assuming such eccentric positions are known as 'adjustable' or 'anatomical' articulators. These articulators vary considerably in their capacity to simulate jaw movements and relationships and may be considered as falling into several classes of instruments.

CLASSIFICATION OF DENTAL ARTICULATORS

1. Simple hinge or plane-line articulators
2. Average value articulators
3. Adjustable articulators which may be either:
    a. simple adjustable or
    b. fully adjustable

A SHORT HISTORY OF ARTICULATORS

As an aid to understanding articulators it will be useful to have an insight into their development. This will be considered on the basis of significant changes rather than a complete history.

The plaster slab

The earliest known device used for relating casts of the upper and lower jaws was by modification of the posterior aspects of the casts to produce a fixed relationship between them. This 'plaster slab' or 'occludator' arrangement is associated with the name of Pfaff (1755) (Fig. 10.1).

Fig. 10.1 Plaster slab articulator.

Simple hinge articulators

It is believed that the simple hinge-like cast relator was invented by Gariot in 1805. Opening and closing movements about a convenient, but not anatomically related, axis were provided for. The Gariot instrument consisted of two metal frames or bows to which the casts could be attached. These were joined by a simple hinge mechanism and a stop or screw to hold the bows a fixed distance apart was provided (Fig. 10.2).

Many forms of this instrument have been, and continue to be, employed. Some forms incorporate, for example, remounting devices and adjustable bearings, but the basic features of the instrument remains essentially similar to that designed by Gariot.

Fig. 10.2 Diagram to show the essential features of the simple hinge articulator. A, Hinge; B, Upper bow; C, Vertical stop mechanism; D, Lower bow.

Average value articulators

In 1840 Evans patented an articulator having a hinge connection between the upper and lower bows and a slot arrangement which allowed a sliding motion at the joint, but it is generally considered that the first instrument incorporating a mechanism meant to reproduce the mandibular movements was that of W. G. Bonwill (1858). Bonwill's 'anatomical' articulator was based on his theory that the distance between the condyles and the mid-incisal point of the mandible was an equilateral triangle of 4 inch side. A sliding ring and spring mechanism about the horizontal 'condylar' element allowed for opening, protrusive and lateral components of movement (Fig. 10.3).

In practical terms, this was the first of the average value articulators and it allowed the possibility of serious points of interference between cusps of teeth to be detected and eliminated, thus permitting a semblance of balanced occlusal relationships to be developed. The 4 inch equilateral triangle concept is now known to be inaccurate and the horizontal condylar mechanism inappropriate but Bonwill's work was significant in recognising the

Fig. 10.3 Essential features of the Bonwill articulator. A, Horizontal sliding mechanism; B, Upper bow; C, Vertical stop mechanism; D, Lower bow.

need to relate articulator design to condylar activity.

Gritman in 1899 produced an articulator having the condylar guides inclined at 15° to the horizontal to allow for the effect of the articular eminence in joint activity.

The Gysi Simplex articulator which was produced in 1914 incorporated curved condylar guidance in recognition of the form of the glenoid fossa, and was provided with an incisal guide pin and an incisal table set at a fixed value of 60° (Fig. 10.4). The incisal guidance mechanism was an important development which significantly assisted setting up of the artificial teeth by stabilising movements of the upper bow of the articulator.

Fig. 10.4 Essential features of the Gysi Simplex articulator. A, Condylar guidance mechanism; B, Upper bow; C, Incisal guide pin; D, Incisal guide plate; E, Lower bow.

A further average value type articulator of interest was that of Monson (1918) which evolved from the concept that the biting surfaces of the upper and lower teeth move over each as over the surface of a sphere of 4 inches radius. The centre of the sphere was considered to be in the region of the glabella. This development represented a philosophical divergence from the accepted role of the condyles in mandibular movement in that it placed the whole emphasis on the teeth as being the guiding influence for mandibular movement once tooth contact occurred. The Monson concept survives in the form of various metal templates, some of which are based on the 4 inch radius sphere, to which artificial teeth are set in an attempt to produce occlusal balance.

Adjustable articulators

While the above instruments simulate movements of the mandible for the 'average' patient, it is clear

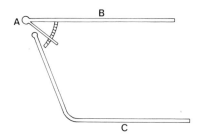

Fig. 10.5 Essential features of the Walker articulator. A, Adjustable condylar mechanism incorporating a vertical stop; B, Upper bow; C, Lower bow.

that the patient as an individual must be catered for in many instances.

W. E. Walker (1897) noted the balance achieved by dentures produced using Bonwill's articulator did not always balance in the mouth of the patient. As a consequence he developed an articulator having individually adjustable condylar guidance (Fig. 10.5).

The Christensen articulator (1901) incorporated adjustable condyle paths which could be set by means of intra-oral registrations of eccentric jaw positions. Christensen also introduced the intra-oral records used to assist the articulator adjustments.

Snow in 1900 produced an articulator similar to the Gritman instrument and introduced the face-bow at this time to relate the intercondylar axis to the maxillae. All adjustable articulators from this time made provision for use of the face-bow.

The Gysi Adaptable articulator (1910) included a curved condylar guidance which was variable vertically and horizontally. Variable intercondylar width was introduced and an incisal guidance mechanism was incorporated (Fig. 10.6). The gothic arch method for establishing the most re-

Fig. 10.6 Essential features of the Gysi Adaptable articulator. A, Adjustable condylar mechanism; B, Upper bow; C, Incisal guide pin; D, Adjustable incisal guide plate; E, Lower bow.

truded relationship of the jaws from which lateral movements could be made was also introduced about this time.

The Wadsworth articulator (1919) had condylar posts which could be moved laterally to match that dimension of the patient and also incorporated removable remounting plates so that casts could be removed from the articulator and replaced accurately as required.

The Hanau articulator (model H) introduced in 1922 and the Dentatus (1944) have condylar adjustments in both the vertical and horizontal (or lateral) planes and incorporate allowance for the Bennett movement. A variable incisal guidance mechanism is also provided on both instruments. The variable condylar path is arranged in such a manner that alteration of the slope of the path does not alter the distance between the upper and lower bows of the articulator. Remounting of casts is provided for by means of replaceable plates which are screwed into position.

Hanau devised a mathematical relationship following experiments with registrations of protrusive and lateral relations between the maxilla and mandible such that:

$$L = \frac{H}{8} + 12$$

where L is the lateral inclination of the condyle path and H is the horizontal inclination. Using this formula the inclination of the condylar guides in the lateral direction can be set when the horizontal inclination has been established using a registration of protrusive relationship. Variation in the lateral condylar inclination varies the amount of Bennett movement provided for.

Many more adjustable articulators have been, and continued to be, produced, and it is likely that developments in this field will continue. Some types have very complex mechanisms and aim to simulate as faithfully as possible the movements of which the temporomandibular joint is capable. Such instruments often require extremely demanding clinical methods to be followed to produce the records necessary for adjustment of the mechanism.

On the other hand, a form of compromise between the average value and the simple adjustable articulator has been provided for by some manufacturers. This type of articulator has a fixed condylar slope generally of the order of 30°, and is provided with an adjustable incisal guidance table. The condylar mechanism may include some provision for Bennett movement. Used in conjunction with a face-bow these articulators are superior to the average value instruments while lacking the capacity for the individual adjustment provided for in other simple adjustable instruments. For removable denture prostheses and particularly those which are soft tissue borne, little advantage will accrue from the use of a highly sophisticated articulator, since the resilience of the tissue underlying such an appliance will usually permit gross movement of the denture in excess of the finer adjustment settings of the instrument.

An instrument of the Dentatus type permitting individual condylar angle variation, Bennett adjustment and incisal guidance adjustment may be regarded as a satisfactory general purpose articulator for removable prostheses. The detailed adjustment capacity of the more complex articulator is more suited for specific clinical methods related to diagnosis and restoration of the occlusion of the natural dentition.

Only an outline of important developments in this large field has been included in the foregoing. The reader is recommended to consult the literature for a fuller treatment of this topic.

FACE-BOW REGISTRATION

The face-bow is a caliper-like device which is used to record the relationship between the intercondylar axis and either the maxillary or mandibular arch. Once established, this relationship can be transferred to an articulator so that casts of the patient's jaws will assume the same relationship to the hinge axis of the articulator as that of the upper or lower jaw of the patient to the intercondylar axis.

Two types of face-bow exist:
1. The simple face-bow
2. The hinge axis face-bow

The simple face-bow

This instrument was introduced by Snow in approximately 1900. Modern simple face-bows are

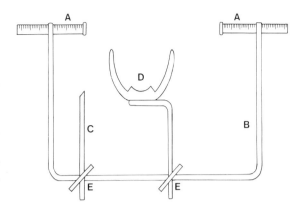

Fig. 10.7 The simple face-bow. A, Calibrated condyle indicators; B, Body; C, Orbital pointer; D, Fork; E, Universal joints.

similar to that of Snow, but with the addition to many of them of an orbital pointer. The pointer serves to identify an anterior point of reference which in conjunction with the condyles forms a horizontal plane of reference.

The face-bow consists of a U-shaped body having calibrated adjustable condyle indicators at each side (Fig. 10.7). The body of the face-bow carries a joint for securing a fork having an offset rod attached, and another for the orbital pointer.

Use of the simple face-bow

This will be considered in some detail as this is the most commonly used face-bow.

The lateral poles of the condyles are located by a combination of estimation of their positions and palpation. The average anatomical position of the condyle is some 12 mm from the posterior point of the tragus of the ear along an imaginary line joining the upper border of the external auditory meatus and the outer canthus of the eye. After determining this point the ball of the finger should be placed over it and the patient asked to make small mouth opening and closing movements when movement of the tissues overlying the lateral pole of the condyle will be appreciated. Some corrections of the position of the finger may be required where variation from the estimated position is present. The site as determined should be marked on the skin of the face using a small self-adhesive paper marker or chinagraph pencil. Both condyles should be located.

The fork of the face-bow is attached to the up-per occlusal rim or, where natural teeth are pres-ent in the upper jaw, to a wax record of the occlusal and incisal surfaces of the teeth. The occlusal rim or wax record is placed in position in the mouth leaving the rod of the fork protruding from the mouth. All joints on the body of the face-bow are loosened and the joint for the face-bow fork is slipped into position. The condylar indi-cators are placed in contact with the previously re-corded marks. An assistant will be required for this procedure. Centring of the face-bow is carried out by ensuring that the condyle indicators show equal graduations while maintaining contact with the skin markers. The fork joint is then tightened.

Where an orbital pointer is used, the patient is instructed to close the eyes while the tip of the pointer is carried towards the lowest part of the orbit (orbitale). The joint on the body for the or-bital pointer is tightened. After slackening off the condyle indicators the face-bow, together with the upper occlusal rim or wax template, is removed from the patient (Fig. 10.8).

Fig. 10.8 The face-bow in position on the face as seen from the lateral aspect. A, Condyle indicator; B, Body of face-bow; C, Orbital pointer; D, Rod of fork; E, Universal joint.

Mounting the models on the articulator

The condyle markers of the face-bow are placed in position on the joint mechanism of the articulator. Provision for face-bow attachment is made on average value and adjustable articulators. The con-dyle indicators are then centred so that equal graduations appear on both indicators.

Fig. 10.9 The face-bow in position on the articulator as seen from the lateral aspect. A, Condyle indicator; B, Body of face-bow; C, Orbital pointer; D, Orbital locator; E, Rod of fork.

Where an orbital indicator has been used the pointer is made to contact the appropriate site near the top of the articulator in order to fix the hori-zontal plane of the record (Fig. 10.9).

Where an orbital pointer is not used, other methods may place the plane of occlusion parallel to the ala-tragus line; or to a line joining the tragus of the ear and the anterior nasal spine; or approx-imately parallel to the base of the articulator.

Once the horizontal disposition is established the face-bow is supported steadily in position. The cast of the maxillary ridge or teeth is firmly seated into position in the upper baseplate carrying the occlusal rim assembly or the wax record as appro-priate. This cast is then luted to the upper bow of the articulator using plaster of Paris. The upper cast has now been attached to the upper bow of the articulator in the same relationship to the hinge of the articulator as the maxilla of the patient bears to the intercondylar axis.

The mandibular cast can then be attached to the lower bow of the articulator by means of a record of retruded jaw relationship obtained as considered in Chapter 9.

The hinge axis face-bow

This instrument was introduced by McCollum in 1930 and is used to determine the centre of ro-tation or hinge axis of the condyles.

The fork of the hinge axis face-bow is attached to the lower jaw (Fig. 10.10) and during opening movements styli which are located in the region of the condyles are adjusted until rotation of the styli is observed without any translation. The points so

Fig. 10.10 Diagram of illustrate the action of the hinge axis face-bow (A). Jaws closed (upper) and open (lower).

determined are marked on the skin as the 'hinge axis'.

Many complex variations of this instrument exist. It is not as commonly used for removable denture prosthetics as the simple face-bow. The validity of the hinge axis concept is considered to be controversial.

THE BASIS FOR SELECTION OF AN ARTICULATOR

This will be considered in terms of the classes of articulator considered above.

Simple hinge articulators

These instruments can only open and close in a hinge-like action. Teeth set up on such an articulator for complete dentures will not always balance in contact positions in the mouth other than the single position in which the casts were related together. This arrangement would be suitable only for a patient whose masticatory and other functional activities are of a simple hinge-like nature.

In complete denture construction the use of a template based on average occlusal contours to which the teeth are set improves the possibility for limited occlusal balance. A range of templates is available, some of which are based on the 4 inch radius used by Monson in conjunction with his articulator. Such methods require posterior teeth of the flat cusp or inverted cusp type to be used so that good conformation of their occlusal surfaces to the template can be developed.

A further technique in which the surface of special occlusal rims are modified by the patient grinding the rims together in the mouth ('chew-in' technique) may be used. This provides a more individual template to which flat cusped teeth may be set to assist in providing balanced contact with the opposing teeth. This method, while occasionally useful, is not commonly used because patients often have difficulties in producing suitable 'templates' during the 'chew-in' phase.

Average value articulators

These articulators provide for 'average' mandibular excursions. Used in conjunction with a face-bow record better results are achievable than with the hinge articulator, but detectable error in eccentric movements of the mandible in relation to occlusal balance will occur in many cases because of variation between the geometry of the instrument and the anatomical form of the patient.

Adjustable articulators

When adjusted to the individual requirements of the patient this class of articulator will provide the best occlusal balance attainable. From the clinical point of view the records required to adjust the articulator in addition to the retruded jaw relationship will include a protrusive registration and a face-bow registration.

Where it is desired to match exactly the occlusal relations of natural teeth which are present, the more complex articulators may need to be considered as the variation in occlusal form of the natural teeth is much wider than that of artificial teeth. In many instances, average value instruments may be used where the numbers and positions of the remaining teeth are such that a clear guide to the position and form of the missing teeth exists. However, in the majority of these cases, an adjustable incisal table is required because the overbite and overjet relations of the natural teeth are frequently outside the range of the fixed incisal guidance instruments.

FURTHER READING

Bergstrom G 1950 On the reproduction of dental articulation by means of articulators. Acta Odont Scand 9 Suppl 4

Posselt U 1968 Physiology of Occlusion and Rehabilitation. 2nd Edn. Blackwell, Oxford

Thorpe R, Smith D E and Nicholls J I 1978 Evaluation of the use of a face-bow in complete denture occlusion. J Prosthet Dent 39: 5

Weinberg L A 1961 An evaluation of the face-bow mounting. J Prosthet Dent 11: 32

Weinberg L A 1963 An evaluation of basic articulators and their concepts. J Prosthet Dent:
Part I   Basic concepts 13: 622
Part II   Arbitrary, positional, semiadjustable articulators 13: 645
Part III   Fully adjustable articulators 13: 873
Part IV   Fully adjustable articulators 13: 1038

11

Principles of tooth selection

INTRODUCTION

The selection of artificial teeth to replace lost natural teeth can be a difficult phase of removable denture production. Where partial dentures are involved, a clear guide may be provided by the remaining natural teeth. For complete dentures and removable partial dentures where many teeth require replacement, in the absence of accurate pre-extraction records no such guide is available. No infallible method of selection exists and the teeth which are to be used must be chosen to harmonise with the aesthetic and functional characteristics of the patient.

The requirements for a patient may have special facets in respect of the anterior and/or posterior artificial teeth and these will be considered separately.

THE SELECTION OF ANTERIOR TEETH FOR REMOVABLE DENTURES

The factors to be taken into account in the selection of anterior teeth include:
1. Size
2. Form
3. Texture
4. Colour
5. Material

Size

Where a removable partial denture is to be produced and a tooth requiring replacement has the corresponding tooth from the opposite side of the arch still *in situ*, determination of the exact size of the tooth required is a simple matter of measurement.

Bodily movement or tilting of the remaining teeth may complicate the use of artificial teeth of the same size as their natural predecessors, and it might be necessary to overlap teeth on the one hand, or provide spacing on the other hand, in order to achieve the degree of balance in size required between the right and left sides of the arch. It is occasionally necessary to use a tooth of a different size to those remaining, but generally the aim is to replace a missing tooth with one of the same size, since it is very uncommon to find corresponding teeth on the left and right sides of the natural dentition which differ in size.

Where no natural anterior teeth remain, the selection of artificial teeth presents the same difficulties as are met in the edentulous patient.

When pre-extraction records are available, they may provide very useful guides to tooth selection. Study models including the patient's natural teeth will give a clear guide to the size and form of the teeth. Clinical photographs can be an equally accurate guide and, while photographs obtained from the family album will rarely provide clear detail of the anterior teeth, they may be very useful as a guide to the relative proportion of the size of the teeth and face of the patient. Other pre-extraction records which can be a helpful guide to tooth size include radiographs of the patient's teeth, and also extracted teeth which have been retained by the patient.

In the absence of any pre-extraction guides, a great deal will depend on the judgement of the dentist. The difficulties experienced during this phase of denture production have resulted in many average value measurements and formulae based on anatomical features being suggested.

General guidelines subject to wide individual

variation suggest that the larger the person, the larger the teeth will be, and that the teeth of women tend to be somewhat smaller than those of men. More specific aspects of anterior tooth selection will be considered in terms of the length and the width of the teeth.

Length

Generally, the incisal edges of the natural central incisors extend below the lowest part of the relaxed lip. For a young person, some 2–3 mm of the upper central incisors may be visible and for an elderly patient only a fraction of a millimetre of tooth may be seen beneath the relaxed lip. There is, of course, wide variation between individuals in this respect.

Some of the factors responsible for differences in the amount of tooth visible include:

1. Age. With increasing age tooth wear tends to shorten the clinical crowns.

2. Length of the upper lip. Where a patient has a short upper lip, up to half the length of the crown of the central incisors may be exposed beneath the relaxed upper lip. On the other hand, a long lip may completely cover the incisors even in a young patient.

3. Overbite. Where a deep overbite exists, more of the upper anterior teeth tend to be exposed.

At the gingival aspect, the high lip line may be taken as a guide. The high lip line is the maximum vertical excursion of the upper lip during functions such as smiling. Thus a combined estimation of the position of the incisal edge and the high lip line will provide a guide to the length of the central incisors.

Alternatively, determination of tooth length may be approached by estimating the width of the anterior teeth and utilising the proportion between the length and width of the teeth provided by the manufacturer for a given tooth form in relation to the length and width of the patient's face. (See Page 188)

Width

There have been many methods suggested for determining the width of the upper anterior teeth. Most methods provide a value for the six anterior teeth together rather than for individual teeth. Some of these methods are listed below:

1. Canine eminence. If this anatomical feature is well defined the distance between lines drawn on the cast of the upper jaw at the distal aspect of the eminences may be taken as the mesio-distal breadth of the upper anterior teeth.

2. Bizygomatic width. It has been suggested that the combined breadth of the six upper anterior teeth may be estimated by dividing the maximum bizygomatic width of the skull by 3.3; and that the width of the upper central incisor is $1/16$ of the bizygomatic width. A face-bow may be used as a caliper in conjunction with a ruler to determine the bizygomatic width. The results of these calculations represent the proportions frequently found in pleasant looking natural dentitions.

3. Cranial circumference. The cranial circumference has been found to have a direct relationship to the width of the six upper anterior teeth in a high proportion of cases. The horizontal circumference of the cranium about a plane passing through the glabella and the maximum occipital point is said to be 10 times the width of the six upper anterior teeth.

4. Corner of the mouth. The distal surface of many natural upper canines is positioned at the corner of the relaxed mouth. The method used to record this position, in a patient lacking natural teeth, requires a properly contoured upper occlusal rim to be in position in the mouth in order to provide correct lip support. The patient is requested to relax with lips in light contact and a pointed instrument is passed to the occlusal rim at each corner of the mouth and a mark recorded on the rim (Fig. 11.1). The distances between these marks following the contour of the rim is taken to represent the width of the six upper anterior teeth.

5. Width of the nose. Parallel lines extended from the lateral surfaces of the ala of the nose onto the properly contoured upper occlusal rim will give an indication of the position of the cusp tip of the upper canine teeth (Fig. 11.2). In practice the distance between the lateral extremities of the ala can be measured with dividers and then transferred to the rim. The mesiodistal width of the teeth between the tip of the cusps of the canine

Fig. 11.1 Marking the position of the corner of the mouth on the occlusal rim.

Fig. 11.2 Establishing the position of the canine teeth. The broken line gives an indication of the position of the distal aspect of the canine. The solid line indicates the position of the tip of the cusp.

teeth is then measured around the contour of the occlusal rim.

6. Lateral surface of the nose. A further, and perhaps more commonly used guide utilising the ala of the nose, requires the projection onto the properly contoured upper occlusal rim of an imaginary line along the lateral surface of the nose, through the centre of the brow-line, and contacting the lateral aspect of the ala. The line on the

occlusal rim gives an indication of the position of the distal aspect of the canine tooth at the point where the projected line passes the occlusal plane (Fig. 11.2).

7. The incisive papilla. It has been demonstrated that a line parallel to the coronal plane and passing through the incisive papilla contacts the natural canine teeth near the tips of the cusps (Fig. 11.3). This may be used as a guide to determining the width of the anterior teeth and positioning the canine teeth when used in conjunction with a properly contoured occlusal rim.

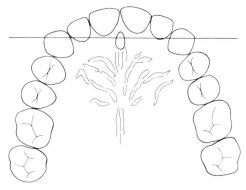

Fig. 11.3 Occlusal view of the upper arch showing the relationship between the incisive papilla and the tip of the cusp of the canines in the coronal plane.

Form

The overall shape of the teeth is important to the development of harmony of form with the face. A method of long standing usage in the selection of aesthetically acceptable tooth form is that developed by J. Leon Williams. The theory introduced by Williams was that the shape of the crown of the upper central incisor corresponded to the outline form of the face. If the outline form of the central incisor is enlarged and the incisal edge placed in the region of the hair line with the neck of the tooth corresponding to the outline of the chin, Williams claimed that the form of the tooth and the face will coincide (Fig. 11.4). He classified the form of the face as square, tapering or avoid — a basic classification which was later added to by combining the basic types to increase the variety of forms (Fig. 11.5).

It has now been demonstrated that the relationship described above occurs only rarely.

Fig. 11.4 Superimposition over the face of an inverted and enlarged form of the crown of the central incisor.

accompanies advancing age, and the softer, more rounded, contours of the teeth of women, are factors to be considered.

The contours of the labial face of the teeth is also important in considering tooth form, and this often relates to the form of the profile of the patient. A patient having a strongly convex profile may require the teeth to have a strongly convex labial surface, for example.

Texture

When viewed in detail most natural anterior teeth possess very complex labial surface features, and these are important to the appearance of the teeth. Smooth surfaced artificial incisors reflect light evenly and have a lifeless appearance because of the lack of a suitable surface texture. In the production of an aesthetically pleasing restoration, artificial teeth which incorporate reproductions of such features as imbrication lines, surface facets, hypoplastic areas, etc., are superior to those having smooth, featureless surfaces.

Artificial teeth should be unobtrusive and the texture of the tooth surface contributes to the harmonious blending of the teeth with the patient's tissues. In this respect surface texture contributes as much as colour selection and

However, it is clear that the application of Williams' method can produce aesthetically satisfactory results.

Age, sex and personality factors have been cited as relevant to selection of tooth form. For example, the wearing down of natural teeth which

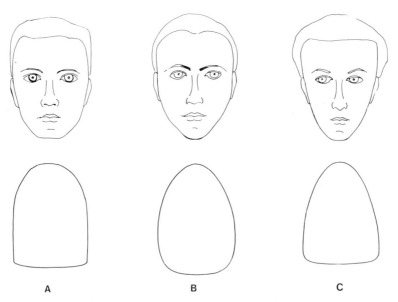

A   B   C

Fig. 11.5 Classification of facial forms as a guide to the selection of tooth form: A, Square; B, Ovoid; C, Tapering.

tooth arrangement to the overall 'natural' appearance of a denture.

Texture is a quality of particular importance in removable partial denture service where anterior teeth are missing unilaterally. The replacement teeth will need to be careful copies of the remaining natural teeth in respect of surface texture as well as colour so that they will not be obviously artificial in appearance.

Colour

The colour variation in natural teeth covers a wide spectrum. There is gradation in the colour over a single tooth which varies from darker near the gingival margin to lighter and more translucent near the incisal tip. In addition there is also variation between teeth — the central incisors generally being lightest in overall colour, the lateral incisors slightly darker, and the canine teeth slightly darker again. The colour, or hue, of the teeth must harmonise with the patient's complexion and in particular with the skin of the face — and to a lesser extent the hair and the iris of the eyes. Skin colour tends to fall into one of three groups having red, yellow or grey tints.

The basic hue of the teeth is a yellow colour, being derived from the dentine. Colour saturation, i.e. the amount of colour per unit area, is a factor of some importance. If the yellow colour is diluted to white, the tooth will appear light in relation to one having a similar basic yellow, but where black is added the result is a darker, more grey tooth. Variation in lightness and darkness is sometimes referred to as brilliance.

Where the complexion is fair or blonde, the tooth colour tends to be light, and for patients having a darker complexion, darker coloured teeth predominate. In the mouth of a patient having a very dark complexion, teeth in which grey tones predominate may appear to be light in colour, and in this respect it is important to appreciate the need for a harmonious balance of basic tooth colour relative to that of the patient's face.

In the natural teeth, the enamel is translucent and provides a thin covering to the dentine near the gingival margin of the crown and a relatively thick covering at the incisal edge. This results in an apparent gradation of colour over the length of the tooth crown. At the incisal edge where there may be no dentine underlying the enamel, the translucence of the enamel results in a greyish appearance which varies in apparent hue depending on the tongue, lip and mouth posture. In the better artificial teeth, this translucence is achieved by the manufacturer, and has the effect of blending the various pigments used in colouring the teeth and also provides for subtle colour variation to occur during functional activity in the mouth, particularly near the incisal edges of the teeth.

It is generally advised that in the selection of the shade for artificial teeth where no natural anterior teeth are present, reference should be made to the skin and also the hair and the eyes. Of these, skin colour is by far the best guide. The hue and saturation of colour in the teeth must harmonise with that of the skin. Hair colour is useful in the younger patient as a guide, but it should be borne in mind that hair colour may be subject to quite rapid change from both natural and artificial causes. The colour of the iris of the eye is sometimes useful in a general sense, but this feature is relatively small in proportion to other colours about the face.

Age has a marked effect on tooth shade. With advancing years tooth wear may result in exposure of dentine which readily takes up extrinsic stains. The reduction in size of the pulp chamber with advancing age produces a yellowing effect because of the increase in the quantity of dentine. Injury to the tooth and repair of the tooth structure also have an effect on the colour of a tooth.

Manufacturers of artificial teeth produce a wide range of shades for their products. While the available range is generally satisfactory for complete dentures, the enormous variation which exists with the natural teeth is not always satisfied by those available for removable partial denture work. In such circumstances it might be necessary to resort to the use of the pigments, stains, etc. which are produced for the purpose of modifying the stock teeth produced commercially. The alternative is to accept the nearest available shade which may not produce an aesthetically harmonious result.

In using the shade guide for artificial teeth as supplied by the manufacturer, the tooth colours are usually observed holding the chosen shade:

1. Outside the mouth against the skin of the face and also near to the eyes and the hair of the patient. This is to establish the basic hue, brilliance and saturation of colour.

2. Under the lip to observe the colour of the tooth in the mouth. Shade selection should be carried out preferably in diffuse daylight, as the light incident on the teeth will influence the apparent colour of the reflected light. The shade guide tooth placed under the lip should be observed with its surface wet.

The selection of tooth shade for an edentulous patient presents a difficult problem and is dependent to a large extent on the artistic interpretation of the dentist. For the partially dentate patient only colour matching is required, and this presents difficulty only when suitably shaded artificial teeth are not available.

Material

Artificial teeth are manufactured in porcelain and in plastic materials. Both types are available in a wide range of sizes, shapes, surface textures and colours. It is not the intention of this section to deal with materials science aspects of the two materials, but it is necessary to touch on these as they affect use of the teeth. Porcelain teeth require mechanical retention to the denture base material, and anterior teeth are usually provided with pins for this purpose. The pins protrude from the tooth and prevent close adaptation of the tooth to the residual ridge, and this is a potential source of difficulty where the space available for placement of the tooth is limited. Where it is necessary to alter the shape of a porcelain tooth it is extremely difficult to polish the material to reproduce the glazed surface which existed prior to alteration.

Plastic teeth are simple to adjust and repolish and do not rely on mechanical retention for attachment to denture base resins. Plastic teeth are also much simpler than porcelain teeth in respect of alteration of surface texture and incorporation of stains, etc. They are therefore much more versatile, and particularly where lack of space for tooth placement is an aspect of the denture being produced.

From the aesthetic and functional points of view, both porcelain and plastic teeth may be regarded as equally satisfactory for replacement of anterior teeth. A table citing the relative merits of porcelain and plastic teeth will be found on page 84.

SELECTION OF POSTERIOR TEETH

The selection of posterior teeth will be considered in relation to:
1. Size
2. Form
3. Colour
4. Material

Size

The selection of the appropriate posterior tooth size is based on the space available for the replacement teeth, and, where upper premolar teeth are involved, the aesthetic requirements must also be considered.

The space available for posterior teeth may be defined in three dimensions:
1. The mesiodistal dimension
2. The occluso-gingival dimension
3. The bucco-lingual dimension

Mesiodistal

For bounded saddles where natural teeth are present in the mouth, the mesiodistal dimension is readily defined as the distance between the distal surface of the mesial abutment and the mesial surface of the distal abutment. It is important that this mesiodistal space is occupied to provide for the development of effective contact points between the denture and the remaining natural teeth in order to minimise the possibility of food packing and the occurrence of stagnation areas about the abutments. Generally, the same number of artificial teeth as that of the natural teeth lost from the dental arch will be provided, but this may not be possible as a result of drifting, tilting or rotation of the remaining teeth and a compromise will be required.

Where complete dentures are concerned, the mesiodistal dimension available for artificial teeth extends between the distal surface of the lower canine and the mesial end of the retromolar pad. Because of the potential displaceability of the thick layer of soft tissue comprising the retromolar pad, artificial teeth must not be placed over that structure as instability of the lower denture will result during chewing when the denture is loaded in this region and the denture consequently is displaced tissuewards. Where the alveolar crest of the lower residual alveolar ridge slopes steeply upwards anterior to the retromolar pad, the mesiodistal dimension for the teeth will need to be reduced. Placing an artificial tooth over such a steeply inclined plane will result in the development of resolved forces during chewing which will tend to displace the denture anteriorly. These principles also apply to the selection of teeth for free-end saddle partial dentures.

Having obtained by measurement the dimension available, reference to a manufacturer's selection guide will give an indication of the teeth available to satisfy this size requirement.

Occluso-gingival dimension

Artificial teeth of similar mesiodistal dimension are available in various lengths. In general, the longest tooth which can be used in the vertical space available should be selected. This is particularly important in respect of the upper premolar teeth, which are often visible during speech, laughing, etc. Where a premolar tooth is used which is significantly shorter than the canine tooth next to it, when viewed from the buccal aspect, the result is aesthetically unacceptable. In removable partial denture treatment where an upper premolar is to be replaced, it may be necessary to substitute a canine tooth for the premolar in order to provide a tooth of adequate length for the aesthetic requirements of the patient.

Bucco-lingual dimension

The bucco-lingual space available for artificial teeth is limited by the cheek and tongue tissues and also by the load bearing capacity of the supporting tissues. In respect of the space between cheek and tongue tissues, earlier artificial tooth forms tended to be of similar dimension to the natural teeth they were intended to replace. This,

however, ignores biomechanical aspects of posterior tooth replacement. The supporting mechanism for natural teeth is well adapted to resist the forces applied to them during functional activity. Artificial teeth which are to be used with soft tissue borne bases utilise the mucosa covering the residual alveolar ridges and palate for support, and this tissue is unable to tolerate without damage the forces capable of acceptance by the natural teeth. Where a removable partial denture is of tooth support design, the capacity of the periodontal ligament of the abutment teeth to support additional denture teeth is such as to require the extra loading to be kept to a minimum. As it is essential to provide adequate contact points between the denture and abutment teeth, the bucco-lingual width of the denture teeth should be kept to a minimum consistent with the other requirements for a particular patient. By this means the surface area of the artificial teeth is reduced, so that higher pressures can be developed for a given force generated by the muscles of mastication over the narrow artificial teeth than would be the case for broader teeth. Thus it is possible that the masticatory ability of the patient wearing dentures having narrow occlusal surfaces might be maintained without overloading the periodontal ligament of the abutment teeth or the mucous membrane underlying the denture base. Further aspects of this facet of posterior tooth selection are considered in the following section.

Form

Early artificial posterior teeth were hand carved from wood, bone or ivory, and even the crowns of natural teeth were used. When porcelain was introduced in France towards the end of the 18th century, very durable artificial teeth simulating natural teeth were produced. The development of porcelain teeth continued through the 19th century using natural teeth as the basis for the form of the teeth. By the end of the 19th century it was realised that natural tooth forms were often quite unsuitable for artificial dentures and there followed efforts by many workers to produce tooth forms aimed at minimising the difficulties experienced. This development has continued up to the present time and various designs have been introduced to aid in stabilising the denture, increasing masticatory efficiency, or minimising trauma to the underlying tissue, or combinations of these objectives.

Some of the developments which have taken place will be described. It is not intended that this represents a review of tooth forms which are or have been available, but the types to be considered are representative of important groups of artificial tooth designs.

Prior to the 20th century, tooth forms were based on 'design' rather than having a basis in relating the factors known to have a relationship to balanced occlusion and articulation.

In 1914, Gysi carved teeth specially for use with his 'Simplex' articulator, on the basis that condylar and incisal guidance angles for most patients required a tooth having a cusp angle of 33°. This represented the first 'anatomical' form of tooth to be produced on the basis of research relating the variable factors involved in articulation (Fig. 11.6).

Fig. 11.6 Bucco-lingual section through 33° molar teeth (Gysi, 1914)

Dr Gysi introduced 'cross-bite' teeth in the 1920's. These teeth were developed because of the realisation that the 33° teeth were not always adequate for a ridge relationship requiring a cross-bite arrangement of the posterior teeth. These teeth (Fig. 11.7) had narrow lower teeth having low cusps for use with a 10° incisal guidance angle. The upper teeth were without a buccal cusp so that a 'mortar and pestle' action was produced.

Sear's Channel Teeth were introduced in 1927. These teeth were produced having a central fossa in the upper teeth which ran mesiodistally through the four posterior teeth. The lowers had a corre-

Fig. 11.7 Gysi's 'Cross-bite' teeth in bucco-lingual section

Fig. 11.8 Bucco-lingual aspect of Sear's Channel teeth

sponding narrow ridge of approximately 1.5 mm width. Freedom from cusp rise on protrusion of the lower teeth was allowed for and the buccal and lingual inclined planes limited lateral gliding (Fig. 11.8).

In 1929 Hall introduced his inverted cusp teeth. These teeth were produced having depressions in the surface and were designed to be set to the surface of a sphere giving freedom of movement in all sliding contacts between the upper and lower teeth. The porcelain surrounding the inverted cusps was intended to act as an effective cutting edge (Fig. 11.9).

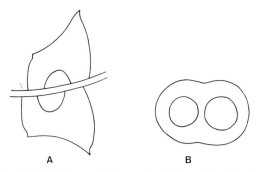

A   B

Fig. 11.9 Hall's Inverted Cusp teeth. A, Bucco-lingual section; B, Plan view of a molar tooth.

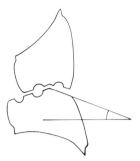

Fig. 11.10 Bucco-lingual section through 20° type teeth

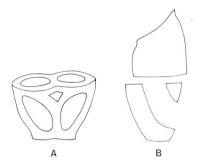

Fig. 11.12 Cook's posterior teeth. A, Viewed from an occluso-buccal aspect; B, Bucco-lingual section.

In 1935 French introduced his 'Modified Posteriors' which were of an inverted cusp style, but having the buccal aspect of the lower teeth removed so that contact occurred only with the lingual aspect of the uppers. French considered this design gave better stability to the lower denture than other occlusal arrangements.

Gysi introduced a further tooth form in 1935 having a low (20°) cusp angle and deep grooves and sulci for a modified inverted cusp effect. This represents a type of design which has been quite widely adopted (Fig. 11.10).

Metal inserts in stylised plastic posterior teeth were introduced in 1946 by Hardy. A zig-zag ribbon of Vitallium was present and raised slightly above the embedding plastic to provide an effective cutting device when opposed by a similar metal ribbon (Fig. 11.11).

Fig. 11.11 Hardy's V.O. posterior teeth. A, Occlusal view; B, Bucco-lingual section. The heavy black line represents the metallic insert.

The development of vacuum firing techniques for porcelain in 1951 enabled much finer detail of cusp geometry, supplementary grooves, etc. to be retained during manufacture of posterior teeth and so improve shearing efficiency.

Cook, in 1952, suggested the use of cobalt chromium lower teeth of inverted cusp form, but incorporating sluiceways on the buccal aspect. These teeth were set against flat porcelain opposing surfaces in the upper teeth (Fig. 11.12).

While being efficient at cutting and dividing food, these teeth suffer from the disadvantage of constantly passing food into the buccal sulcus from which it may be difficult for the patient to remove, and also having a tendency for some foods to clog the sluiceways.

Bader in 1957 introduced a 'cutter-bar' which was a metal bar replacing the lower second premolar and the first and second molars. The bar was opposed by flat porcelain upper teeth (Fig. 11.13).

With the exception of the higher cusped 'anatomical' type teeth which simulate the natural teeth in a general way, many of the above tooth types have been developed for complete denture production. In removable partial denture work the cuspal inclines and arrangement of the remaining natural teeth will determine contact movements paths between the opposing teeth where some anterior and posterior teeth remain. Where only anterior teeth are present the incisal guidance angle will to a large extent determine the form of posterior tooth to be used. The closer the incisal guidance approaches zero, the wider the choice of posterior tooth form becomes and non-anatomical tooth forms may be considered.

If a deeper overbite exists, higher cusped teeth will be required where posterior occlusal balance is sought. However, it must be appreciated that high cusped teeth transmit relatively high lateral

Fig. 11.13 Bader Cutter-bar

Table 11.1 Advantages and disadvantages of porcelain and acrylic resin teeth.

Property	Acrylic resin	Porcelain
Rate of wear	May be rapid	Very slow
Brittleness	Tough and will not chip	Brittle and may chip
Ease of adjustment	Easily ground and repolished	More difficult to grind and repolish
Density	1.18 g/cm³	2.35 g/cm³
Aesthetics	Can be excellent	Can be excellent
Ease of modification	Simple to characterise using stains, etc.	Difficult to characterise
Noise during use	Little impact sound on contact	Sharp impact sound
Retention to base	Potential for chemical bond	Mechanical bond only
Transmission of occlusal forces	Considered to transmit reduced forces	Considered to transmit all forces

stresses to the denture base and the underlying supporting tissues, and this is to be avoided wherever possible — particularly where the residual alveolar ridge shows substantial atrophy. In general terms, the lower the crest of the residual alveolar ridge is in relation to the surrounding sulcus, the lower the cuspal angle of the teeth selected should be. Also, as pointed out previously, stresses on the underlying supporting tissue will be minimised by narrowing the occlusal table provided.

Colour

In selecting the colour of posterior teeth for removable partial denture work, the shade of the remaining natural teeth should be matched. Where an exact shade is not available, it is considered preferable to err on the side of selecting the nearest shade on the dark side of that required. Where a lighter option is used, the aesthetic effect may undesirably draw attention to the artificial replacement even when only posterior teeth are involved.

For complete denture prostheses the same shade of posterior tooth should be selected as that chosen for the anterior teeth.

Material

With the exception of the tooth forms described above as being made of metal, most types of posterior teeth are available in both porcelain or plastic (acrylic resin). No general rules are available in respect of the choice between porcelain and acrylic resin except that relating to the available interridge distance. Where this is minimal acrylic teeth will be required as excessive grinding of porcelain posterior teeth will remove the diatoric holes provided for retention of the tooth to the baseplate. Because of the relatively rapid rate of wear of acrylic resin posterior teeth, some operators would contend that the resultant changes in occlusion would mitigate against their use. Patients seeking replacement dentures and who have acrylic resin teeth on their existing dentures may not readily tolerate a replacement denture having porcelain teeth. The simplicity of adjustment of acrylic teeth is often the major factor in their choice by many operators.

The advantages and disadvantages of porcelain and acrylic resin teeth are listed in Table 11.1.

FURTHER READING

Brewer A 1970 Selection of denture teeth for esthetics and function. J Prosthet Dent 23: 368

Frush J P and Fisher R D 1956 How dentogenic restorations interpret the sex factor. J Prosthet Dent 6: 160

Frush J P and Fisher R D 1956 How dentogenics interprets the personality factor. J Prosthet Dent 6: 441

Frush J P and Fisher R D 1957 The age factor in dentogenics. J Prosthet Dent 7: 5

Ray G E 1963 Artificial posterior teeth. Dent Pract Dent Rec 14: 31

Saleski C G 1972 Colour, light and shade matching. J Prosthet Dent 27: 263

Sears V H 1957 The selection and management of posterior teeth. J Prosthet Dent 7: 723

Wehner P J, Hickey J C and Boucher C O 1967 Selection of artificial teeth. J Prosthet Dent 18: 222

PART II

Special Aspects Relating to Partial Denture Treatment

12

Introductory considerations

DEFINITION

Of the many definitions which have been proposed for removable partial dentures, the following is felt to be the most apt:
'A removable partial denture is an appliance which restores a partial loss of natural teeth and associated tissues and which receives its retention and support from the natural teeth and/or from the mucous membrane.'

This definition is based on one given by Craddock, modifications having been introduced to meet the requirements of British terminology.

TREATMENT OBJECTIVES

As noted in Chapter 6 — Diagnosis and treatment planning — the provision of a removable partial denture is one of the ways of providing treatment for the partially edentulous condition. If, instead, a decision is made to provide no replacement of the missing teeth, it should be borne in mind that a number of problems may develop. These are as follows:

1. Increased alveolar resorption

It has been claimed that the lack of any appreciable degree of loading stimulus will cause the alveolar processes in the edentulous regions to resorb at a faster rate than that which occurs when a denture has been fitted.

Gross alveolar resorption, which particularly tends to occur in the mandible, will reduce the prognosis for successful provision of a denture at a later date.

2. Reduction in masticatory efficiency

Manly and Braley have shown that the loss of the third molars reduces the masticatory function of a full complement of natural teeth by 10%. Additional removal of the first molars brings the value down by a further 20%.

Although the majority of individuals can manage to chew most foods satisfactorily when only one or two posterior teeth have been lost, additional loss may produce a noticeable fall in masticatory efficiency.

Where multiple loss has occurred, the patient may complain of dietary limitation and there is also a possibility that digestive disturbances will arise.

3. Effect on aesthetics

Tooth loss can affect aesthetics in two ways. Firstly, there will be an obvious loss of aesthetics where normally visible teeth are absent from the dentition. This will be most noticeable where anterior teeth are missing but the effect may extend into the premolar regions. Secondly, the support for the lips and cheeks which the teeth provide will be lost. Loss of either anterior or posterior teeth may be evident because an inward collapse of lips or cheeks has occurred.

4. Effect on speech

The various consonants and vowels of the alphabet are produced by placing the lips or tongue in certain positions relative to the teeth, so developing definitive air channels. For example, 'F' and 'V' are made by bringing the lower lip into apposition with the upper anterior teeth (Fig. 12.1). As a consequence, loss of the upper anterior teeth will inevi-

Fig. 12.1 Sagittal section of the oral cavity showing the position of the lower lip relative to the upper anterior teeth in the formation of the 'F' and 'V' sounds.

tably interfere with the formation of the 'F' and 'V' sounds. Similarly, loss of other teeth from the arches can affect the quality of production of other speech sounds.

It is common to find, though, that in a relatively short time after tooth loss has occurred, a degree of adaptation will develop by, for instance, modification in tongue position, so lessening the effect on phonetics. It is, in fact, unusual for a patient to attend with a complaint of poor phonetics arising from a partial loss of the natural dentition. Even so, there may well be a residual effect on the quality of speech where multiple tooth loss has occurred and the provision of a denture in such cases can produce a noticeable improvement.

5. Effect on the integrity of the dentition

There is little doubt that the loss of a single tooth from the intact natural dentition can lead in some instances to general malocclusion and the loss of the integrity of both dental arches.

There is a natural tendency for the teeth adjacent to the space created by tooth loss to tilt and drift into that space. This results in the opening up of contact areas between teeth in more remote positions in the arch, inviting food packing and plaque accumulation with consequential increase in the risk of caries and periodontal damage arising. Where tilting occurs, the affected teeth become subject to non-axial loading from the opposing dentition. This can hasten periodontal breakdown with thickening of the lamina dura, loss of

bone from the alveolar crest and deepening of the periodontal pockets. The teeth in the opposing jaw which are situated opposite to the space will now lack occlusal stimulation. As a consequence, they tend to over-erupt into the space and the effects thus extend to the opposing jaw.

Eventually, where multiple tooth loss has occurred, disruption of tooth contact between the opposing jaws may reach the point where mandibular overclosure develops. When this happens the temporomandibular joints may be affected. A detrimental effect on aesthetics may also arise as the mandible moves upwards and forwards into its new stop position.

Over-eruption of unopposed teeth may leave little or no room for the positioning of artificial teeth where the provision of a removable partial denture is attempted in such a case. In addition, the tilting of isolated teeth may make the positioning of retentive clasp units on such teeth very difficult.

At times, conditions will become so severe that further extractions must be carried out before the provision of a removable partial denture becomes a feasible proposition.

6. Attrition of the remaining dentition

As the volume of the natural dentition is reduced by tooth loss, the remaining teeth will bear an increased masticatory load. Especially in those instances where tooth contact only occurs on the anterior teeth, there is a risk that gross attrition will occur in these teeth. Where this eventuality arises, treatment may necessitate the application of relatively complex procedures.

7. Effect on the neutral zone

Where any sizeable edentulous area is left unrestored for a period of time, it will be found that the tongue tends to occupy a part of the space vacated by tooth loss. Likewise, the cheeks and lips will tend to move inwards into the space.

The size of the neutral zone (or zone of minimum conflict) will thereby be decreased and this may make the placement of teeth in the zone more difficult in any subsequent denture construction. An increased risk of denture instability so arises.

8. Effect on masticatory movements

As tooth loss occurs, the necessity to chew on a reduced complement of the dentition may lead to the development of atypical masticatory movements. Facial pain may arise as a consequence of the onset of temporomandibular joint disturbance. Increased difficulty may also be experienced in registering the correct fully retruded jaw relationship where denture construction is subsequently carried out.

The formidable size of the above list of the possible consequences of a failure to restore a partial loss of the natural dentition clearly indicates the need for some form of replacement therapy to be applied in most instances. Where it is decided that this shall be achieved by the provision of a removable partial denture, the objectives may be summarised as follows:
1. Restoration of appearance.
2. Restoration of masticatory efficiency.
3. Restoration of speech to a normal quality.
4. Maintenance of the health and integrity of the soft and hard tissues of the oral cavity.

It is likely that a patient would place these four treatment objectives in the order given above in terms of priority. The dental surgeon, though, should place treatment objective No. 4 at the top of the list of priorities. In that way he will be best able to satisfy the prime aim of partial denture prosthesis as advocated by De Van: 'our objective should be the perpetual preservation of what remains rather than the meticulous restoration of what is missing'.

A well-designed partial denture may meet this objective excellently, for instance by splinting together the remaining natural teeth and by providing functional stimulus to the edentulous tissue areas. The need for such a biological concept of partial denture provision should be the uppermost consideration in all stages of design and construction.

CLASSIFICATION

Classification of partial dentures may serve one or both of two possible functions:
1. Provide a simple or 'shorthand' description of the features of a case, in terms of the disposition of the natural teeth and edentulous tissue areas in the arch.
2. Provide a guide to denture design, or at least be linked to design.

Many proposals have been made for schemes of classification. Of these, two have been selected for consideration on the basis of their frequency of application:

The Kennedy system

First introduced in 1928, this system fulfils only the first of the above functions but is very widely used. It may be said to provide only a description of the unrestored natural dentition rather than relate to the partial denture which is to be provided. Four classes are described:

Class I — The edentulous areas are bilateral and lie posterior to the standing teeth (Fig. 12.2).

Class II — The edentulous area is unilateral and lies posterior to the standing teeth on that side (Fig. 12.3).

Class III — The edentulous area is unilateral and has standing teeth both anterior and posterior to it (Fig. 12.4).

Class IV — A single edentulous area lies anterior to the standing teeth (Fig. 12.5).

In addition to the basic class descriptions, modifications are also described for each of the first three classes. These are numbered according to the number of additional edentulous areas which are present, one additional edentulous area being termed: Modification 1, two additional edentulous areas; Modification 2, and so on. Examples of cases showing modifications are shown in Figures 12.6 and 12.7.

No modifications are possible in the case of Class IV dentitions as the presence of any additional edentulous areas would bring such a case within the definition of one of the first three classes.

The Craddock system

This system meets in particular the second of the possible functions of systems of classification. It is based on earlier proposals of Bailyn and is linked to the means which are to be adopted for supporting

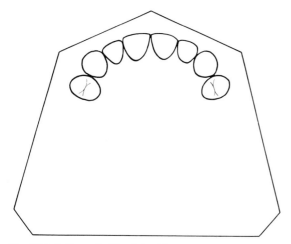

Fig. 12.2 A Kennedy Class I dentition.

Fig. 12.3 A Kennedy Class II dentition.

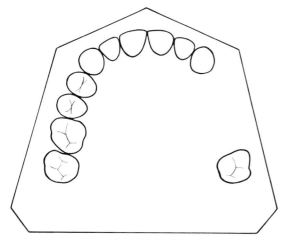

Fig. 12.4 A Kennedy Class III dentition.

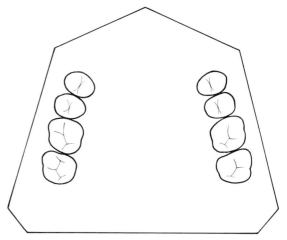

Fig. 12.5 A Kennedy Class IV dentition.

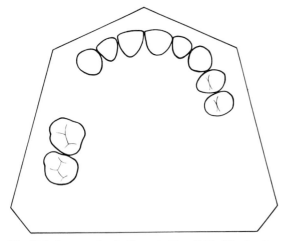

Fig. 12.6 An example of a Kennedy Class II Modification 1 dentition.

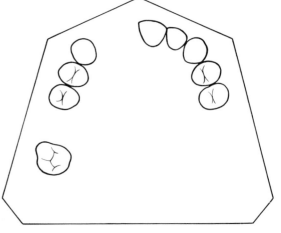

Fig. 12.7 An example of a Kennedy Class II Modification 2 dentition.

the partial denture on the oral tissues. Three classes are described:

Class I — Denture entirely supported on the abutment teeth.

Class II — Denture entirely supported on the mucous membrane.

Class III — Denture support provided by both the abutment teeth and the mucous membrane, neither tissue being judged able to bear the applied load alone without sustaining damage.

The existence of various systems of classification necessitates that in all cases where reference is made to a class a prefix must be applied to indicate the system which is being referred to. For example, one should refer to a 'Kennedy Class I' case and not just a 'Class I' case.

FURTHER READING

Craddock F W 1951 Prosthetic Dentisty: A Clinical Outline. Henry Kimpton, London

De Van M M 1952 The nature of the partial denture foundation. Suggestions for its preservation. J Prosthet Dent 2: 210

Kennedy E 1942 Partial Denture Construction. Dental Items of Interest Publishing Co Inc, New York

Lawson W A and Bond E K 1969 Speech and its relation to dentistry. Dent Pract Dent Rec 19: 150

Manley R S and Braley L C 1950 Masticatory performance and efficiency. J Dent Res 29: 448

13

Component elements

INTRODUCTION

The component elements which may be present in a removable partial denture are as follows:
1. Saddles
2. Rests
3. Direct retainers
4. Indirect retainers
5. Connectors
6. Stress-breakers

All partial dentures contain at least two of these elements — saddles and connectors. The presence of additional elements will confer increasing complexity on the appliance up to the point where all six elements may be present.

SADDLES

A saddle is that element of a partial denture which carries the artificial teeth. It also performs major functional and aesthetic roles in providing replacement for lost alveolar tissues.

Saddles can be classified as being either bounded or free-end. A bounded saddle has abutment teeth present at both extremities of the saddle. A free-end saddle has only a single abutment tooth at its mesial end.

Support for a saddle may be obtained from the abutment teeth, or from the mucosa underlying the saddle, or from a combination of both. The saddle may be made totally in a polymeric material such as acrylic resin or in a combination of a metal such as cobalt-chromium alloy and a polymer.

The extension adopted for a saddle is dependent on its mode of support. Where the saddle is to be wholly or partly supported on the mucosa then the maximum possible area of mucosa should be covered. This is necessary in order to keep the load borne by each unit area of mucosa to a minimum, so reducing the risk of evoking a pathological response in the loaded tissues. Where, instead, the saddle is to be supported on the abutment teeth, the extension developed can often be less, the outline here being dictated by the need to provide replacement for lost alveolar tissues.

RESTS

A rest is an extension from a partial denture which is positioned on the surface of a standing tooth capable of providing resistance to displacement of the rest in a tissue-wards direction. Where tooth morphology is favourable, a rest may be placed on an unprepared tooth surface. In many instances, though, preparation of the tooth will be necessary if optimal resting action is to be obtained.

Rests are made in metal, as non-metallic materials such as acrylic resin lack the strength and abrasion resistance in thin section needed for this application. They may be wrought or cast in construction, the preference being for cast rests as this allows the development of a better fit where an irregularly shaped rest seat is present.

There are three types of rests:
1. Occlusal rests — used on posterior teeth.
2. Cingulum rests — used on anterior teeth.
3. Incisal rests — used on anterior teeth.

Occlusal rests

Occlusal rests are normally positioned on the mesio-occlusal or disto-occlusal fossa of a posterior tooth. They find wide application in the construction of tooth-supported and tooth-and-mucosa-supported partial dentures.

Their outline form is triangular in shape, the base of the triangle lying along the marginal ridge of the tooth, with the apex positioned near the centre of the tooth. Bucco-lingually, the rest should fill all the available space between the buccal and lingual cusps. The rest is joined to the denture by means of an attachment tag which may either enter the polymeric portion of an adjacent saddle or may be an integral part of a cast metal framework for the denture.

The occlusal morphology of a rest should resemble that of the tooth on which it is placed and should take due account of the occlusion with the opposing dentition. Its thickness must be adequate to provide resistance to distortion and fracture.

Cingulum rests

Cingulum rests can be placed on anterior teeth where a well-developed cingulum is present. This condition is most commonly met in upper central incisors and upper and lower canines. Upper lateral incisors may also present a suitable surface for their placement in some cases. Where the morphology of the tooth is such that a comparatively horizontal surface is present at the superior aspect of the cingulum, then the rest may be placed directly on the tooth surface without preparation (Fig. 13.1).

Problems may be encountered, though, where such direct placement of cingulum rests is used. Firstly, the rest presents a positive build-up on the tooth surface in an area of high tongue activity and so may give rise to tongue irritation. Secondly, unless the surface on which the rest is placed is at right angles to the long axis of the tooth (and this finding is rare), a horizontal force component will arise by inclined plane action when the rest applies

Fig. 13.2 Cingulum rest utilising a prepared rest seat in a lower canine.

load to the tooth. This may cause horizontal tooth movement, which is clearly undesirable. Thirdly, inadequate space may be present for a rest where the anterior tooth relationship is close.

In most cases where a cingulum rest is to be used, preparation of the tooth is thus needed so that a horizontal facet is available for load application (Fig. 13.2).

The use of a rest seat preparation also reduces the build-up effect of the rest on the tooth surface and thus aids tongue comfort.

Cingulum rests, especially those fitted into prepared rest seats, are nearly always cast.

Incisal rests

Incisal rests can be placed on any anterior tooth. They may, though, give rise to aesthetic problems and for this reason their application tends to be limited to those teeth for which the use of cingulum rests is normally not feasible (e.g. lower incisors). They may take various forms:

Form 1. An extension of metal-work on the lingual or palatal surface of an anterior tooth to provide a thin cover over the whole incisal surface of the tooth (Fig. 13.3). This provides a very positive resting action, but presents an unaesthetic show of metal.

Form 2. A rest seat may be prepared at the mesial or distal incisal corner of a tooth to present a horizontal facet for resting, the metal rest restor-

Fig. 13.1 Cingulum rest placed on the unprepared surface of a lower canine. A, Cingulum rest; B, Attachment tag.

Fig. 13.3 Sagittal view of an incisal rest of form one used on a lower incisor. A, Incisal rest; B, Lingual plate.

Fig. 13.4 Anterior view of an incisal rest of form two used on a lower incisor.

ing the cut-out portion of the tooth (Fig. 13.4). Attachment of the rest would normally be via lingual or palatal metalwork. Again, aesthetic problems arise.

Form 3. Where the antero-posterior dimension of the tooth is adequate, a corner rest seat can be prepared as in Form 2, but with maintenance of the labial enamel surface (Fig. 13.5).

Fig. 13.5 Plan view of an incisal rest of form three used on a lower incisor. A, Labial surface; B, Lingual surface.

Fig. 13.6 Anterior view of incisal rests of form four on $\overline{21|12}$. Metal covering the incisal edges of the teeth has been extended interproximally on to small areas of the labial surfaces to form embrasure hooks.

Form 4. Incisal edge metal coverage as in Form 1 may be extended into the interproximal embrasures and onto a small area of the labial surface of adjacent teeth. Such a development is termed an embrasure hook (Fig. 13.6). When properly designed, embrasure hooks serve to splint teeth together and prevent their labial displacement. As with cingulum rests, all forms of incisal rests are normally prepared by casting.

The functions of rests

Function 1. Where a clasp arm is to be placed on a tooth, the presence of an associated rest serves to locate correctly the clasp arm on the tooth in its intended position.

Function 2. A rest can serve as a means of transferring vertical load borne by a denture saddle

onto a standing tooth. It can thereby develop a tooth-supported or tooth-and-mucosa-supported characteristic in a saddle.

If it can be arranged that the vertical load applied by the rest to the tooth is transmitted along the long axis of the tooth, a favourable response by the periodontal attachment of the tooth is likely. If, instead, an off-centre load is transmitted to a tooth by a rest, a rotatory torque will arise and this may be less well tolerated by the periodontal attachment. This point should be borne in mind during the planning of the form and positioning of rests so that the risk of causing periodontal damage will be minimised.

The problem of off-centre loading is particularly encountered where occlusal rests are used. Where design features permit, consideration should be given to the placement of two occlusal rests on a tooth, situated on opposing fossae. A condition approaching axial loading will thereby be achieved. Where only a single rest is to be used, the off-centre loading it gives rise to will be reduced by extending the rest as near to the centre of the tooth as is possible. It will also help if rests are sited in relation to the saddle in such a manner that resistance to tilting of an abutment tooth is present. With bounded saddles, rests should be placed on the fossae of the abutment teeth adjacent to the saddle. The saddle will then be able to act as a brace, resisting tilting of the teeth (Fig. 13.7).

With a free-end saddle, the rest should be placed on the fossa of the abutment tooth remote

Fig. 13.7 Positioning the rests for a bounded saddle. The saddle resists tilting of the abutment teeth in the directions indicated by the arrows. A, Rest; B, Saddle.

Fig. 13.8 Positioning the rest for a free-end saddle. The contiguous tooth resists tilting of the abutment tooth in the direction indicated by the arrow. A, Rest; B, Saddle.

from the saddle. The tendency for tilting of the abutment tooth which the rest gives rise to will then be resisted by the contiguous tooth, or by another saddle where one is present (Fig. 13.8)

In certain circumstances it may be possible to extend a rest to cover the whole occlusal surface of a posterior tooth. Such a development is referred to as an onlay. Optimal load transfer along the long axis of the tooth will so be obtained. Use of onlays is, however, only feasible where there is a need for the appliance to provide an increase in vertical dimension, either on isolated teeth or over the whole dentition. If used in other circumstances onlays would produce an unacceptable decrease or even obliteration of the freeway space. In addition, onlays should only be used where the patient is prepared to follow a very strict regime of oral hygiene as full coverage of an occlusal surface produces a considerable increase in caries risk.

Function 3. A rest can serve as a means of transferring horizontal (mainly lateral) loads from a denture saddle to a standing tooth.

The extent to which such a transfer of load arises will depend upon the form of the rest seat in which the rest is fitted. Where the rest is placed on a flat surface, only minor resistance to horizontal movement will arise from friction. Use, instead, of a saucer-shaped form of rest seat will produce moderate load transfer, whilst maximum load transfer will arise if a box form of rest seat is used (Fig. 13.9).

Varying the form of the rest seat thus provides a means of controlling the degree to which horizontal (mainly lateral) loads can be transferred from a denture saddle to a rested tooth.

Function 4. Where a rest is placed on a surface of an abutment tooth adjacent to a saddle, and rest and saddle are in continuity, the space between the saddle and the abutment tooth will be covered. This lessens the risk of food packing into the space, with corresponding reduction in the risk of plaque retention and gingival irritation.

A similar benefit can arise where adjacent rests are joined to create a bridge spanning an interdental space (Fig. 13.10).

Fig. 13.10 Adjacent rests on 7| and 5| joined to bridge the inter-dental space.

Interdental spaces of two to three millimetres are not uncommon. They are too small to allow placement of a saddle carrying an artificial tooth, and yet if left unrestored can be a source of irritation to the patient as a consequence of food packing.

Function 5. By appropriate shaping, a rest may serve to improve the occlusion with the opposing dentition (Fig. 13.11).

This need particularly arises where tilting of teeth has occurred and is seen most commonly in the relationship of isolated third molars.

Function 6. A rest may act as an indirect retainer (see page 104).

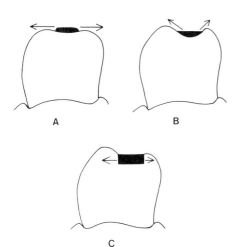

Fig. 13.9 Rest seat forms. A, Flat form; B, Saucer-shaped form; C, Box form.

Fig. 13.11 Occlusal rest on a lower molar shaped to improve the occlusion with the opposing upper molar.

Function 7. A rest may provide reciprocation for a retentive clasp arm (see page 100). This is seen most commonly where a cingulum rest on a canine acts as reciprocation for a gingivally-approaching retentive clasp arm placed on the labial surface of the tooth.

Function 8. A rest may serve to prevent supra-eruption of the tooth on which it is placed, where no opposing tooth is present to perform this function.

DIRECT RETAINERS

Direct retainers are those elements of a removable partial denture which serve to provide resistance to bodily translation of the denture away from the supportive tissues, when it is subject to the action of gravity or functional forces.

They may be classified as follows:

1. Elements utilised in single unit dentures:
   a. Clasp units
   b. Precision attachments
2. Elements utilised in sectional dentures:
   a. Hinged flanges
   b. Two-part structures

Clasp units

Introduction

In a clasp unit, retention is obtained by positioning a flexible metal arm, arising from a suitable portion of a partial denture (e.g. a rest), so that at least part of the arm lies in an undercut zone on a natural tooth (Fig. 13.12).

When a force arises which causes displacement of the denture, the portion of the arm below the survey line has to flex outwards. This results in

Fig. 13.13 Anterior view of a retentive clasp arm on a lower premolar. A, Position of the arm at the survey line; B, Position of the arm with the denture in the fully fitted position; C, Extent of flexure of the arm necessary for it to pass over the survey line.

the arm applying inward pressure to the tooth, leading to the development of frictional resistance between the arm and the tooth which hinders further displacement. The retaining force will progressively increase as displacement occurs, up to the point where the arm leaves the undercut zone (Fig. 13.13).

Classification of clasp arms

Clasp arms can be divided into two main classes:

1. Those which approach the undercut from the occlusal (or incisal) surface of a tooth. These are termed occlusally-approaching or supra-bulge clasps (Fig. 13.12).

2. Those which approach the undercut from the gingival aspect of a tooth. These are termed gingivally-approaching or infra-bulge clasps (Fig. 13.14)

Sub-classification of clasps is usually based on the development of a link between the form of the survey line on a tooth and the correspondingly appropriate form of clasp. There are two such systems which are commonly used, the Ney system and the Blatterfein system.

Fig. 13.12 Lateral view of a clasp unit on a lower molar. A, Rest; B, Attachment tag; C, Survey line; D, Retentive portion of clasp arm positioned in undercut.

Fig. 13.14 A gingivally-approaching or infra-bulge clasp arm

Fig. 13.15 Ney Class I survey line and clasp. A, Rest; B, Clasp arm.

Fig. 13.17 A Ney Class III survey line and clasp. A, Rest; B, Clasp arm.

The Ney system. Three basic survey lines are described, along with an appropriate clasp form for each one.

The Class I survey line runs diagonally across the tooth surface, its situation relative to the intended rest position being shown in Figure 13.15.

For this survey line, the use of a cast occlusally-approaching arm is suggested, the terminal third of the arm entering the undercut.

The Class II survey line also runs diagonally across the tooth surface, but as a mirror image of the Class I line. Here, the use of a gingivally-approaching clasp arm is suggested (Fig. 13.16).

Fig. 13.18 Survey lines on a tilted premolar. The survey line is low on side A and high on side B

Fig. 13.16 Ney Class II survey line and clasp. A, Rest; B, Clasp arm.

The Class III survey line is parallel to the occlusal surface and lies just below it. For this survey line, the use of a wrought, occlusally-approaching arm is suggested, with the terminal two-thirds of the arm entering the undercut (Fig. 13.17).

Variants of the Ney Class I type of clasp are also described, these being termed back-action, reverse back-action and ring clasps. Back-action and reverse back-action clasps are described for use on premolar and anterior abutment teeth, especially in association with a free-end saddle. They are indicated where the tooth concerned is tilted such

that a high survey line is present on one side of the tooth and a low survey line on the other side (Fig. 13.18). The survey line on side A is too low to allow placement of a retentive clasp arm on that surface without encroaching on the gingival margin. The survey line on side B is too high to allow engagement of the undercut by a short arm placed only on that surface.

Such a condition can best be met by using an arm that extends around three surfaces of the tooth (e.g. lingual, distal and buccal), the attachment to the denture arising from the end of the arm. Where the attachment is placed lingually, the unit is referred to as a back-action clasp (Fig. 13.19). Where, alternatively, the attachment is

Fig. 13.19 Ney back-action clasp. A, Retentive portion of the clasp arm; B, Lingual attachment of the clasp arm.

Fig. 13.20 Ney reverse back-action clasp. A, Retentive portion of the clasp arm; B, Buccal attachment of the clasp arm.

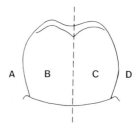

Fig. 13.22 Reference zones used in the Blatterfein system. A, Saddle; B, Near zone; C, Far zone; D, Contiguous tooth.

placed buccally, the unit is referred to as a reverse back-action clasp (Fig. 13.20).

The third variant of the Ney Class I clasp, the ring clasp, is described for use on upper or lower molars which are standing alone, no saddle being required posterior to the tooth. Like the back-action and reverse back-action clasps it is used where the survey line is high on one side of the tooth (normally buccally for an upper molar and lingually for a lower molar) and is low on the other side.

It has two occlusal rests, embraces three surfaces of the tooth and is attached to the denture at the mesial rest. An optional strengthening element may be added, joining the mesial and distal rests on the side of the tooth having the low survey line (Fig. 13.21).

The Blatterfein system. In the Blatterfein system four types of survey lines are described, along with an indication of suitable clasps for use with each type.

The position of each type of survey line is described in relation to two zones, developed by bisecting the tooth along its long axis. The half of

Fig. 13.23 Blatterfein typical or medium survey line. A, Rest.

the tooth adjacent to the saddle is termed the near zone and that adjacent to the contiguous tooth is termed the far zone (Figure 13.22). The four types of survey lines which are described are as follows:

1. The Typical or Medium Survey Line. This extends from the mid-point between the occlusal surface and the gingival margin in the near zone, to a point two-thirds of the distance from the occlusal surface to the gingival margin in the far zone (Fig. 13.23).

Clasps suggested for use where such a survey line is present include occlusally-approaching and gingivally-approaching arms of the Ney Class I and Class II types.

2. The Atypical A or Diagonal Survey Line. This runs diagonally across the tooth surface from a high position in the near zone to a low position in the far zone (Fig. 13.24).

If it is desired to use a cast occlusally-approaching arm where such a survey line is

Fig. 13.21 Ney ring clasp. A, Retentive portion of the clasp arm; B, Optional strengthening element; C, Saddle.

Fig. 13.24 Blatterfein atypical A or diagonal survey line. A, Rest.

Fig. 13.25 Recurved form of cast occlusally-approaching clasp arm used in association with a Blatterfein diagonal survey line. A, Rest.

Fig. 13.26 Blatterfein atypical B or high survey line. A, Rest.

present, the arm needs to be of a recurved form to enable the undercut to be engaged at a suitable level (Fig. 13.25).

Gingivally-approaching arms may also be used.

3. Atypical B or High Survey Line. This line is parallel to the occlusal surface and lies close to it (Fig. 13.26). Wrought, occlusally-approaching arms of the Ney Class III type may be used where this survey line is present. Alternatively, if accompanied by a low survey line on the opposite side of the tooth, clasps of the Ney back-action, reverse back-action or ring type can be used as appropriate.

4. Atypical C or Low Survey Line. Here, the survey line is parallel with the occlusal surface, but lies just above the level of the gingival margin (Fig. 13.27).

This type of survey line contraindicates the placement of a retentive clasp arm on the tooth surface concerned, as the arm would need to be

Fig. 13.28 Developing direct retention by the use of a gingivally-approaching clasp arm and a Class V gold inlay. A, Rest.

placed too close to the gingival margin for safe application. Where all the usable surfaces of a tooth present survey lines of this type, it is necessary to seek alternative means of obtaining retention. These methods include:

1. Placement of a crown on the tooth to artificially develop undercuts.

2. Placement of a Class V gold inlay. A dimple is cut in the inlay and a ball head on a gingivally-approaching arm positioned to engage the dimple (Fig. 13.28).

3. An extended arm clasp may be used where the contiguous tooth offers favourable conditions for retention (Fig. 13.29).

4. Undercut may be developed by adjusting the contour of the tooth by grinding. Caution is essential in applying this procedure as if the enamel cap of the tooth is penetrated a considerable increase in caries risk will arise. A simpler alternative method of developing undercut is to change the contour of the tooth by positive addition to its surface. This can be achieved using acid etch composites, a procedure which is currently under evaluation. Initial results have been promising, although the life expectancy of the additions is still in doubt.

Fig. 13.27 Blatterfein atypical C or low survey line. A, Rest.

Fig. 13.29 Developing direct retention by the use of an extended arm clasp engaging undercut on the contiguous tooth. A, Rest.

The functions and design features of clasp units

To achieve optimal efficiency, a clasp unit must be designed to take account of its intended function or functions. These are as follows:

Support. In all cases where a clasp arm is to be placed on a tooth, some form of rest should be placed on the tooth to locate correctly the clasp arm in its designated position.

Retention. As previously noted, retention is obtained by the placement of a flexible element of a clasp arm into undercut. This must be done in such a manner that three criteria will be satisfied:

1. Sufficient undercut must be engaged to ensure that the required degree of retention is obtained.

2. The force which arises when the clasp arm flexes during insertion and withdrawal of the denture must be within the level of tolerance of the periodontal attachment of the clasped tooth, otherwise damage to the attachment will occur.

3. The force which arises when the clasp arm flexes during insertion and withdrawal of the denture must also be less than that which would cause permanent deformation of the arm to occur.

Satisfying these criteria requires the engagement of an undercut appropriate to the length, cross-section, form and material of construction of the arm. Measurement of undercuts should always be made by use of appropriate undercut gauges in the cast surveyor. As an approximate guide only, cast occlusally-approaching clasps in cobalt-chromium alloy should engage only 0.25 mm undercut. Cast occlusally-approaching clasps in gold alloy may engage 0.50 mm undercut, as may wrought occlusally-approaching clasps in stainless steel or cast gingivally-approaching clasps in cobalt-chromium alloy. Wrought occlusally-approaching clasps in gold alloy may engage 0.75 mm undercut if of adequate length (on a molar, for example) and this undercut may also be engaged by gingivally-approaching clasps in gold alloy.

Bracing. Bracing is the provision of resistance to lateral displacement of the denture and is a function performed jointly by the rest and by the clasp arms in a clasp unit. All clasp arms will provide some degree of bracing. For an occlusally-approaching arm, bracing will be at a maximum at the rigid portion close to the origin and will de-

crease along the arm to the free end. The bracing provided by a gingivally-approaching clasp arm will normally be much less than that of an occlusally-approaching clasp arm since only the flexible terminal portion of the former lies on the tooth. The required level of bracing in a clasp unit may be achieved by the action of the rest plus that arising from one or more arms placed for retention, where these are of the occlusally-approaching type. Where a gingivally-approaching clasp arm is being used for retention, it is usually necessary to place an occlusally-approaching arm on another surface of the tooth to achieve an adequate level of bracing in the unit. Such an arm will lie above the survey line.

Both bracing and retention should be opposed across the arch to obtain optimal value –– where retention or bracing is obtained on the buccal surface of the teeth on one side of the arch, it must also be obtained on the buccal surface of the teeth on the other side of the arch. Alternatively, lingual or palatal retention or bracing on one side should be accompanied by lingual or palatal retention or bracing on the other side.

Reciprocation. In all cases where a retentive clasp arm is positioned on one surface of a tooth, then some suitable element must be provided on the opposite surface to act as a reciprocating balance. This is necessary since if the flexible retentive arm was accidentally bent by the patient (e.g. when cleaning the denture) the arm could apply a constant force to the tooth when the denture was in position. Such a force could give rise to tooth movement or damage the periodontal attachment of the tooth, and these are not intended functions of a partial denture. The provision of a reciprocating element provides opposition to the potential displacing force and avoids the risk of tooth movement or other damage occurring.

Reciprocation may be provided by another retentive clasp arm or by a bracing arm. In the case of anterior teeth, a rest may be used and for both anterior and posterior teeth where a connector lies on a tooth surface it may also function as a reciprocator.

Biological acceptability. It is important that the clasp unit be designed on biologically sound principles if it is to function satisfactorily. As previously noted, it must avoid excessive force application to the tooth by ensuring that form and undercut engagement are correctly linked. It must cover the minimum tooth substance compatible with other requirements, so as to reduce the risk of food stagnation to a minimum. The arm should be kept free of the gingival margin of the tooth by at least 2 mm to minimise the risk of it causing gingival trauma. In all cases where an arm needs to cross the gingival margin (in the gingivally-approaching type) the arm should be relieved from direct contact with the gingival tissues.

Attachment to denture. Adequate attachment must be provided between the clasp unit and the rest of the denture. This is normally achieved by means of a tag, which is either firmly embedded in the polymeric area of a saddle or is attached by soldering, welding, or unit cast construction to a metal framework, where one is being used.

Mechanical acceptability. The dimensions of the elements making up a clasp unit must be adequate to achieve a structure which will be resistant to permanent deformation and fracture. Only materials possessing adequate mechanical properties should be used and their handling should be such that optimal properties will be achieved. This will include the application of appropriate heat-treatment procedures where gold alloys are used. Where fabrication is by casting, porosity must be avoided. Where fabrication is by wrought work, care should be taken not to leave plier marks or other imperfections on the metal work as these can act as stress-concentrators and increase the risk of fracture occurring.

Precision attachments

Introduction

Precision attachments consist of two units, one being attached to an abutment tooth, the other being attached to the denture saddle. When the two units are fitted together they provide direct retention by means of a combination of friction and spring action.

Relative to the use of clasp units as tooth-bearing direct retainers, precision attachments may be said to offer certain advantages:

1. They can provide excellent transfer of vertical and horizontal loads from the denture saddles to the abutment teeth on which they are placed.

2. Good aesthetics are obtainable, with no clasp arms being visible, for instance.

3. They may be more hygienic, with minimal external components present to trap food and accumulate plaque.

4. They are generally well tolerated by patients, as their form normally avoids irritation of the tongue, lips or cheeks.

5. Unlike the position with clasp units, use is not dictated by the presence or absence of undercuts on a tooth.

Disadvantages which may arise from the use of precision attachments include the following:

1. Their application is usually much more time-consuming in both the clinical and laboratory areas. In addition, the intrinsic cost of many of the attachments is high. Thus their use may need to be limited by economic considerations.

2. Placement of an attachment on an abutment tooth may necessitate the removal of a considerable amount of sound tooth substance.

3. Special problems can arise where a precision attachment is to be used to provide retention of a free-end saddle. If an attachment is used which provides a rigid link between the saddle and the abutment tooth, then destructive overload of the periodontal attachment of the abutment tooth can occur. Instead, it is usually recommended that an attachment of a more complex (and hence expensive) type should be used which provides some form of flexible link between the saddle and the abutment tooth, as well as providing direct retention. Attachments of this type are referred to as stress-broken attachments. Doubt has been expressed about their ability to maintain their initial flexibility over a long period of wear.

Classification and form

A primary classification of precision attachments may be made on the basis of the site of attachment to the abutment tooth:

Class 1 — Coronal attachments

Class 2 — Root-face attachments

For Class 1, sub-classification may be made on the basis of the site at which retention is achieved:

Class 1A — Extra-coronal attachments

Class 1B — Intra-coronal attachments

Fig. 13.30 The Roach ball extra-coronal attachment. A, Sleeve set in the saddle; B, Rod set in an inlay; C, Plan view of the attachment.

For Class 2, sub-classification may be made on the form of the attachment:

Class 2A — Stud type

Class 2B — Bar type

It is usual for precision attachments to be purchased in a pre-fabricated form. A wide range of attachments is available within each of the above classes. In this text it is only possible to provide examples of the attachments in each class. A more detailed consideration will be found in specialist texts.

Class 1A — Extra-coronal attachments. Here, the retentive element lies external to the crown of the abutment tooth. An example is provided by the Roach ball attachment (Fig. 13.30).

A rod, arising from an inlay set in the abutment tooth, carries a ball at its free end. A sleeve is set into the associated end of the saddle. As the denture is inserted the sleeve slides over the ball and develops frictional grip retention.

Class 1B — Intra-coronal attachments. These are generally much more complicated in form than the extra-coronal attachments. The female unit of the attachment is set within an abutment inlay or crown and presents a dovetailed slot. The male unit presents a correspondingly-shaped projection and is attached to the denture saddle. When the two units slide into each other they provide frictional grip retention, which may be augmented in some types by a spring action. An attachment of this type is illustrated in Figure 2.8C.

A large restoration, such as a three-quarter crown, is required to provide adequate retention of the restoration carrying the female unit. When, as is usual, a number of such units are to be used for denture retention, they need to be accurately paralleled by use of a surveyor technique at the stage of placement within the wax patterns of the abutment retainers.

Class 2A — Stud type attachments. As a preliminary to the use of such attachments, root treatment of the abutment tooth is carried out and the crown is cut off near to the level of the gingival margin. They are particularly indicated for use where the periodontal status of the root is adequate but the condition of the crown is judged to be unsuitable to allow placement of a coronal attachment. A cast metal post and diaphragm are prepared for the root, the diaphragm offering retention for the base unit of the stud, either via use of soldering or by screw attachment.

As an example of the form of a stud attachment, the Dalbo is illustrated in Figure 2.8A. The male unit is attached to the root face diaphragm and carries a ball-shaped head. The female unit is placed within the denture saddle and has a hemispherical cavity to provide frictional fit on the ball head of the male unit. Vertical slits in the female unit allow a degree of flexibility and provide grip action as the two units are fitted together.

Class 2B — Bar type attachments. As in the use of attachments of the Class 2A type, abutment teeth are root filled and the crowns removed near to gingival level. Posts and diaphragms are again prepared.

The attachment takes the form of a bar which extends between and is attached to each of two di-

Fig. 13.31 Dolder bar attachment. A, Bar unit A; B, Bar unit B; C, Plan view of bar unit A attached to diaphragms on $\overline{3|3}$.

aphragms. An example of an attachment of this type is provided by a Dolder bar. This is most commonly used to link the root faces of two lower canines, as illustrated in Figure 13.31.

Unit A bar is pear-shaped in section, 3 mm deep and 2.2 mm wide. It is fitted so that its base lies just in contact with the oral mucosa between the diaphragms to which it is attached. Unit B is carried within the denture saddle. It clips into position over Unit A, the side pieces extending below the points of maximum convexity of Unit A, so gaining retention.

Sectional dentures utilising hinged flanges

Retention is here obtained by using a combination of lingual (or palatal) and labial connectors, the latter being positioned to engage tissue undercuts. If such a combination of connectors was employed in single-unit denture construction, undercuts would prevent seating of the denture. By joining the labial connector to the denture by means of a hinge at one end, and by using a clasp fastener at the other end, the labial connector can be hinged outwards to allow seating of the rest of the denture and can then be closed. Such a system is utilised in 'Swinglock' dentures, an example being illustrated in Figure 13.32.

The labial connector may be made in the form of a metal bar, or may be made in acrylic resin (at least in part) and be brought as a veneer around the gingival margins of standing teeth. Such a

Fig. 13.32 Denture of the 'Swinglock' type, showing the labial connector in the open position. A, Clasp fastener; B, Hinge.

veneer is sometimes said to serve as a periodontal splint. It also provides replacement for gingival tissues where these have been lost by gingival recession or periodontal surgery.

It is important that the denture be properly supported by use of rests, otherwise damage to the tissues covered by the labial connector is liable to occur when the denture receives functional loading. The maintenance of scrupulous oral hygiene by the patient is also essential if tissue damage is to be avoided.

Sectional dentures utilising two-part construction

Here, retention is obtained by designing the denture in two parts, each part having a different path of insertion. When fitted together in the oral cavity and united by means of a locking device, the two parts confer mutual retention on each other.

The principle can be applied to produce small dentures whose extent is limited to a single bounded saddle and the associated abutment teeth. As an example of its use, a case involving replacement of $\lceil$56 will be considered.

If a single unit denture is to be designed to provide replacement of these teeth, it will necessitate interproximal undercuts being blocked out to develop a path of insertion.

Safety factors will also indicate a need for the denture to be extended to the other side of the arch, possibly involving teeth in the design remote from the replacement area.

As an alternative, a two-part denture can be constructed. Each part has a separate path of insertion, enabling it to engage fully the undercut on the proximal surface of the adjacent abutment tooth. A bracing spur extends from the main body of each part to contact the remote surface of the distant abutment tooth (Fig. 13.33 B & C).

Fixation of the two parts is usually achieved by the use of a bolt. The sleeve of the bolt runs through the plastic work attached to one part and the shank engages a hole prepared in the other part. The relationship of the parts to the bolt is shown in plan view in Figure 13.33 A.

The bolt shank can be turned through 90° and may then be withdrawn from the retaining hole.

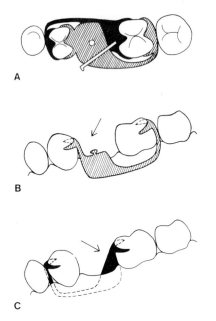

Fig. 13.33 Two-part denture providing replacement of ⌐56. A, Plan view of the assembled denture showing the bolt action; B and C, Component parts of the denture. The arrows indicate the path of insertion of each part.

The two parts of the denture can then be removed for cleaning. In the fitted position, the handle of the shank is positioned to be flat along the surface of the acrylic flange.

INDIRECT RETAINERS

Indirect retainers are those elements of a partial denture which provide resistance to the rotation of the denture about fulcrum axes. Such axes will be present in all instances where rests have been included in the design to produce a tooth or tooth-and-mucosa-supported type of denture. Theoretical aspects of indirect retention in relation to partial denture design are considered in Chapter 14, page 120. Here, consideration will be limited to the form and position of the various types of indirect retainers that are used. They can be divided into two groups according to positioning:

Group A — those indirect retainers that are positioned on the standing teeth and which may be used in either the upper or lower jaw. They include:

1. Rests
2. Tooth-bearing direct retainers
3. Continuous clasps
4. Cummer arms
5. Tooth-bearing connectors

Group B — those indirect retainers that are positioned on mucous membrane. These should only be used in the upper jaw. They include:

1. Palatal arms.
2. Palatal-bearing connectors.

Rests

The various types of rests (occlusal, cingulum and incisal) may all function as indirect retainers when placed on the opposite side of the fulcrum axis to that on which the displacing saddle is situated. Their form is considered in detail on pages 92–94.

An example of their application is seen in the design of a partial denture for a Kennedy Class IV upper dentition, as shown in Figure 13.34.

During the mastication of sticky foods, there will be a tendency for the saddle to move away from the underlying tissues, the denture rotating about an axis joining the rests placed for saddle support. This tendency for rotation can be resisted by placing occlusal rests bilaterally on the posterior aspects of the last standing teeth. The posterior rests are joined to the saddle by means of antero-posteriorly directed bars lying on the palate.

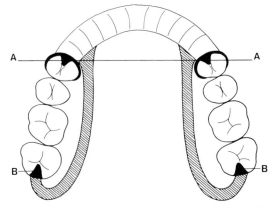

Fig. 13.34 Indirect retention for a Kennedy Class IV dentition achieved by posterior placement of occlusal rests. AA, Axis of rotation developed by the rests supporting the anterior saddle; B, Posteriorly placed occlusal rest.

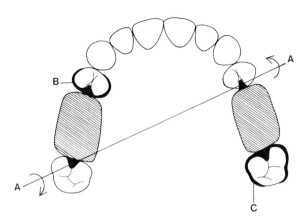

Fig. 13.35 Indirect retention for a Kennedy Class III dentition achieved by tooth-bearing direct retainers. AA, Axis of rotation; B, Clasp unit on 4|; C, Clasp unit on |7.

Tooth-bearing direct retainers

Clasp units (see page 96) and precision attachments (see page 101) may also function as indirect retainers. To perform this function they are placed on the same side of the fulcrum axis as that on which the displacing saddle is situated.

This can be seen in the design of a partial denture for a Kennedy Class III, Modification 1 dentition replacing 65|56 (Fig. 13.35). Consider the potential axis of rotation passing through 7|4. During the chewing of sticky foods, the posterior end of the saddle carrying |56 may tend to rise away from the supporting tissues, the denture rotating in a counter-clockwise direction about the axis. This can be resisted by the placement of a direct retainer (for example, a clasp unit) on |7. Similarly, a clasp unit placed on 4| will resist a clockwise rotation about the same axis which tends to occur where the anterior end of the saddle carrying 65| is subject to a displacing force, pulling it away from the underlying tissues. The indirect retainer action obtained in this way by the placement of tooth-bearing direct retainers should be regarded as an auxiliary feature to their main function of providing direct retention. Where a need arises in partial denture design for elements to be placed specifically to act as indirect retainers — mainly encountered in the design of partial dentures for Kennedy Class I and Class IV dentitions — it is rare for tooth-bearing direct retainers to be used.

Fig. 13.36 A continuous clasp positioned on 321|123

The continuous clasp

Often referred to as the Beech or Kennedy continuous clasp, this consists of a continuous band of metal positioned on or above the survey lines of the lingual or palatal aspects of the anterior dentition (Fig. 13.36).

The ends of the clasp may join a major connector (for example, a lingual bar, as illustrated in Figure 13.36) or may extend posteriorly to terminate in the denture saddles. It is often chosen to provide indirect retention in the Kennedy Class I situation. Here, the need often arises for an element to be placed forward of the axis of rotation to provide resistance to rotatory displacement of the free-end saddles. A continuous clasp can perform this function with maximum mechanical advantage since it extends anteriorly to the limit permitted by the arch form. Also, since it acts on the whole anterior dentition rather than on a single tooth, the risk of it producing tooth movement is minimised.

In addition to acting as an indirect retainer, a continuous clasp can provide other functions:

1. It transfers part of the vertical and horizontal loads borne by the saddle on to the covered anterior dentition. It thus lessens the load applied to the abutment teeth, with corresponding reduction in the risk of the abutment teeth sustaining periodontal damage.

2. It can act as an auxiliary connector of saddles, assisting the major connector, for example a lingual bar, in performing this function. This may allow the cross-sectional area of the major connector to be reduced, so aiding its tolerance by the environmental tissues.

3. Where splinting of anterior teeth is required, a continuous clasp can serve as a useful point for the origin of embrasure hooks.

Despite its functional advantages, the continuous clasp also presents a number of possible

Fig. 13.37 Shaping a continuous clasp to aid acceptance by the tongue. A, Preferred form; B, Deprecated form.

disadvantages which must be taken into consideration before a decision is made to include it in the design of a partial denture. These are as follows:

1. It may give rise to problems of tolerance. Usually, this is associated with tongue irritation, but speech problems may also occur. Acceptance by the tongue will be aided by the use of a deep and relatively thin form in preference to the use of a shallower and thicker form (Fig. 13.37). Upper and lower margins of the clasp should blend in to the tooth form and not present a ledge to the tongue.

2. The occlusal relationship of the anterior teeth (deep overbite combined with shallow overjet) may be such as to provide inadequate space for placement.

3. Where the anterior teeth are lingually or palatally inclined, there may be insufficient room above the survey lines to allow placement of a continuous clasp.

4. Placement may be difficult where the teeth only present short clinical crowns.

5. Aesthetic problems arise if the teeth are spaced. However, where a single diastema is present, this problem can be overcome by division of the continuous clasp (Fig. 13.38).

6. When long, there is a risk that a continuous clasp will be distorted by the patient during the cleaning of the denture.

Fig. 13.38 Division of a continuous clasp to avoid the display of metal through a diastema.

Cummer arms

The Cummer arm consists of a metal bar extending anteriorly from a suitable component of the denture (usually a saddle or connector) to termin-

Fig. 13.39 Indirect retention for a Kennedy Class I dentition achieved by the use of Cummer arms on 3|3.

ate on the unprepared palatal or lingual surface of an anterior tooth. They are used bilaterally. The only teeth really suitable for their placement are periodontally sound upper canines, although they are occasionally used on lower canines. If used on other anterior teeth they are very liable to cause tooth movement.

Like the continuous clasp, they may be chosen for use as specific indirect retainers in the design of partial dentures for Kennedy Class I dentitions. An example of their application is shown in Figure 13.39.

They are less effective than the continuous clasp as an indirect retainer since they are positioned closer to the axis of rotation. They share with the continuous clasp the disadvantage of liability to distortion during cleaning of the denture. Their use is only indicated where long free-end saddles are present and a continuous clasp cannot be used because of the existence of a close incisor relationship.

Tooth-bearing connectors

Two of the tooth-bearing connectors which are used in the design of lower partial dentures offer the advantage of providing auxiliary indirect retention where this is required. They are:
1. The lingual plate
2. The modified continuous clasp.

The form and positioning of these connectors is considered on page 112.

Their auxiliary indirect retainer action can be

utilised with benefit when designing lower partial dentures for the Kennedy Class I dentition. They will share the effectiveness of indirect retainer action of the continuous clasp since like that clasp they extend as far anterior of the axis of rotation as the arch form permits.

Palatal arms

The palatal arm consists of an extension from a saddle or palatal connector, usually made in metal, which extends anteriorly forward of the fulcrum axis to lie on the anterior part of the hard palate. They may be used unilaterally or bilaterally to provide indirect retention for free-end saddles. An example of their use is shown in Figure 13.40. As

Fig. 13.40 Indirect retention for a Kennedy Class I dentition achieved by the use of palatal arms.

the arms extend on to the rugae they often give rise to irritation of the tongue and may also interfere with phonetics.

Palatal-bearing connectors

Certain of the palatal-bearing connectors used in the design of upper partial dentures can provide the auxiliary function of indirect retention. These are:

1. The anterior palatal bar. This can be used to provide indirect retention where free-end saddles are present.

2. The posterior palatal bar. This can be used to provide indirect retention where a single anterior saddle is present (Kennedy Class IV dentition).

The form and positioning of palatal bars is considered on page 108.

The palatal plate connector can also be used to provide indirect retention by extending it to lie either anterior to the axis of rotation (for free-end saddles) or posterior to the axis of rotation (for a single anterior saddle) see Figure 13.41.

CONNECTORS

Connectors are those elements of a partial denture which are used to unite other components to form a unit appliance.

Fig. 13.41 Indirect retention achieved by the use of palatal plate extensions. A shows extension of the palatal plate anterior to the axis of rotation for a Kennedy Class I dentition. B shows extension of the palatal plate posterior to the axis of rotation for a Kennedy Class IV dentition.

They are classified as minor or major connectors according to their length or area of tissue covered. Minor connectors are considered in Chapter 14, page 124. In this section, consideration will be limited to major connectors whose main role is that of joining saddles. They are always designed to be rigid in nature.

They can be divided into two main groups on the basis of the jaw in which they are to be used and then subdivided on the basis of their form and positioning:

Group A — Major connectors used in a maxillary denture:
1. Posterior palatal bar
2. Middle palatal bar
3. Anterior palatal bar
4. Palatal plate

Group B — Major connectors used in a mandibular denture:
1. Lingual bar
2. Lingual plate
3. Labial or buccal bar
4. Modified continuous clasp

The posterior palatal bar

This bar lies on the posterior part of the hard palate. It arises from saddles or direct retainer units on each side of the arch and extends posteriorly in a smooth curve to terminate at the vibrating line. An example is shown in Figure 13.42.

The antero-posterior dimension of the bar will depend upon the number of teeth being replaced

Fig. 13.42 A posterior palatal bar used to connect saddles replacing 6|6.

by the denture and on the physical properties of the alloy used for constructing the bar, the aim being always to achieve rigid connection. It will rarely exceed 1 cm.

Anterior and posterior margins of the bar should be thinned down to taper into the palate, without developing cutting edges. This will help to avoid irritation of the tongue. The posterior margin, which lies at the vibrating line, should be developed to provide a post-dam as utilised in complete dentures. Other margins of the bar should be provided with a minor dam line, approximately 0.5 mm deep, to aid peripheral seal and reduce the risk of food passing to the fitting surface aspect of the bar.

The posterior palatal bar has the merit of being positioned in an area of the palate where tongue activity is at a minimum. For that reason it is usually well tolerated by patients. Tolerance will also be aided by use of a thickness not exceeding 1 mm. Increased rigidity, where necessary, should be gained by increasing antero-posterior dimension rather than by increasing thickness.

Despite the merit of tolerance provided by the position of a posterior palatal bar, the latter feature can also lead to a problem. This arises from the fact that the bar is positioned on a relatively compressible tissue base. When load is applied to the saddles of the partial denture it may be found that antero-posterior rocking of the appliance occurs as a consequence of depression of the posterior palatal bar into the underlying tissues. This movement of the bar will be increased if the bar is not a perfect fit on the tissues in its original fitted position. Such lack of fit may occur as a consequence of casting shrinkage and will be accentuated if the bar is long.

Since the posterior palatal bar terminates at the vibrating line, its position enables it to function as an indirect retainer, resisting rotation of the denture originating from anterior saddles. Its effectiveness in performing this function must, however, be questioned in view of the displaceable nature of the palatal tissues on which it is placed.

The posterior palatal bar may also serve as a means of transferring part of the vertical and horizontal load borne by the denture to the palatal tissues. It may thus be said to have auxiliary supporting and bracing functions. Again, these will be limited in value by the displaceable nature of the covered tissues.

The middle palatal bar

This bar lies on the central portion of the hard palate. The anterior border lies just posterior to the commencement of the rugae on the hard palate. Its path across the palate between saddles or direct retainer units on each side of the arch is more direct than that of a posterior palatal bar. The antero-posterior dimension of the middle palatal bar is usually a little greater than that of a posterior palatal bar. Its form is illustrated in Figure 13.43.

As with the posterior palatal bar, anterior and posterior borders of the middle palatal bar should be thinned to blend in with the palatal tissues. Its situation does not allow the development of a full post-dam and a minor dam line, approximately 0.5 mm deep, is provided along both the anterior and posterior margins to aid the development of peripheral seal.

Its more direct course across the palate relative to that of a posterior palatal bar results in less liability for casting shrinkage and hence a better fit is seen in most instances. Also, the palatal tissues underlying the middle palatal bar are usually of a less displaceable character than those under a posterior palatal bar. The problem of antero-posterior rock in function that arises in a posterior palatal bar is thus rarely encountered with a middle palatal bar. The nature of the foundation tissues also

Fig. 13.43 A middle palatal bar used to connect saddles replacing 54|45.

enables the middle palatal bar to perform effectively auxiliary supporting and bracing functions. Its more anterior placement in the palate does, though, result in it being a less effective indirect retainer for anterior saddles than the posterior palatal bar, and it is also more likely to give rise to tongue irritation. Despite this, the middle palatal bar is generally well tolerated.

The anterior palatal bar

This bar lies in the anterior, rugal area of the hard palate. In crossing the palate to link saddles or direct retainer units, it should be positioned in the valleys between rugal elevations as far as possible. This is necessary since it lies in an area of high tongue activity, and if placed upon rugal elevations it may give rise to tongue irritation and phonetic disruption. The need to position it between rugal elevations often necessitates it following a more tortuous path across the palate than that seen with middle or posterior palatal bars. The bar should be as shallow as mechanical considerations will permit.

It is rarely used as a sole connector, normally being used in association with a posterior palatal bar. In view of the problems which may arise from its placement in an area of high tongue activity, it should only be used where special indications apply, which include the following:

1. Where it is needed to develop a connector system of adequate rigidity. Where only one or two short saddles are present and cobalt-chromium alloy is to be used in fabrication of the connector, a posterior palatal bar used alone will often provide adequate rigidity. Where long saddles, or a greater number of saddles than two is present, the use of an extra connector may be required to achieve adequate rigidity. The 'ring' form of connection developed by using a combination of anterior and posterior palatal bars results in a considerable increase in the rigidity of the structure, relative to that obtainable from a single connector. Such a double connector system will nearly always prove to be necessary where gold alloy is used in construction of the connectors.

2. Where it is needed to act as an indirect retainer for posterior saddles. This need may arise where the occlusal relationship of the anterior

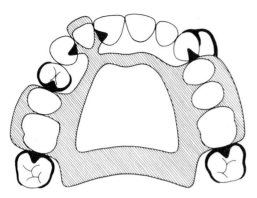

Fig. 13.44 Anterior and posterior palatal bars used to form a 'ring' connector system for a denture replacing 652|456.

teeth prevents use of a continuous clasp or Cummer arms.

3. Where it is needed to provide a convenient point of attachment for an anterior saddle, as illustrated in Figure 13.44.

The palatal plate

Although no strict dividing line exists between the terms 'bar' and 'plate' as applied to palatal connectors, the term plate is usually reserved for those cases where the connector covers an appreciable area of the hard palate. Often, the area of coverage would be similar to that which would occur in a hypothetical design involving simultaneous use of all three palatal bar connectors.

The use of a palatal plate is illustrated in Figure 13.45.

Fig. 13.45 A palatal plate connector used in a mucosa-supported denture replacing 6 1|1 6.

Relative to the use of bar connectors, the plate connector has the biological disadvantage of covering a greater area of the hard palate. Where the palatal tissues are covered, they lack the natural stimulus provided by the tongue and salivary flow, with risk of the development of an adverse tissue reaction. Against this must be weighed the advantages arising from increased palatal coverage:

1. An increased proportion of the vertical and horizontal loads which are applied to the denture can be borne by the palate. Where tooth or tooth-and-mucosa-supported designs are being used, such load transfer to the palate can reduce the risk of overloading of the abutment teeth occurring. It also introduces the posibility of using totally mucosa-supported designs in the maxillary denture.

2. It may be possible to achieve adequate rigidity in the connector system using a polymeric denture base material. In distinction, palatal bars are always made in metal. Use of a polymeric denture base material for construction of the connector offers advantages in terms of weight, colour and cost.

Wherever possible, a palatal plate should extend posteriorly to the vibrating line and a post-dam should be developed. Along other palatal margins a shallow dam should be developed, approximately 0.5 mm deep, to aid the development of peripheral seal. The health of the palatal gingival tissues will benefit from the use of designs which avoid coverage of the gingival tissues, as seen in the 'Every' or 'spoon' designs. Comfort will be aided by making the plate as thin as is compatible with achieving the required rigidity. This favours the use of a metal in the construction of a palatal plate connector.

The lingual bar

The lingual bar connects saddles or retainer units on each side of the lower arch, being positioned in close proximity to the lingual alveolar tissues. The bar is usually oval in cross-section, approximately 3 mm deep and 1.5 mm thick, although occasionally a bar of a half pear-shaped section is used.

The bar should be positioned so that its upper border is at least 2 mm below the gingival margins of the standing teeth and its lower border is not

Fig. 13.46 Sagittal section in the lower incisor region illustrating the form and position of a lingual bar. A and B should be equal to or exceed 2 mm.

Fig. 13.47 Sagittal section in the lower incisor region illustrating the necessary position of a lingual bar when the incisors are retroclined.

less than 2 mm above the floor of the mouth, as illustrated in Figure 13.46.

Where a lingual bar is to be used, a space of a least 7 mm must thus be present between the gingival margins of the standing teeth and the floor of the mouth. Where the available space is less than 7 mm, the use of a lingual bar is contraindicated and an alternative type of connector must be selected. Where the available space exceeds 7 mm, it is advisable for the bar to be placed as low as possible as this lessens the risk of the bar causing irritation to the tongue.

A lingual bar may be wrought using stainless steel or gold alloy or may be cast in cobalt-chromium alloy or gold alloy. The bar should be relieved from contact with the under-lying tissues by a small gap. This allows for minor movements of the bar to occur during the functioning of the denture without causing trauma to the underlying tissues. Except for the provision of this relief the bar should be positioned to follow closely the contours of the lingual alveolus. There should be no unplanned space between the upper portion of the bar and the alveolar tissues, as a space here would permit food packing. Similarly, there must be no unplanned space between the lower portion of the bar and the alveolar tissues, or the tip of the tongue may enter this space and be irritated. Tongue thrusting into a lower space could also cause displacement of the denture.

One contra-indication to the use of a lingual bar has already been noted, that of lack of the necessary space between the gingival margins of the standing teeth and the floor of the mouth. Another arises where retroclination of the lower dentition is present. Like all rigid connectors, a lingual bar must not enter an undercut. Retroclination of the anterior dentition would necessitate the bar being

placed away from the alveolar tissues to achieve a free path of insertion (Fig. 13.47) and a lingual bar in this position would almost certainly cause tongue irritation.

Likewise, a grossly undercut lingual alveolus contraindicates use of a lingual bar.

On biological grounds, the lingual bar can be considered to be the most satisfactory of the available types of lower connectors. It avoids contact with the standing teeth and their gingival tissues and when correctly positioned should not give rise to tissue trauma. It does, however, have one major disadvantage and this is a liability of causing irritation to the tongue. Patients have likened their experience when wearing a denture bearing a lingual bar to that of a horse with a bit in its mouth!

In an attempt to lessen tongue irritation, proposals have been made that a sub-lingual positioning should be adopted for the bar. In this case it is usual to use a bar of the half pear-shaped form, the larger element of the bar being positioned at the base and under the tongue, as illustrated in Figure 13.48. Care must be taken to ensure that the base of the bar is kept above the functional level of the floor of the mouth, otherwise severe irritation of the tissues could arise.

Fig. 13.48 Sagittal section in the lower incisor region illustrating the form and position of a sub-lingual bar.

Fig. 13.49 Sagittal section in the lower incisor region illustrating the form and position of a lingual plate.

The lingual plate

The lingual plate joins saddles or direct retainer units on each side of the lower arch, being positioned in contact with both the lingual surfaces of the anterior teeth and the lingual aspect of the alveolar processes (Fig. 13.49). In the region where it crosses the gingival margins of the standing teeth, it should be relieved from direct contact with the tissues by, for example, the placement of foil on the master cast.

The upper border of the plate must be above the survey lines and should extend to a level approximately 2 mm below the incisal edges of the standing teeth, except where full coverage is required for the development of incisal rests or embrasure hooks. The lower margin of the plate should leave a gap of at least 2 mm above the functional level of the floor of the mouth.

Although biologically less satisfactory than a lingual bar since it covers the gingivae, the lingual plate is usually well-tolerated by patients. It is particularly indicated for use in those cases where inadequate space exists to permit placement of a lingual bar. The lingual plate also offers another advantage relative to a lingual bar in that the increased dimension of the plate in a vertical direction enables polymeric materials such as acrylic resin to be used in its construction. In distinction, the lingual bar is always made in metal. An economic advantage can so arise, although it should be noted that a metal plate will be more rigid and usually evokes less adverse reaction in the covered soft tissues. With the exception of the relieved gingival margin area, it is essential that a lingual plate should be a close fit on the covered tissues. Otherwise, problems related to food packing may arise.

As with the lingual bar, use of a lingual plate is contraindicated where the anterior teeth are retroclined or a grossly undercut lingual alveolar process is present.

The labial or buccal bar

This connector is normally only chosen for use where a lingual connector is contraindicated due to retroclination of the dentition.

In form, fitting and construction, it is similar to a lingual bar except for being placed external to the arch. It is spaced from the gingival margins of the standing teeth and the base of the labial sulcus in a similar manner to a lingual bar (Fig. 13.50).

Fig. 13.50 Sagittal section in the lower incisor region illustrating the form and position of a labial bar.

As the labial bar lies external to the arch it lies on an arc of greater radius than its lingual counterpart. To achieve the required rigidity, increase in cross-section is necessary relative to that of a lingual bar. This is usually achieved by increase in bar depth rather than thickness. Care must be taken in its placement to avoid contact with the labial and buccal frenae. It should also be provided with slightly more relief from contact with the underlying tissues than is necessary for a lingual bar. Increased relief is especially necessary over the canine eminences.

The labial bar often gives rise to aesthetic problems. It may also cause irritation to the lips and cheeks. On that basis its use is usually reserved for those cases where no alternative is possible.

The modified continuous clasp

This connector is similar in form to the continuous clasp (see page 105) but its dimensions, especially its thickness, are increased to develop a level of rigidity enabling it to act as sole connector be-

Fig. 13.51 Sagittal section in the lower incisor region illustrating the form and position of a modified continuous clasp.

tween saddles or direct retainer units on each side of the arch (Fig. 13.51). Relative to the lingual plate, it has the merit of avoiding coverage of the gingival margins. It can, though, only be used where the teeth have long clinical crowns, as this allows the necessary rigidity to be achieved without undue increase in thickness. Achieving the necessary rigidity will also be aided by the use of an alloy of high modulus of elasticity, such as cobalt-chromium alloy, in its construction.

Of the three lingually-positioned lower connectors, the modified continuous clasp is used much less frequently than the lingual bar or the lingual plate because of the rarity of cases presenting with the necessary length of clinical crowns. One special indication for its use arises where gingival surgery has been carried out, creating the required length of clinical crowns. Often, in such cases, inadequate room remains to permit placement of a lingual bar and coverage of the gingival tissues with a lingual plate may be considered to be undesirable.

STRESS-BREAKERS

Stress-breakers are those elements of partial dentures which are interposed in a connector system in order to introduce a controlled and intentional degree of flexibility into the structure. Their most common application arises in the design of dentures carrying free-end saddles, where they are used to vary the rigidity of the connection between the saddle and the retainer unit. The principles concerning their application for this purpose are considered in Chapter 21.

Stress-breakers can be classified according to their mode of action:

Type 1 — Those utilising a hinge or moveable joint.

Type 2 — Those utilising flexible connection.

Type 1 Stress-breakers

These can be used in association with either precision attachments or clasp units as tooth-bearing direct retainers.

An example of their use with precision attachments is seen in the Crismani combined unit (Fig. 13.52). The alternative use of a Type 1 stress-breaker in conjunction with the use of a clasp unit for the provision of direct retention can be exemplified by the Wipla Unit, shown in exploded view in Figure 13.53.

Fig. 13.52 The Crismani combined unit. A, Dovetailed element providing intra-coronal attachment to an abutment tooth; B, Spring-controlled hinged element attached to a free-end saddle; C, Movement about the hinge.

Fig. 13.53 The Wipla hinge unit. A, Back plate attached to the tag of the clasp unit; B, Axis of rotation of the unit in the direction indicated by the arrow; C, Free ends of arms attached to the metalwork of the free-end saddle.

Type 2 Stress-breakers

These are normally used in association with clasp units as direct retainers. Various forms are possible of which the following are commonly applied:

1. Torsion bars

These may be used in the design of a lower partial denture carrying bi-lateral free-end saddles. Bars extend anteriorly from the clasp units on each side to join a lingual bar near the mid line (Fig. 13.54).

Flexibility can be controlled by varying the cross-section of the torsion bars, the method of construction (cast or wrought) and the material of construction (normally gold alloys or cobalt-chromium alloys).

Disadvantages are associated with the use of the torsion bar structure in that the double bar system is liable to trap food and cause irritation to the tongue.

Fig. 13.54 Torsion bar stress-breaker used in a lower partial denture replacing $\overline{65|56}$.

2. Partial division of connectors

The principle can be applied in both upper and lower dentures. For example, in a lower denture, a lingual plate may be partly divided by an antero-posterior slot. The upper portion of the plate is attached to the retainer unit on the abutment tooth and the lower portion is attached to the saddle (Fig. 13.55). A degree of flexibility between the retainer unit and the saddle is so developed.

Fig. 13.55 A lower partial denture framework with partial division of a lingual plate to achieve stress-breaking.

3. Mesial placement of occlusal rests

This offers the simplest available approach to stress-breaking. The degree of stress-breaking achieved is, though, much less than that available where more complex devices are employed. It may be used in the design of either upper or lower dentures.

By positioning the rest of the clasp unit on the mesial instead of on the distal fossa of the abutment tooth and by using a minor connector to link the rest to a major connector (for example, a lingual bar) some flexibility may be introduced into the clasp unit/saddle link (Fig. 13.56).

Fig. 13.56 A lower partial denture with mesial placement of occlusal rests to aid stress-breaking.

FURTHER READING

Basker R M and Tryde G 1977 Connectors for mandibular partial dentures: use of the sublingual bar. J Oral Rehab 4: 389

Bates J F 1963 Cast clasps for partial dentures. Int Dent J 13: 610

Bates J F 1975 Removable Partial Denture Construction. 2nd Edn. Wright, Bristol

Blatterfein L 1951 A study of partial denture clasping. J Amer Dent Assoc 43: 169

Craddock F W 1946 Labial bar partial dentures. N Z Dent J 42: 67

Dolder E J 1961 The bar joint mandibular denture. J Prosthet Dent 11: 689

Every R G 1949 The elimination of destructive forces in replacing teeth with partial dentures. N Z Dent J 45: 207

Henderson D 1973 Major connectors for mandibular removable partial dentures. J Prosthet Dent 30: 532

Lee J H 1963 Sectional partial dentures incorporating an internal locking bolt. J Prosthet Dent 13: 1067

Osborne J and Lammie G A 1974 Partial Dentures. 4th Edn. Blackwell Scientific Publications, Oxford

Planned Partials 1951 The J M Ney Company. Hartford, Connecticut

Preiskel H W 1979 Precision Attachments in Dentistry. 3rd Edn. Henry Kimpton, London

Quinn D M 1981 Artificial undercuts for partial denture clasps. Brit Dent J 151: 192

Schuyler C H 1953 Analysis of the use and relative value of the precision attachment and the clasp in partial denture planning. J Prosthet Dent 3: 711

Stileman R D W 1951 Spoon dentures. Brit Dent J 91: 294

Walter, J D 1980 Partial denture technique.
Brit Dent J:

Part 3. Supporting the denture	148 : 13.
Part 5. Connectors.	148 : 133.
Part 6. Resistance to displacement.	148 : 189.
Part 7. Sectional dentures.	148 : 257.

14

Designing partial dentures

INTRODUCTION

Before the designing of a partial denture is commenced, it is essential that all the necessary information should be available. Details of the required information are to be found in Chapter 5. Included is a full knowledge of the clinical condition of the patient. On that basis it is essential that partial denture designing should be undertaken by the dental surgeon responsible for the patient's care. It is both unwise and unfair for partial denture designing to be delegated to a dental technician who will not be in possession of the necessary clinical findings.

Caution must also be sounded concerning the design procedure which is adopted. All too often this has involved scanning through the pages of a text book until an example of design is found where the missing teeth coincide with those in the case under consideration. A request is then made to the technician to produce a denture of similar design. Such a procedure is dangerous since it cannot take into consideration the ruling clinical conditions of the case and may result in irreparable tissue damage.

The only approach which is acceptable is that of designing from first principles. This involves going through a series of stages in a step-by-step manner. If the order and nature of these stages is understood, even the beginner should experience no difficulty in producing successful partial denture designs.

DESIGN STAGES

There are five stages involved in partial denture design:

1. Classify and outline the saddles.
2. Provide support.
3. Provide direct retention.
4. Provide, where necessary, indirect retention.
5. Unite the various components of the denture with connectors.

Classify and outline the saddles

Note should be made of the number of saddles which are present, their length and their disposition in the arch. Each saddle should first be classified as being either bounded or free-end. A second stage in the classification of each saddle is then to decide on the way that the load borne by the saddle is to be transferred to the available supporting tissues. This secondary classification of the saddles is very important since it will influence procedures in a number of the subsequent stages of design and will also play a major part in deciding the success of the denture.

With bounded saddles, the choice lies between:
1. Tooth support.
2. Mucosa support.
3. Combined tooth-and-mucosa support.

With free-end saddles, the choice is limited to:
1. Mucosa support.
2. Combined tooth-and-mucosa support.

The factors taken into consideration when deciding the secondary classification of saddles are:

1. An estimate of the response to loading of the available supporting tissues.

2. The jaw for which the denture is to be provided (i.e. maxilla or mandible).

3. The length of the saddles.

4. The number of saddles to be carried by the denture.

Factor 1

Information on the likely response to loading of the abutment teeth and of the mucosa and underlying bone in the saddle areas will be available from visual, tactile and radiographic examination of the oral tissues. Where the abutment teeth are periodontally sound, a bounded saddle may be tooth-supported. This is preferred where possible since it develops optimal masticatory efficiency.

The second alternative, that of making a bounded saddle mucosa-supported, should be considered where the periodontal condition of the abutment teeth is suspect and where it is judged that the tissues underlying the saddle would respond favourably to load-bearing. The latter requirement would be met by:

1. The presence under the saddle of a healthy mucosa of normal and even thickness.

2. The alveolar bone in the saddle area possessing a dense cortical plate overlying well-developed trabeculae in the cancellous bone.

3. The absence of a history of rapid alveolar bone resorption in the saddle area.

The third alternative of choosing a combination of tooth-and-mucosa support for a bounded saddle is to be deprecated. It introduces the problem of providing equitable distribution of loading between the two supporting tissues and is rarely necessary in the bounded saddle situation.

When deciding on the secondary classification of free-end saddles, it should be noted that ideally they should be mucosa-supported. This avoids the risk of overloading of the abutment tooth and uneven loading of the soft and hard tissues in the saddle area which tooth-and-mucosa support may cause. The ideal situation may, though, only be attainable by the introduction of undue complexity into the design. In such cases the compromise approach of using combined tooth-and-mucosa support may be selected. This should only be considered if the periodontal condition of the abutment tooth is satisfactory.

Factor 2

In the mandibular denture, it is desirable that bounded saddles be made tooth-supported. This is necessitated by the very limited area of mucosa which is available in the mandible to provide support. If bounded saddles in the mandible are made mucosa-supported, they are liable to be traumatic to the underlying tissues. Where the abutment teeth of a mandibular bounded saddle are judged to be unable to carry the load that will be transferred to them by the saddle, it may be necessary to extract one or more of the teeth until tooth support becomes feasible.

In the maxilla, different conditions prevail, since here the hard palate provides a sizeable area of mucosa which can be used to help support the denture. Hence either tooth support or mucosa support is acceptable for bounded saddles in the maxilla.

Factor 3

Where long bounded saddles are present on a maxillary denture, they are often better made mucosa-supported to avoid the risk of overloading of the abutment teeth.

Factor 4

The presence of multiple bounded saddles in a maxillary denture often indicates the desirability for them to be made mucosa-supported to avoid over-complexity in denture design.

On completion of the classification of the saddles they should then be outlined. In the case of saddles of the mucosa-supported or tooth-and-mucosa-supported classes, the outline developed should be that which will provide coverage of the maximum possible area of mucosa. Labially, buccally and lingually, flanges should be extended to lie at the base of the sulcus defined by a functionally moulded impression. This ensures that the load applied to each unit area of covered mucosa will be of minimal value. The risk of evoking a pathological response in the covered tissues is thereby reduced.

With tooth-supported saddles, the need for maximal mucosal coverage to spread the applied load over the mucosa does not apply. Here, saddle outline is dictated by aesthetic needs. The extension developed is that necessary to provide restoration of alveolar form and will be proportional to the degree of alveolar resorption that has occurred in the area.

In the case of all classes of saddle, the outline decided by application of the above considerations may need to be modified by two further criteria:

1. Aesthetics

Aesthetic considerations may necessitate the use of an open-face structure in the anterior maxillary area of a denture, even where other factors indicate the use of a labial flange.

2. Undercuts

Note must be made of the presence and extent of undercuts in areas where flange extensions of saddles are to be positioned. The flange outline developed must allow free insertion and withdrawal of the denture.

Provide support

To be successful, a partial denture must be satisfactory at the time of insertion and must maintain that condition throughout its normal period of life expectancy. Providing proper allowance for support during the designing of a partial denture is essential if this requirement is to be met. Within a year or two of the insertion of a partial denture, it is usual to find that some degree of alveolar resorption has occured under the saddles. Unless proper provision has been made for support this may allow the fitting position of the saddles to change. When this occurs, the artificial teeth carried by the saddles may lose contact with the opposing dentition, so impairing masticatory efficiency. A further serious consequence of a change in the position of the saddles is that it may be accompanied by a change in position of other denture components (eg, connectors or clasp arms). Because of this, these other components may become traumatic to the soft and hard tissues which they contact. Improperly supported dentures which give rise to this phenomenon have rightly been termed 'gum strippers'. To avoid the risk of such consequences occurring, the following procedures should be applied:

Provision of support for bounded saddles

Where bounded saddles are to be mucosa-supported, the whole denture — including the saddles — should cover the maximum possible area of mucosa compatible with other requirements. It should be remembered that it is normally only in the maxilla (via use of the hard palate) that sufficient area of mucosa will be available to allow bounded saddles to be made mucosa-supported without risk of undue trauma to the mucosa arising.

Where tooth support of bounded saddles is required, this is achieved by the placement of a rest on each of the abutment teeth. To ensure that the load borne by the saddle will be transferred fully to the abutment teeth, the rests must provide a rigid attachment between the saddle and the teeth. This requirement is met by placing each rest on the portion of the abutment tooth immediately adjacent to the saddle, as illustrated in Figure 14.1.

The form and positioning of the various types of rests that may be used to achieve tooth support on both anterior and posterior teeth are considered in Chapter 13. By their correct use, tooth support of the saddles of a partial denture can be achieved where this is desired.

Additional support for the denture may arise from components other than the rests. For example, this will occur where connectors are placed on the hard palate or on the anterior teeth. Used

Fig. 14.1 Tooth support in the bounded saddle of a mandibular partial denture replacing $\overline{67}$ achieved by placing occlusal rests on the disto-occlusal fossa of $\overline{5}$ and the mesio-occlusal fossa of $\overline{8}$.

alone, such auxiliary supportive devices will not ensure that the saddles are tooth-supported. They should be regarded as an addition to, and not a substitute for, the use of rests to achieve tooth support in the saddles.

Provision of support for free-end saddles

Irrespective of whether the saddle is to be made mucosa-supported, or tooth-and-mucosa-supported, it must cover the maximum possible area of mucosa. In the case of a maxillary denture, buccal flanges should extend to the full depth of the sulci, the tuberosities should be fully covered and the posterior extension lie in the pterygo-maxillary fissures. With a mandibular denture, buccal and lingual flanges should extend to the full depth of the sulci, with emphasis on achieving full engagement of the postero-lingual areas. Posteriorly, the saddles should extend over at least the anterior one-third of the retro-molar pads.

With a saddle which is to be tooth-and-mucosa-supported, there is an additional requirement for a rest to be placed on the single abutment tooth. It is usually desirable that this rest should be placed on the mesial aspect of the abutment tooth. This applies unless the design includes the use of a stress-breaker interposed between the rest and the saddle. In that case the placement of the rest on the distal aspect of the abutment tooth is permissable.

Further information on the rationale for rest placement and on the types of stress-breakers that may be used in this situation appear in Chapter 13. Reference should also be made to Chapter 21 which deals with the specific problems presented by partial dentures which carry free-end saddles.

Provide direct retention

Direct retention is one of the means by which a partial denture is provided with resistance to displacement. When a patient who is wearing a partial denture chews foods, especially those of a sticky consistency, forces arise which tend to cause a bodily translation of the denture away from the supportive tissues. Forces giving rise to translation may also be developed by the action of the oral and facial musculature during activities such as speech and laughter.

If translatory displacement occurs, it can clearly be a source of embarrassment to the patient. In addition, the repetitive unseating and reseating of the denture which occurs can cause trauma to both the soft and hard tissues contacted by the denture.

The function of direct retention is to develop forces which oppose those tending to cause translatory displacement. Where the sum of the retentive forces equals or exceeds that of the displacing forces, translation of the denture will be inhibited. The development of direct retention to the level where this is achieved is an essential feature of partial denture design. The methods available for achieving direct retention are as follows:

1. Utilisation of the forces responsible for achieving retention in complete dentures.

2. Frictional resistance to displacement arising from the development of tight contacts between the artificial teeth and the natural abutment teeth.

3. Placement of direct retainers on the abutment teeth.

It should be noted that in a given denture it is sometimes possible to achieve adequate direct retention by the use of only one of these methods. Most dentures, though, will require the use of a combination of two or more of the available methods.

Method 1 of providing direct retention

Included here are:

1. Use of the physical forces arising from the presence of a saliva film between the denture and the underlying soft tissues.

2. The engagement of undercuts in the tissues underlying the saddles.

3. Shaping of the denture so that the environmental musculature will provide a positive retentive force.

4. The force of gravity in a mandibular denture.

The level to which these forces can be developed in a partial denture is often quite low relative to that achievable in a complete denture. This applies particularly to the development of the physical forces which will be limited by the decreased area of tissue coverage in a partial denture and by the presence of the natural teeth which interfere with the development of a full peripheral seal. Thus, in only a very limited number of cases will this method, used alone, provide adequate retention in a partial denture. It may be considered in the case of a maxillary denture which carries only mucosa-supported free-end saddles. In the case of all partial dentures, though, this method will contribute to the overall retention which is achieved.

Method 2 of providing direct retention

This method can assist the development of direct retention where the partial denture carries one or more bounded saddles. Maintenance of the force will be assisted by the use of porcelain artificial teeth in preference to the use of acrylic teeth, since this will reduce the degree of wear which occurs at the contact points.

Methods 1 and 2 used in combination will provide adequate retention for many maxillary partial dentures which carry only mucosa-supported saddles. Success will be aided by the presence of multiple bounded saddles.

Method 3 of providing direct retention

The direct retainers which are used may take the form of either pre-formed (precision) attachments or clasp units. The various types which can be used are considered in Chapter 13.

Their use will prove to be necessary in nearly all instances where a partial denture carries tooth-supported or tooth-and-mucosa-supported saddles. As previously noted, this will apply to nearly all mandibular dentures and to a proportion of maxillary dentures.

When considering the placement of tooth-borne direct retainers, it should be borne in mind that each saddle needs to be provided with adequate direct retention. That requirement can best be met by placing a direct retainer on each abutment tooth and this is done wherever possible. Certain conditions may be encountered, though, where departure from that principle is indicated. These are as follows:

1. Where the abutment tooth concerned is a central or lateral incisor, the placement of a clasp unit on the tooth as a direct retainer would gen-

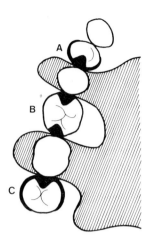

Fig. 14.2 An example of a case in which adequate retention for two short saddles may be obtained by placing direct retainers on only the terminal abutment teeth (A and C). Abutment tooth B carries rests to aid the development of tooth support in both saddles but carries no direct retainer.

erally prove to be unacceptable on aesthetic grounds.

2. Where it would involve the placement of a clasp unit as a direct retainer on an abutment tooth which possesses no usable undercuts. In that case an adjacent tooth may offer more favourable conditions for placement of the clasp unit.

3. Where it would involve the introduction of unnecessary complexity into the design of the partial denture, with associated increased risk of causing caries or periodontal breakdown of the abutment tooth. This arises where two short tooth-supported saddles are separated by a single abutment tooth (Fig. 14.2).

In all instances an attempt should be made to keep the distance between a saddle and its direct retainers to a minimum. This is necessary since the principles of the action of levers shows that the more remote a retainer is placed relative to the saddle the less effective will it be in providing retention for that saddle.

Provide, where necessary, indirect retention

Indirect retainers are used to assist direct retainers in resisting displacement of partial dentures in function. As noted above (page 119), when a patient who is wearing a partial denture chews sticky foodstuffs, forces arise which tend to cause the saddles to be displaced away from the underlying

Fig. 14.3 Plan view of a mandibular partial denture carrying saddles replacing 7̄6̄|6̄7̄. Clasp units have been placed on 5̄|5̄ and a lingual bar used as the major connector. Rotation of the denture may occur about axis AA in the directions indicated by the arrows.

tissues. Direct retention is provided to prevent this translatory displacement. Where the denture has been provided with rests to develop the necessary support in the second stage of design it will, however, be found that a second method of displacement is possible. This is by rotation of the denture about one or more axes developed by the supporting rests in the manner of a see-saw. The portion of the denture which lies on the saddle side of the axis will move away from the supporting tissues. At the same time, the portion of the denture which lies on the opposite side of the axis to that of the saddle will be depressed tissuewards. This situation is depicted in Figure 14.3, which presents a plan view of a mandibular partial denture being provided for a dentition of the Kennedy Class I type.

In the opening movement of the masticatory cycle, a force may arise which will cause the saddles to move away from the underlying tissues. The denture may then rotate about an axis passing through the rests on 5̄|5̄ and the portion of the lingual bar which lies anterior to this axis will correspondingly be depressed tissuewards.

If such rotatory displacement is able to occur it will clearly be a source of embarrassment to the patient. In addition, it may well give rise to severe tissue trauma. It is to prevent such rotation that indirect retainers are used.

The procedures involved in this stage of partial denture design are as follows:

Procedure 1

Examine the cast and note the elements already provided in the preceding design stages. Where rests have been provided in Stage 2 of design, potential axes of rotation will exist which may be defined as follows:

1. A line joining any two rests which have been provided for support of the denture.
2. Where a tooth-and-mucosa-supported free-end saddle is present, a line passing along the crest of the ridge underlying the saddle and passing through the rest on the abutment tooth.

The number and disposition of the potential axes of rotation must be noted. Examples of the application of this procedure are shown in Figures 14.4 and 14.5. The direction in which rotation can occur about a potential axis of rotation should also be noted (i.e. clockwise or counter-clockwise). Where more than one saddle is present on a partial denture the combined action of the saddles can lead to two-way rotation being possible about a given axis of rotation. For example, if reference is made to the diagonal axis passing through 4| and |7 in Fig. 14.4, it will be seen that where forces arise which tend to cause the anterior end of the saddle carrying |56 to move away from the underlying tissues, the denture will rotate in a counter-clockwise direction about this axis. If, instead,

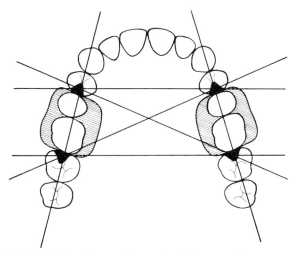

Fig. 14.4 The six potential axes of rotation present in a maxillary partial denture with two tooth-supported bounded saddles replacing 65|56. Occlusal rests have been placed on 74|47.

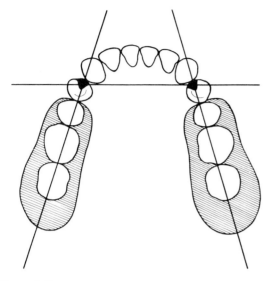

Fig. 14.5 The three potential axes of rotation present in a mandibular partial denture with two tooth-and-mucosa supported free-end saddles replacing 765|567. Occlusal rests have been placed on 4|4.

forces arise which tend to cause the posterior end of the saddle carrying 65| to move away from the underlying tissues, the denture will now rotate in a clockwise direction about the axis.

Procedure 2

Examine the disposition of rests provided in Stage 2 of design and of any tooth-borne direct retainers provided in Stage 3 of design, in relation to the axes of rotation.

Decide whether or not these elements will provide resistance to rotation about all the existing axes. In reaching that decision it should be noted that resistance to rotation can be provided by:

1. A rest placed on the opposite side of the axis of rotation to that on which the displacing saddle is situated. For example, in Figure 14.4, clockwise rotation of the denture about the axis passing through 4| and |7 will be resisted by the rest placed on |4. Likewise, anti-clockwise rotation about that axis is resisted by the rest on 7|.

2. A tooth-bearing direct retainer placed on the same side of the axis of rotation as that on which the displacing saddle is situated. Referring again to the axis passing through 4| and |7 shown in Figure 14.4, a direct retainer on 7| will resist clock-

wise rotation and a direct retainer on |4 will resist anti-clockwise rotation about the axis.

When Procedure 2 is applied to dentures which are being designed for dentitions of the Kennedy Class II and Class III types it is usual to find that the elements already provided render the denture resistant to rotation about any potential axes of rotation. In that case no further action is necessary in Stage 4 of design.

With dentitions of the Kennedy Class I or IV types, though, application of Procedure 2 will usually demonstrate the existence of one or more axes where resistance to rotation will not be provided by the elements already placed. As an example of this finding, consider a dentition of the Kennedy Class I type as depicted in Figure 14.6.

When the three axes are examined in turn it will be found that the elements already present provide resistance to rotation about each of the antero-posterior axes. This does not apply, though, to the lateral axis passing through the rests on 4|4. Clockwise rotation of the denture about this axis is possible. The direct retainers on 4|4 will resist the tendency for rotation to some extent, but may be unable to prevent it fully because of their proximity to the axis of rotation.

In all such cases where residual potential axes of

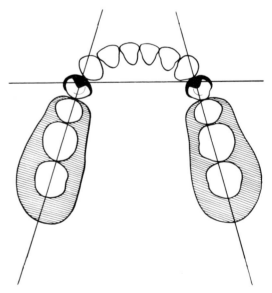

Fig. 14.6 Potential axes of rotation in a mandibular partial denture with two tooth-and-mucosa supported free-end saddles replacing 765|567. Clasp units to provide support and direct retention have been placed on 4|4.

rotation are found to be present, the provision of indirect retainers is necessary to provide resistance to rotation about these axes. This is effected in Procedure 3.

Procedure 3

Where a need for the addition of indirect retainers has been demonstrated in Procedure 2, a decision must now be made on:
1. The type or types to be used.
2. Where they should be placed.

Decision 1. As previously noted, resistance to rotation about potential axes may be achieved by the use of either tooth-borne direct retainers or rests. Where the former are to be used they are conventional in form. Where indirect retention is to be achieved by rests then this action can be obtained by placement of conventional rests of the occlusal, cingulum or incisal type. Alternatively, certain other elements can be used to achieve the necessary resting action. For example, certain types of connectors when positioned on the hard palate will serve as indirect retainers of the rest type. The necessary resting effect can also be obtained by the use of elements designed specifically to act as indirect retainers, e.g. continuous clasps or the Cummer arm. These find application particularly where placement on the anterior teeth is required.

Reference should be made to Chapter 13 for details of the form and positioning of the various types.

Decision 2. In all instances, indirect retainers should be positioned the maximum possible distance from the potential axis of rotation. This will ensure by lever action that they obtain maximal mechanical advantage. In the case of a maxillary denture, indirect retainers may be placed on either the hard palate or the teeth. With a mandibular denture, only tooth-bearing indirect retainers should be used.

When dealing with a potential axis of rotation developed by the placement of two rests, the best position for placement of an indirect retainer may be found as follows: Determine the mid point of the axis between the two rests. From that point draw a line at right angles to the axis until the line intersects the dentition. The point of intersection

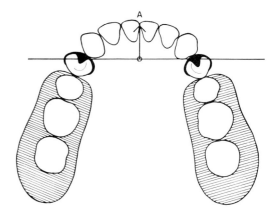

Fig. 14.7 Optimum position for the placement of an indirect retainer in the denture illustrated in Figure 14.6 is indicated by the arrow at point A.

represents the best position for placement of an indirect retainer.

If this procedure is applied to the case previously illustrated in Fig. 14.6, it will be found that the point of intersection lies in the vicinity of $\overline{1|1}$ (Fig. 14.7).

Where this procedure is applied to dentitions of the Kennedy Class IV types, it may be found that the line drawn from the mid point of the axis will fail to interest the dentition. In such a case the indication is for the placement of bilateral indirect retainers, situated as posteriorly as possible (Fig. 14.8.).

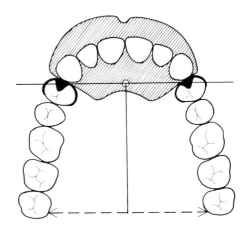

Fig. 14.8 Optimum positions for the placement of indirect retainers in a maxillary partial denture replacing $\underline{321|123}$ are indicated by the arrows. Clasp units to provide support and direct retention have been placed on $\underline{4|4}$.

Unite the various components of the denture with connectors

At the conclusion of the fourth stage of partial denture design, the placement of a series of isolated components will have been planned. In all cases the saddle areas will have been outlined. In some cases rests will have been placed on teeth to provide support for the denture along with the possible placement of direct and indirect retainers. The final stage in denture design involves the placement of connectors to unite these isolated components into a single entity.

Connectors are classified as being either major or minor according to their length or the area of tissue which they cover. Major connectors include those used to join saddles and they are always rigid in nature. Minor connectors have an auxiliary connecting role, as where a support/retention unit on a tooth needs to be joined to a major connector (Fig. 14.9). They are also usually made to be rigid, but occasionally an intentional degree of flexibility is introduced into their structure by the inclusion of a stress-breaker. The form and function of stress-breakers is considered in Chapters 13 and 21. In the present chapter, further consideration will be limited to rigid connectors. The normal requirement that connectors should be rigid stems from the need for a partial denture to be able to function as a single unit. When forces are applied to any part of the denture it is usually deemed desirable that the denture should be able to transfer the forces to all the soft and hard tissues which it contacts. That aim can best be achieved by the use of rigid connectors.

The various types of major connectors which can be used to join saddles are considered in Chapter 13. The choice lies between four connectors which can be used in a maxillary denture and four which can be used in a mandibular denture:

Maxillary connectors
1. Anterior palatal bar
2. Middle palatal bar
3. Posterior palatal bar
4. Palatal plate

Mandibular connectors
1. Lingual bar
2. Lingual plate
3. Labial or buccal bar
4. Modified continuous clasp

It should be noted that in some cases the use of two or more of the available range of connectors may be desirable in a single denture.

The factors that should be taken into consideration when selecting the appropriate connector or connectors to use in a denture are as follows:

1. The patient's history of partial denture wearing (if any).
2. Biological features related to the area of tissue which will be covered by the connector.
3. The material of construction which is to be used.
4. Whether the denture is to be provided for the maxilla or for the mandible.

Fig. 14.9 An example of the use of a minor connector. A clasp unit on $\overline{5}$ is being joined to a major connector (lingual bar) in a mandibular partial denture.

Factor 1

Where the history reveals that a particular form of connector has been successful both in terms of patient tolerance and tissue reaction, it is usually desirable for the same form of connector to be used in the replacement denture. Where the converse is true, change to an alternative form of connector should be considered.

Factor 2

The use of a bar type of connector relative to the use of a plate will normally result in an appreciable decrease in the area of tissue covered by the connector. Since tissue coverage is always accompanied by the risk of evoking a pathological response in the area concerned, reducing area of coverage can be beneficial to tissue health. In the case of a maxillary denture, reduced coverage of the palate may also reduce impairment of the patient's taste sensation. These features favour the choice of a bar connector where possible. Against this must be weighed the fact that plate connectors, by virtue of their greater tissue coverage, offer superior support to the denture than that achievable by the use of bar connectors. The auxiliary support offered by plate connectors may be an essential feature of some denture designs, as where all the saddles in a maxillary denture are to be made mucosa-supported.

Factor 3

Choice of the material of construction is closely linked to that of the type of connector to be used. To achieve the necessary rigidity in a bar type of connector, it must be made in metal. It may be cast in a gold alloy or cobalt-chromium alloy or be fabricated by wrought work using a gold alloy or stainless steel. Plate connectors can also be made in metal, but here, because of the greater area of coverage, it may also be possible to achieve the necessary rigidity by use of a plastic such as acrylic resin. The use of a plastic in place of a metal for the construction of a plate connector offers a clear economic advantage. In addition, it will decrease the weight of the denture and thus favour retention in the case of a maxillary denture.

In terms of the preservation of tissue health, however, the use of metal for the construction of plates is to be preferred. Tissues which are covered by a metal plate usually maintain a healthier state with less pathological reaction than that seen where a plastic plate is used. In part, this may be due to a different response by the tissues to the chemical nature of the overlying materials. The much greater value for the coefficient of thermal conductivity of metals relative to that of plastics may also play a part in the observed difference. Yet another factor which may help to explain the difference in tissue response is the comparative rigidity of the two structures. The modulus of elasticity of cobalt-chromium alloy, for example, is approximately sixty times that of acrylic resin.

Even a thin lingual plate constructed in cobalt-chromium alloy will be more rigid than the thickest tolerable form of acrylic lingual plate. During the normal functioning of the denture far less flexing of a metal plate will occur than is the case with a plastic plate, and consequently less mechanical irritation of the tissues is likely to arise.

Where bar connectors are to be used, selection of the appropriate connector system will be influenced by the modulus of elasticity of the metal to be used in their construction. The modulus of elasticity of cobalt-chromium alloys is approximately twice that of gold alloys. As a consequence, where a maxillary denture carries only two short, laterally-positioned bounded saddles, adequate rigidity can often by achieved by the use of a posterior palatal bar as sole connector if cobalt-chromium alloy is used. Where, instead, the same denture is to be constructed in a gold alloy, the use of a combination of anterior and posterior palatal bars will usually be necessary to achieve the same rigidity.

Factor 4

The general preference for use of bar connectors rather than plate connectors wherever possible has already been noted. It applies equally to dentures being provided for the maxilla or for the mandible.

Where a plate connector is to be used in a maxillary denture, it is desirable that it should be constructed on the principles advocated by Every. Important amongst these principles is that of developing a self-cleansing gap of approximately 4 mm between the palatal plate and the palatal aspects of the gingival margins of the standing teeth. This helps towards the maintenance of the health of the periodontal tissues of the teeth. Alternative designs which involve colleting of the palatal plate around the standing teeth carry a greater risk of producing an inflammatory reaction in the gingival tissues.

A simplified version of the 'Every' palatal plate connector is seen in the 'spoon' form. This can be used where a maxillary partial denture is being constructed for a Kennedy Class IV dentition and not more than two adjacent teeth are to be replaced. As a 'spoon' connector avoids contact with any of the standing teeth it has biological merit, but it suffers the disadvantage of achieving only limited retention and stability. The development of an acceptable level of retention will be favoured by the presence of a 'U' shaped palate relative to that of a 'V' shaped palate. It is more successful in children and adolescents than in adult patients, probably because younger patients find it easier to develop control of the denture by tongue action.

When selecting the connector to be used to join saddles in a mandibular denture, the biological superiority of the lingual bar should always be borne in mind. Against this, must be weighed the fact that it may give rise to tongue irritation in some patients. The risk of this occurring can be reduced by positioning the bar as low as possible in relation to the floor of the mouth. The adopting of a sub-lingual position for the bar may also aid its acceptance.

The lingual plate is usually well tolerated by patients, especially when made in metal and carefully contoured to simulate the form of the natural teeth which it covers. However, the lingual plate crosses the gingival margins of the teeth it covers and this always carries the risk of producing periodontal damage.

The buccal or labial bar is poorly tolerated by many patients on both aesthetic and functional grounds, and its use should be restricted to those cases where there is no alternative. This is usually due to the presence of a retroclined dentition.

The modified continuous clasp is rarely selected for use. It is indicated where the teeth upon which it is to be positioned have long clinical crowns, where the health of the gingivae of those teeth contraindicate their being covered, and yet inadequate space is available for use of a lingual bar.

FURTHER READING

Barbenel J C 1971 Design of partial denture components. J Dent Res 50: 586

Bates J F 1968 Studies in the retention of cobalt-chromium partial dentures. Brit Dent J 125: 97

Collett H A 1951 Principles of partial denture design. Dent Dig 57: 24

Dyer M R Y 1972 The 'Every' type acrylic partial denture. Dent Pract Dent Rec 22: 339

Firtell D N 1968 Effect of clasp design upon retention of removable partial dentures. J Prosthet Dent 20: 43

Kratochvil P J 1963 Influence of occlusal rest position and clasp design on movement of abutment teeth. J Prosthet Dent 13: 114

Krogh-Poulsen W 1954 Partial denture design in relation to occlusal trauma and periodontal breakdown. Int Dent J 4: 847

McCracken W L 1960 Partial Denture Construction. Mosby, St Louis

Neill D J and Walter J D 1977 Partial Denture Prosthetics. Blackwell Scientific Publications, Oxford

Osborne J and Lammie G A 1974 Partial Dentures. 4th Edn. Blackwell Scientific Publications, Oxford

Tomlin H R and Osborne J 1961 Cobalt-chromium partial dentures. Brit Dent J 110: 307

Walter J D 1979 Partial denture technique. Brit Dent J:
Part 1. Introduction 147: 241
Part 2. The purpose of the denture: choice of material 147: 302

Wilson J H 1949 Partial denture construction — some aspects of diagnosis and design. Dent J Austral 21: 347

15

The impression stage of treatment

PRIMARY IMPRESSIONS

Introduction

Primary impressions are used in the preparation of study casts which play a vital role in the planning and construction of a removable partial denture. After a record has been made of the patient's jaw relationship, the casts will be mounted on an anatomical type of articulator and the occlusion and articulation of the dentition will be examined. The casts will also be surveyed as an essential preliminary to denture design. These procedures are considered in Chapter 5, which deals with the examination of the patient.

When diagnostic uses of the study casts have been completed, they will then be utilised in the construction of special trays.

To perform the above functions satisfactorily, it is essential that study casts provide an exact copy of the oral tissues. This will only be possible if the primary impressions meet the required level of accuracy. It will, for instance, be impossible to obtain an accurate picture of the occlusal relationship of the teeth if imperfections are present on the occlusal surfaces because air inclusions were present in the impressions. Primary impression taking should thus be approached with an appreciation of the care and attention to detail which is necessary for success.

Choice of trays

Stock trays of the 'box' form are normally used to obtain primary impressions of a partially edentulous patient. The trays are available made in either metal or a polymeric material, the preference being for metal trays because of their greater rigidity.

Where a choice is available of trays with or without perforations, the former are to be preferred as the perforations aid the retention in the trays of certain impression materials, such as alginate.

Stock trays are available in a range of sizes. Selection of the size to use should be based on finding trays which provide a spacing which is as even as possible from the tissues to be recorded in the impression and which cover the required tissue area to an optimal extent. Where doubt exists as to which tray to use, it is suggested that a better result will usually be obtained by selecting a tray which is slightly oversize in preference to one which is undersize.

Preparation of trays

It is rare to find a stock tray which fully meets the size requirements noted above. This helps to explain why it is usually necessary to use a two-stage impression procedure, the construction of a special tray being interposed between the primary and secondary impression stages. Even so, every effort should be made to obtain accuracy in the primary impression stage. This aim can often be helped by modifying stock trays prior to their use. Where, as is commonly the case, a hydrocolloidal or elastomeric impression material is to be used to take the primary impression, tray modification can be made by the use of impression compound. Additions of impression compound may be made to the tray to increase peripheral extension in any area where the tray itself fails to provide the required tissue coverage. This need will often be found to arise in the upper labial sulcus region and posteriorly in both upper and lower trays.

Where long edentulous regions are to be recorded in the impression, especially where free-end saddles are involved, it is beneficial to place softened impression compound in the tray in the areas concerned. The tray is then inserted and border moulding is carried out. The compound impression is examined and any areas where compound has flowed into regions of standing teeth are trimmed back to leave only the impression of the edentulous regions. The compound should also be trimmed to remove any undercuts which have developed.

Impression compound may also be applied to any areas of the trays where an excessive spacing is seen to be present between the tray and the underlying tissues. The area where this form of modification is most commonly required is in the palatal region of an upper tray.

To avoid the risk of distortion of an impression occurring during and subsequent to the impression-taking procedure, steps must be taken to ensure that an adequate bond is developed between stock trays and the impression material which is used. This is especially important where hydrocoloidal or elastomeric impression materials are being used as such materials do not themselves bond to trays. The required bonding is achieved in two ways. Firstly, by the use of perforations in the trays which offer a mechanical lock for the impression material. Secondly, an adhesive may be applied to the tray surface before the tray is filled with the impression material. The adhesive used should be of a type specifically intended for use with the chosen impression material. Studies have shown that perforations in a tray provide an effective means of resisting the shear stresses which arise during removal of an impression, but are poor in resisting tensile stresses. The latter deficiency can be overcome by the application of an appropriate adhesive to the tray. Thus, the combined use of perforations and an adhesive is advisable to provide full security of retention of the impression material in the tray.

Choice of impression material

Impressions of the oral tissues of partially edentulous patients usually involve a need to reproduce a multitude of undercuts, particularly found in relation to the standing natural teeth. Reproduction of these undercuts will be facilitated if an impression material of the elastic type is used. Alternative impression materials of the plastic or brittle types can be used, but are rarely selected because of the difficulty in use they present in the multiple undercut situation.

Elastic impression materials can be divided into two main groups, each of which can be further subdivided:

1. Hydrocolloids
   a. Reversible — agar-agar
   b. Irreversible — alginate
2. Elastomers
   a. Polysulphides
   b. Silicones
   c. Polyethers

Some of these materials are available in a range of viscosities. For example, polysulphides are available in light, medium and heavy-bodied forms, the light form often being intended for application to the tissues by a syringe, the other forms being applied via a tray. Silicones are available in a putty form and a lower viscosity form.

Of the above materials, alginate is selected most frequently for use in primary impression taking. It is relatively cheap to purchase, easy to manipulate and if used with the application of appropriate precautions will, in most instances, produce excellent results. Alginate does, though, present two major disadvantages. Firstly, it is very liable to distort if abused, both during and subsequent to impression taking. Secondly, it shows a relatively low resistance to tearing when withdrawn from moderate to severe undercuts. Where the latter problem is encountered, improved resistance to tearing will be obtained if one of the elastomeric materials is used. Of the three types of elastomers which are available the preference is usually for the use of silicones in obtaining primary impressions.

Impression taking procedure

As alginate is commonly selected as the material to be used in primary impression taking, the procedure for using this material will be discussed in some detail. Where alternative materials are being used some modification in the procedure will be necessary, particularly in relation to the preparation of the impression material for use.

The procedure for alginate should be applied in a step-by-step manner, as summarised below:

1. Read carefully the instructions provided by the manufacturer of the brand of alginate being used. Note in particular features such as powder/water ratio and the temperature of the water to use.

2. Ensure the bowl and spatula to be used are clean and free of any extraneous matter. Place the measured amount of powder in the bowl and add the correspondingly measured amount of water. Start mixing slowly and then, when the powder particles have been wetted, mix more vigorously. Avoid a beating action which may incorporate air. Mix for the period indicated by the manufacturer (commonly of the order of 30 seconds). Some brands of alginate incorporate a coloured indicator and show by colour change of the material the point where mixing is complete.

3. Use the spatula to place the mixed alginate into the impression tray. Bare areas of the tray should be filled to the level of the margins and any areas where additions of impression compound have been applied should be covered by at least a 3 mm deep layer of alginate.

4. An optional procedure is now to apply some of the excess mix over areas of the tissue surfaces where trapping of air is liable to occur. Such areas include the occlusal surfaces of the teeth, the palate and any grossly undercut regions labially, buccally or lingually. Speed is essential where this procedure is used as oral temperature accelerates setting of the alginate and the main mass of alginate within the tray must be positioned before setting commences, or distortion of the impression is likely to occur.

5. Adopt the correct stance relative to the patient for the impression concerned (upper or lower), as described in Chapter 8. Rotate the tray into correct position over the oral tissues and apply pressure until excess material is observable all round the periphery. Apply border moulding movements of cheeks, lips and tongue as required by the impression concerned. Await the expiration of the

setting time indicated by the manufacturer. During the setting period support the upper tray in position by light pressure to counter gravity. The lower tray only requires downward pressure to resist displacement by the tongue, but support for the mandible should be provided by placement of the operator's thumbs under the lower border of the mandible in about the premolar area on each side. It is very important that there should be no change in the pressure applied to either the upper or lower tray as setting of the alginate proceeds, otherwise distortion of the impression is liable to occur. Do not attempt to remove the impression until excess material around the periphery shows setting has occurred by the development of elastic solidity. Little, if any, harm will arise by leaving the impression in situ for a minute or so after setting. In contrast, if an attempt is made to remove the impression before setting and the development of elasticity has fully occurred, distortion of the impression will be inevitable.

6. Release the impression from its seating position by the application of a rapid pull away from the tissues. This is necessary since alginate has greater elasticity when subjected to a rapid displacing force than when a slow displacing force is applied. Once the impression has been released from undercuts, rotate it carefully out of the mouth.

7. Rinse the impression in cool running water to remove saliva and mucus from its surface. Removal of mucus in particular will be aided by a preliminary rinse in an antiseptic solution having an associated detergent action, such as 'Savlon'. Use an air syringe to displace water from areas of the impression where natural teeth have been reproduced.

Examine the impression carefully for any imperfections such as the presence of air inclusions or inadequate coverage of the required tissue area. The margins of the impression, except posteriorly, should show a peripheral roll developed by border moulding.

Where any imperfections are found to be present the impression must be repeated until a satisfactory result is obtained.

Impressions should be immersed in an antiseptic solution such as 'Savlon' for the recommended period before cast production is carried out.

Preparation of study casts

As the study casts will be used to analyse the occlusion and articulation of the natural dentition and will also be surveyed, it is essential that they possess adequate surface hardness and abrasion resistance. This can best be achieved by the use of an artificial stone in their construction.

Where the primary impressions have been taken in alginate the impressions should be cast up within half an hour of being taken. Otherwise, a dimensional inaccuracy is liable to develop as a consequence of syneresis or imbibition. Impressions should be protected from change in the interval between being taken and cast up by being covered with a damp napkin.

Appropriate precautions should be taken in the casting-up process to avoid errors such as air inclusions or distortion of the impression material.

Where alginate has been used, the impression material should be removed from the study casts in not less than half an hour nor more than one hour after casting-up commenced. If removal of the impression material from the casts is attempted before the elapse of half an hour there is a considerable risk that any teeth being reproduced will fracture. Where the impression material is left in contact with the cast for more than an hour, the alginate may absorb water from the cast and lead to the development of a weak, chalky surface on it. Also, developing rigidity and forcible contraction of the alginate increases the difficulty of removing the alginate from the cast and the risk that tooth fracture will occur in this procedure.

Prescription writing

Two main requirements will arise at this stage:

Preparation of study casts

The material to be used in the casting-up of the impressions should be indicated. This will normally be an artificial stone.

Preparation of special trays

The information provided should include:
1. *Extension.* Lines should be marked on the study casts to indicate the required extension. The lines should be approximately 2 mm short of the sulcus buccally, labially and lingually, with appropriate allowance for frenae. The posterior border of an upper tray shoud be a straight line between the pterygo-maxillary fissures and the posterior border of the lower tray should extend approximately half way across the retromolar pads.

2. *Spacing.* The thickness of spacer to be used should be indicated. This will usually be two sheets of baseplate wax (approximately 3 mm) where alginate is to be used as secondary impression material. The spacer can be a little thinner than this where an elastomeric impression material is to be used.

3. *Material of construction.* It is essential that a special tray which is to be used to take a secondary impression should be rigid and resistant to warpage at oral temperatures. This can best be achieved by the use of a polymeric material such as acrylic resin. Either the self-curing or heat-curing types may be used.

4. *Perforations.* An indication should be given as to whether or not perforations are to be provided in the tray. Perforations are essential for alginate and desirable for elastomers.

SECONDARY IMPRESSIONS

Introduction

Secondary impressions are taken in order to prepare the casts on which denture construction will be carried out. This may include the construction of a cast or wrought metal framework, where dimensional accuracy is critical. It is thus essential that secondary impressions should provide an exact negative form of the oral tissues they record. The procedure followed should be based on the need to achieve this requirement.

Choice of trays

It is recommended that special trays be used to take secondary impressions in partial denture construction. The general advantages which arise from the use of trays of this type have been indicated in Chapter 8. In addition, in partial denture prosthesis, certain design features demand a knowledge of the exact position of the functional sulcus relative to the gingival margins of the standing teeth. For example, a decision on the use of a lingual bar or a lingual plate as connector for a lower partial denture will be influenced by knowledge on this point. It is only by the use of a special tray that such features can be reliably determined.

The special trays should be constructed using a material which can provide the required structural rigidity without necessitating undue bulk. The material used must also be resistant to warpage at oral temperatures and allow easy modification of peripheral form by trimming, should this prove to be necessary. As previously noted, acrylic resin in either the heat-curing or self-curing form, provides a material which adequately meets these needs.

Choice of impression material

In recording the oral tissues of a partially edentulous patient at the secondary impression stage it is usual to apply a minimum pressure impression procedure (considered in Chapter 8).

If digital pressure on the tray is kept to the minimal value necessary to ensure correct seating of the impression, the pressure applied to the tissues will be dependent on the viscosity of the impression material which is used. The materials chosen for use are normally taken from the 'elastic' range considered above (see page 128).

Of these materials, the hydrocolloids are generally of low viscosity. The heavy-bodied polysulphides offer maximum viscosity, other materials providing intermediate values.

By selection of an appropriate impression material the operator has a means of controlling the level of pressure which will be applied to the tissues in the impression-taking procedure. This choice is of particular value when dealing with dentures carrying free-end saddles and is considered further in Chapter 21. In these circumstances it may also be decided that a true pressure or mucodisplacive type of impression is indicated, which may be achieved by the use of impression composition. Special impression procedures such as

this will be further considered in a later section (see page 133).

In most instances, an 'elastic' type of impression material will be used and of the available materials alginate will be prime choice, as at the primary impression stage. An alternative material may be chosen where relatively severe undercuts are to be reproduced, to avoid the problem of tearing of alginate. Silicones are chosen most commonly to meet this need, the preference being for use of the paste type rather than the combined use of a putty form, followed by use of a low-viscosity surface layer. The latter procedure has been subjected to criticism on the basis of possible development of internal stress with consequential distortion of the impression.

Impression taking procedures

The special trays to be used are first tried in and checked for satisfaction. They should cover the entire tissue areas to be reproduced in the impressions and their margins should relate correctly to the levels of the functional sulci. If any areas of over-extension are found to be present the trays should be trimmed to the correct level. If any deficiencies of extension are noted these can be corrected by the application of green-stick impression compound in the areas concerned. Where long edentulous tissue areas are present, especially when free-ended, the application of carefully positioned wax stops to the fitting surface of the tray in a crest-of-ridge position will aid correct location of the trays.

Where, as is usual, alginate is to be used as the secondary impression material, the impression-taking procedure should follow that outlined above (page 128). Where other materials are being used the procedure followed will be similar except for the preparation for use of the material. In all cases the instructions for proportioning and mixing of the material provided by the manufacturer of the product concerned should be followed.

Cast production

Choice of the material to be used in the preparation of the working or master casts from secondary impressions is based on the constructional procedures to be used in denture construction. Where a polymeric denture base such as acrylic resin is to be used, the casts should be prepared using a prosthetic grade of artificial stone. Where, though, the denture design involves the use of a metal framework, especially where this is to be pre-pared by casting, it is advisable to use instead a die grade of artificial stone. The additional surface hardness of the latter material reduces the risk of cast damage occurring in the procedures associated with the construction of a metal framework.

Where alginate has been used to take the secon-

Details of partial denture design:

Upper Denture:

Rests ....

Clasps ....

....

....

Connectors ....

Other Instructions ....

....

....

....

....

Lower Denture:

Rests ....

Clasps ....

....

....

Connectors ....

Other Instructions ....

....

....

....

....

....

Fig. 15.1 Prescription form for partial dentures.

dary impressions, precautions must be taken in the casting-up procedure, as detailed on page 130.

Prescription writing

The requirements which may arise at this stage are:

1. The design of a metal framework

Where the construction of a metal framework is required, detailed instructions must be given. This can best be provided by means of a diagram, accompanied by information on each of the component elements. Use of a prescription form such as that illustrated in Figure 15.1 will facilitate this process. It is also helpful to the technician if the required design for the framework is drawn on the study casts. This can provide more definitive information on the required position of elements such as palatal connectors than is afforded by a two-dimensional drawing on the prescription form.

2. Occlusal rims

These may be required in certain cases for use in the subsequent clinical stage of registration of the patient's jaw relationship. Whether or not they are required is dependent on the number and distribution of tooth contacts which are present, and this will be discussed further in Chapter 16.

Where occlusal rims are required, the prescription for them should indicate:

1. The material or materials to be used in baseplate construction, with required extension.
2. Whether placement of strengthening elements or retainers is required.
3. The material to be used in rim construction.

SPECIAL IMPRESSION PROCEDURES

Pressure or muco-displacive impressions

In certain circumstances a decision may be made to take an impression which records the tissues under loading conditions which simulate those arising in masticatory functioning of the appliance. The rationale for this procedure is considered in Chapter 21, where the problems presented by dentures carrying free-end saddles are discussed.

Two approaches are possible when obtaining pressure impressions in the partially edentulous condition:

1. Pressure may be applied evenly over the whole area to be recorded by the impression. This can be most readily achieved by the use of impression composition as impression material. Since undercuts are likely to be associated with standing teeth, accuracy of reproduction of these undercuts will only be obtained if a sectional approach is used. The impression is built up in sections, each having a different path of insertion allowing withdrawal from associated undercuts. As each section is added it is positioned in relation to other sections by means of notches, which allow accurate re-assembly of the sections following withdrawl from the mouth. For more detailed information of this procedure a specialist text should be consulted.

2. Pressure application may be concentrated on the edentulous areas to be recorded by the impression, a lower level of pressure being applied to the standing teeth. This procedure may be selected since it is the edentulous tissue areas which will be liable to show any gross level of displacement under pressure, displacement of the teeth being limited to the movement permitted by the periodontal attachment tissues. The advantage of this procedure is that the recording of the undercuts on the teeth is facilitated by the ability to use an elastic impression material in the tooth-bearing section of the impression.

A suitable combination of impression materials to use in this procedure is provided by impression compound in the edentulous areas and alginate in the tooth-bearing areas. A special tray is used and compound applied initially in the edentulous regions. Any excess that has flowed into the tooth-bearing section is trimmed back and then, as a second stage, the tooth-bearing section is recorded in alginate. To avoid the problem of a parting line between the two impression materials the alginate may be extended as a wash over the compound portion if desired.

At each of the stages of impression taking, manual pressure is applied to the tray to an extent which is felt will match that developed in the functioning of the appliance.

Impression procedures for relining partial dentures

The relining of mucosa-supported partial dentures is a rarely applied procedure because of the technical difficulties which can arise. These are associated with the multiple undercuts which are usually present. In the original construction of the denture, interproximal undercuts will have been blocked out to allow insertion of the denture along the chosen path. If a reline impression is taken in the denture, the impression material will flow into any interproximal undercuts. Unless special steps are taken this material entering the undercuts will be reproduced in the relined denture and insertion will be impossible. For this reason, remaking rather than relining of mucosa-supported dentures is often advocated.

Although relining of mucosa-supported dentures may be deprecated, the same is not true of tooth-supported and especially tooth-and-mucosa-supported dentures.

Relining of removable partial dentures of the tooth-and-mucosa-supported type, which normally carry free-end saddles, is a frequent requirement. Where a metal base is included in the design, relining can only be applied to those saddles where the metal work has been relieved from direct contact with the tissues. The lack of adhesion between metals and polymeric materials such as acrylic resin, debars the addition of a thin polymeric film on a metal base.

Where the relining of free-end saddles on a tooth-and-mucosa-supported partial denture is required, the following procedure may be used:

1. Examine the extension of the saddle areas and correct this if found to be necessary.

2. Remove any undercuts present on the fitting surface aspects of the saddles.

3. Take a reline impression in the saddle areas. Zinc oxide-eugenol impression paste is frequently used as the impression material at this stage. Alternatively, Kerrs Korecta Wax No. 4 may be used, with application of wax in stages until full surface coverage of the saddle area is achieved and excess wax appears all round the margins. In taking the impression it is important that pressure should only be applied to the anterior framework aspect of the denture to ensure it seats correctly in a fully-fitting position on the standing teeth. Manual pressure should not be applied to the saddle areas, nor should the patient be requested to apply biting pressure on the denture.

When the denture is re-inserted following the completion of the laboratory procedure of relining of the saddles, it will usually be found that some degree of occlusal disharmony will be present, premature contact occuring on the posterior teeth. This must be corrected by selective grinding of the dentition until the required occlusion has been developed.

This procedure for relining the free-end saddles of a partial denture may be used in those instances where antero-posterior rocking of the denture is found to occur about an axis joining the occlusal rests, when pressure is applied in a tissueward direction on the free-end saddles. The circumstances which give rise to instability of this type are considered in Chapter 21.

Relining may be necessary for the 'completed' denture prior to it being worn by the patient or the need may be found to arise at any or all of the subsequent six-monthly review appointments of the patient.

An alternative procedure which may be used to overcome the problem of antero-posterior rocking of the denture is to use a techniques based on that proposed by Applegate. This is termed the 'Altered Cast' technique and can only be used during the original construction of the denture. If relining is subsequently found to be necessary during the period of wear of the appliance, another procedure such as that described earlier will need to be used.

In the altered cast technique, a conventional metal framework for the denture is first prepared on a cast taken from an impression in which an impression material of a relatively low order of viscosity was used, such as alginate. Baseplates are now attached to the metal-work in the saddle areas to fully cover the required tissue areas of the saddles and so that they are relieved from the tissue contact by a gap of approximately 2 mm.

Kerr's Korecta Wax No. 4 is now painted on the fitting surface aspect of the blaseplates to a depth of 2 mm. The denture is inserted with pressure applied only on the anterior tooth-bearing area of the metal framework. Wax additions and re-insertion are carried out until over-all coverage of the tissues in the saddle regions has been achieved and excess wax has flowed out around all the margins.

In the laboratory, the original cast is now sectioned to remove those portions of the cast which originally reproduced the tissues under the saddles. The section lines used for a lower cast are shown in plan view in Figure 15.2. The framework is then positioned on the remaining portion of the cast and new saddle areas are poured up in the saddle impression zones to reform the cast. Setting up of the teeth and finishing of the denture are then carried out on the altered cast. A particular

Fig. 15.2 Plan view of a lower cast showing the section lines used in the Applegate 'altered cast' technique.

advantage of this procedure is that as the teeth are set up on the altered cast no occlusal disruption arises. Against this must be considered the demanding nature of the procedure from both the clinical and laboratory aspects, which restrict its application.

FURTHER READING

Beckett L S 1955 Partial denture impressions. Dent J Austral 27: 135

Grant A A and Walsh J F 1975 Reducing cross-contamination in prosthodontics. J Prosthet Dent 34: 324

Henderson D 1966 Writing work authorizations for removable partial dentures. J Prosthet Dent 16: 696

Holmes J B 1970 The altered cast impression procedure for the distal extension removable partial denture. Dent Clin North Amer 14: 569

Kramer H M 1961 Impression techniques for removable partial dentures. J Prosthet Dent 11: 84

McCrorie J W 1982 Corrective impression waxes. A simple formula. Brit Dent J 152: 95

Osborne J and Lammie G A 1954 The manipulation of alginate impression materials. Brit Dent J 96: 51

Wilson H J and Smith D C 1963 Bonding of alginate impression materials to impression trays. Brit Dent J 115: 291

16

The jaw registration stage of treatment

INTRODUCTION

In the provision of removable partial dentures, the jaw registration stage has to be applied at two treatment stages:

1. To allow the study casts to be mounted on an articulator in the correct relationship. This is an essential precursor to the stages of occlusal analysis and partial denture design.

2. To allow the working casts to be mounted on an articulator in the correct relationship, prior to setting-up of the artificial teeth.

Often, the same or similar procedures will be used to effect jaw registration in both these stages. However, one essential difference is that where a cast metal framework has been prepared for a denture this will be used, where appropriate, as a baseplate for the registration procedure in the second stage.

In all cases the jaw registration stage requires:
1. Establishing the correct vertical dimension.
2. Establishing the correct horizontal relationship.

Additional records will be required where complex analysis of the dentition is indicated. These involve a face-bow and protrusive or lateral records of jaw relationship. In all cases the procedures adopted should be based on the principles of registering jaw relationships considered in Chapter 9.

ESTABLISHING THE CORRECT VERTICAL DIMENSION

Three types of case may be encountered, each requiring a separate approach:

1. Cases in which natural tooth contact occurs at a vertical dimension providing an acceptable freeway space.

2. Cases in which natural tooth contact occurs at a vertical dimension providing an excessive freeway space.

3. Cases in which no natural tooth contact occurs.

Cases in which natural tooth contact occurs at a vertical dimension providing an acceptable freeway space

Where a stable contact of upper and lower natural teeth occurs at a vertical dimension at which an adequate and yet not excessive freeway space is present (normally 2–4 mm), the registration should be established at this contact height in the subsequent stage of establishing the horizontal relationship.

Cases in which natural tooth contact occurs at a vertical dimension providing an excessive freeway space

Here, the vertical dimension should be established at a value increased on that of tooth contact by an amount necessary to bring the freeway space down to an appropriate value. This may be achieved by the use of a wax wafer interposed between the teeth, the thickness of the wax being varied until the required freeway space has been achieved. It is desirable that the wax wafer registration should include a metal plate, cut to lie within the arch of the teeth and with the wax affixed to it peripherally. This considerably reduces the risk that distortion of the registration will occur in the interval preceding mounting of the casts. The use of a wax wafer registration is only feasible where the number and disposition of standing teeth are such that the wafer will locate precisely on the study casts. This normally necessitates the presence of contacting teeth in both the premolar and molar regions on each side of the arch. Where this condition is not met, the registration is carried out using occlusal rims, the height of rim/rim or rim/tooth contact being varied by addition or subtraction of wax until the required freeway space has been developed.

Cases in which no natural tooth contact occurs

Where no contact of natural teeth occurs on mandibular closure, the registration must be made via the use of occlusal rims in one or both jaws as necessary. The height of the occlusal surfaces of the rims is adjusted until contact of rim and teeth and/or rim and rim occurs at a vertical dimension providing the required freeway space. A particular type of case of this category which is frequently encountered is that where an edentulous maxilla opposes a partially edentulous mandible, the standing natural teeth being the six lower anteriors. Establishing vertical dimension in this type of case requires initially that the upper occlusal rim be developed as in a complete denture case. Wax is added or subtracted from the labial and buccal aspects of the rim until it is judged that correct lip and cheek support has been developed. The occlusal surface of the rim is then developed so as to lie at the required level relative to the upper lip and so that it is parallel to the inter-pupillary and ala-tragal lines. The mandible is then closed to bring the standing anterior teeth in contact with the occlusal surface of the rim and the freeway space (if any) which is present at this contact height is measured relative to the rest vertical dimension. The contact relationship between the upper rim and the lower standing teeth is then adjusted until the required freeway space has been achieved. This will usually necessitate softening the rim surface in the area where the teeth contact to allow the teeth to indent the rim, so developing an overbite. Occasionally, where excessive freeway

space is found to be present, it will instead be necessary to increase the depth of the upper rim until contact occurs at an acceptable value of freeway space.

ESTABLISHING THE CORRECT HORIZONTAL RELATIONSHIP

Two methods may be used to establish the correct horizontal jaw relationship. Selection of the method to use in an individual case is based on an assessment of the inter-cuspal relationship of the dentition which is present.

1. Where the number and disposition of the standing teeth in both jaws are such that when the mandible closes in a retruded relation, a definitive and regular inter-cuspal relationship develops at the correct occlusal vertical dimension, this horizontal contact relationship should be the one which is registered.

2. In all other cases, the relationship which is registered should be that of retruded jaw relationship (centric jaw relationship), as utilised in complete denture construction.

Establishing horizontal jaw relationship by use of the inter-cuspal relationship of the natural dentition

The procedures that can be used to obtain the registration are as follows:

1. Hand occlusion of the casts

In a small number of cases, it will be found that when upper and lower casts are placed into occlusion by hand they will locate in a constant and definite manner. A check should be made that the relationship of the casts so developed parallels that observed in the natural dentition in the closed relationship. Where this condition is satisfied, no further registration procedure need be applied. The method has the advantage that no registration material lies between the teeth, hence the risk of the recording being made at an increased vertical dimension is avoided.

2. Use of a wax wafer registration, a zinc oxide-eugenol impression paste registration, or a buccal plaster record

Where an adequate number of teeth are present (which usually involves bilateral contact of premolars and molars), and yet the casts will not themselves locate in a definitive position, a wax wafer registration may be used. The wax wafer should be stabilised by incorporation of a metal plate, as previously noted in the consideration of the development of the vertical relationship. The wax horseshoe is thoroughly softened and then placed between upper and lower teeth. The mandible is closed in a retruded position until the maximal inter-cuspal relationship of the teeth is achieved. The wafer is removed from the mouth, chilled in cold water and then buccal excess wax trimmed off until the remaining portion of the registration lies within the cuspal arch. The trimmed wafer is then replaced in position on the teeth and repeated mandibular closure applied to ensure that a consistent intercuspal relationship has been recorded. Removal of buccal excess wax facilitates observation of this relationship and also aids correct positioning of the wafer on the casts in the subsequent procedure in which the casts are mounted on an articulator.

A disadvantage arising from the use of a wax wafer registration is that the wax always has a positive thickness — it is impossible to expel wax from between teeth which would otherwise come into full contact in the absence of the wafer. The registration is thus obtained at a slightly increased vertical dimension relative to that of tooth contact. Some operators prefer to use zinc oxide-eugenol impression paste instead of wax for the registration, since this may reduce the increase in vertical dimension which arises. Such a registration can best be obtained by using a wire carrier frame covered with gauze to facilitate positioning of the paste between the arches. A low-viscosity type of zinc oxide-eugenol impression paste should be used in the procedure. The paste is mixed and a thin layer placed over the gauze. The frame is immediately placed around the lower teeth and the mandible is closed until maximal intercuspal relationship is achieved. This position must be maintained until the paste is fully set.

Yet another alternative is the use of a buccal plaster record. Here, the patient is requested to close into the position of maximal intercuspal relationship. With maintenance of this jaw relationship, a mix of impression plaster at the 'putty' stage is massaged into the right and left buccal sulci to lie over the contacting teeth. When the plaster has set, the right and left records are removed and may subsequently be positioned on the casts to provide the required location. In theory, the method is excellent in that no increase in vertical dimension should occur. Some difficulty may be encountered, though, in achieving full location of the plaster records on the casts and this problem restricts the use of this procedure.

3. Use of occlusal rims

Where an insufficient number of teeth are present to allow the registration to be made by procedures 1 or 2, the use of occlusal rims will be necessary in one or both jaws. Where the occlusal surface of a rim opposes standing teeth, a layer of modelling wax approximately 2 mm deep is added to the occlusal surface of the rim and the wax is thoroughly softened by use of a hot wax knife. The rim is seated in the mouth and mandibular closure applied until maximal intercuspal contact of opposing natural teeth occurs. Where the occlusal surface of a rim opposes that of another rim in the opposing jaw, the registration procedure used should follow that utilised in complete denture construction. A notch is cut in one rim surface (usually the upper one) and about 2 mm of wax is cut away in the opposing area of the lower rim to provide an escape way for excess wax. A pillar of softened modelling wax is now built on to the lower rim opposite the notch, providing a volume of wax which is just a little more that that estimated as necessary to fill the notch and make up the cut away portion of the rim. The rim is inserted and mandibular closure applied until maximal intercuspal contact of the opposing natural teeth occurs.

Where the registration is being carried out to allow mounting of working casts on an articulator and the denture design includes use of a cast metal framework, the reader is reminded that the metal framework should be used as the baseplate on which any necessary occlusal rim areas are constructed. This will ensure that a baseplate of optimal retention and stability is used in the registration and avoid the risk of one potential error — that of baseplate distortion — arising in the registration procedure.

Establishing horizontal jaw relationship at the position of mandibular retrusion

Where the contact of standing teeth does not provide adequate indication of horizontal jaw relationship at the required occlusal vertical dimension, the registration procedure should parallel that utilised in complete denture construction. This need will arise in cases of the second and third types considered on page 136 in relation to the establishment of the correct occlusal vertical dimension.

The registration is based on achieving retruded jaw relation (centric jaw relation) at the established vertical dimension of occlusion. A common procedure utilised to develop the required position of mandibular retrusion is to ask the patient to curl their tongue upwards and backwards until the tip lies in contact with the posterior palatal tissues. Other procedures may sometimes prove to be necessary (see Chapter 9). Repeated mandibular closure should be applied and a note made via rim marking or otherwise that a reproducible position of full retrusion is being achieved. Location of this position is then obtained, usually by use of softened modelling wax added to appropriate areas of a wax wafer or occlusal rim. A wax/tooth relationship or a rim/rim relationship (via use of notching) is recorded as previously described. Care should be taken that the previously developed occlusal vertical dimension is not disrupted in this process.

Although modelling wax provides a satisfactory means of recording jaw relationships in most cases, alternative procedures are desirable where a free-end saddle is present in the lower jaw, especially where it extends to the premolar region. If, in the recording procedure, pressure is applied to the occlusal surface of a rim overlying a lower free-end edentulous span, the rim will descend tissuewards due to displacement of the underlying soft tissues. The registration will thus be recorded in a position of tissue displacement. No such displacement will occur when the registration is subsequently placed on the cast and the position of upper and lower casts will be different than that present in the oral cavity at the time of registration. If the casts are mounted on an articulator using such a registration and the artificial teeth are set up, premature contact of the posterior teeth will be seen at the trial denture stage. To overcome this problem it is necessary to record the relationship applying minimum load to the free-end saddle area of the rim. This can best be achieved by reducing the level of the free-end saddle rim until it is free of contact with the opposing teeth or opposing occlusal rim surface by about 2 mm. Notches are cut in the lower occlusal rim surface to provide location and then impression plaster at the 'putty' stage is placed over the rim and mandibular closure applied to achieve retruded jaw relation. This position is maintained until the plaster has set. When the casts are assembled by use of such a record their relationship will now coincide with that present intra-orally.

Whatever method of recording of the vertical and horizontal jaw relationships is selected for use, always assemble the casts via use of the record obtained and check for coincidence between the relationship of the casts and that seen by examination of the oral tissues. This should be done while the patient is still in the chair so that any errors noted can be corrected at that visit.

ADDITIONAL RECORDS FOR OCCLUSAL ANALYSIS

Where study casts are to be mounted on an adjustable articulator to allow full occlusal analysis, the following additional records will be required.

A face-bow record

In the partially edentulous situation, the method used to locate the face-bow fork orally in relation to the maxilla will depend upon the number of standing teeth present in the maxilla. Where teeth are present in the anterior and both posterior segments, the link may be achieved by allowing the teeth to indent softened modelling wax wrapped around the face-bow fork. Where this condition is not satisfied, the fork will be attached to a maxillary occlusal rim.

Other features of the procedure for obtaining the record and for using it to mount the maxillary cast will be as described in Chapter 10.

A protrusive and/or right and left lateral records of jaw relationship

These will allow setting of the condylar inclinations of the articulator.

Where standing teeth are present in both jaws in the anterior and right and left posterior segments, the registration(s) may be obtained using a wax wafer alone. The wax should be about 3 mm thick initially and be wide enough to allow upper and lower teeth to indent the wax in a position where the mandible is either about 4 mm anterior or lateral to the position of retruded jaw relation. Where insufficient standing teeth are present to meet this requirement, the registration(s) is made using a wax wafer placed between occlusal rims in one or both jaws as necessary. Location of the wafer on the occlusal surfaces of the rims is achieved via the cutting of notches in the rim surfaces.

The further procedure for obtaining the records and for using them to set the condylar inclinations of the articulator are as described in Chapter 10.

SELECTION OF TEETH

It is usual to select the artificial teeth for denture construction at the conclusion of the jaw registration stage of treatment. In partial denture prosthesis, especially where natural teeth are present both anteriorly and posteriorly, selection of the artificial teeth can be a much simpler task than that which may face the operator in complete denture prosthesis. Examination of the standing teeth and of the edentulous spaces will provide guidance on the size, form, texture and colour of anterior teeth to be used and on the size, form and colour of posterior teeth to be used.

Where standing teeth are absent in either the anterior or posterior regions, it may be necessary to select appropriate teeth using the guiding principles considered in Chapter 11. In all cases,

though, the colour of the standing teeth should be used as a guide to selection of the colour of the artificial teeth.

In relation to the selection of the material from which the artificial teeth are made, the choice rests between acrylic resin and porcelain. In partial denture prosthesis, there is much to be said in favour of the selection of porcelain teeth. When set in opposition to natural teeth, porcelain posterior teeth will resist occlusal wear much better than acrylic resin teeth. Where a partial denture is to be mucosa-supported, as in the use of maxillary dentures of the 'Every' form, the development and maintenance of good contacts between the natural and artificial teeth is essential to obtain adequate retention. Such contacts will be better maintained in the service life of the denture where porcelain teeth have been used because of their better wear resistance. Unfortunately, the irregular nature of the occlusal surfaces of natural teeth combined with the fact that there is often minimal space available between the occlusal surface of an artificial tooth and the underlying edentulous ridge often necessitates considerable grinding of the artificial teeth in the setting-up process. The mechanical system of retention which is necessary in porcelain artificial teeth (normally diatoric holes in posterior teeth and pins in anterior teeth) limits the degree of grinding which can be applied to such teeth without loss of the retention occurring. Thus, despite the theoretical advantages offered by porcelain teeth, it is often necessary to use acrylic resin teeth in partial denture prosthesis.

As part of the selection process it is important that the patient should be questioned as to any special wishes they may have. For example, they may request the use of facsimile restorations to duplicate the original natural dentition. Any special requests which the patient may make in relation to tooth arrangement should also be noted at this stage.

PRESCRIPTION WRITING

The information necessary to allow the technician to proceed to the stage of preparing trial dentures is as follows:

1. The type of articulator to be used.

2. An indication that the maxillary cast should be mounted via use of a face-bow record where one has been taken.

3. A request that the mandibular cast be mounted in relation to the maxillary cast utilising the record of vertical and horizontal relationship provided.

4. Requirements in relation to the setting of the condylar inclinations where an adjustable articulator is to be used and protrusive and/or right and left lateral records of jaw relationship have been taken.

5. Details of the required setting of the angle of the incisal guidance table where a fully adjustable or semi-adjustable articulator is to be used.

6. Full details of the artificial teeth which have been selected for use, along with any required modifications to the teeth (e.g. facsimile restorations).

7. Guidance on any special features of tooth arrangement not provided by occlusal rims (e.g. rotation or overlapping of individual teeth).

FURTHER READING

Beckett L S 1954 Accurate occlusal relations in partial denture construction. J Prosthet Dent 4: 487

Beyron H L 1954 Characteristics of functionally optimal occlusion and principles of occlusal rehabilitation. J Amer Dent Assoc 48: 648

Block L S 1952 Preparing and conditioning the patient for intermaxillary relations. J Prosthet Dent 2: 599

Mc Cracken W L 1958 Functional occlusion in removable partial denture construction. J Prosthet Dent 8: 955

Silverman M M 1953 The speaking method in measuring vertical dimension. J Prosthet Dent 3: 193

17

The principles of tooth arrangement

INTRODUCTION

Tooth arrangement should aim at aiding the achievement of the objectives of removable partial denture provision. As noted in Chapter 12, the objectives may be summarised as follows:
1. Restoration of appearance
2. Restoration of masticatory efficiency
3. Restoration of speech to a normal quality
4. Maintenance of the health and integrity of the soft and hard tissues of the oral cavity.

Achievement of the first of these objectives will mainly be influenced by the arrangement of any anterior teeth carried by the partial denture, while achievement of the second objective will mainly be dependent on the arrangement of any posterior teeth carried by the denture. Objectives three and four can be helped by appropriate placement of anterior teeth and/or posterior teeth.

For convenience, the principles of arranging the anterior teeth and the posterior teeth will be considered in separate sections. It should be realised, however, that many partial dentures replace both anterior teeth and posterior teeth. Where this applies, the arrangement of the anterior and posterior teeth should be integrated to create a harmonious unit with the standing natural dentition.

ARRANGEMENT OF THE ANTERIOR TEETH

Where some anterior teeth only are to be replaced

Here, the arrangement of the teeth to be replaced should simulate that of the standing natural anterior teeth in relation to length and axial inclination.

In general, the development of a symmetrical arrangement about the mid-line is desirable. Special note should be made of any aging features which are present in the natural dentition such as incisal wear and gingival recession at the necks of the teeth. Where present, these features should be simulated in the setting of the replacement teeth.

Wherever possible, the development of tight contact points between the natural and replacement teeth should be obtained. In the case of mucosa-supported dentures, friction at contact points can play a significant role in the achievement of retention.

Often, it will be found that the natural standing teeth will not be all the same colour. The optimal aesthetic result will usually be achieved by selecting replacement teeth for the span concerned with a colour which presents a compromise between the colours of the abutment teeth.

Occasionally, colour matching from the available range of stock teeth is difficult, perhaps because of the presence of abnormally stained natural teeth. Where necessary, teeth of the required colour can be individually prepared in the laboratory using dentine-type acrylic resins of an appropriate shade. Alternatively, stock teeth may be modified by the application of surface stains.

Where all the anterior teeth are to be replaced

Here, the anterior teeth should be arranged in a manner similar to that used in complete denture construction. An upper occlusal rim should be available, the labial surface of which has been contoured to indicate the required setting of the teeth to achieve correct lip support. The occlusal plane of the rim should have been developed to indicate

Fig. 17.1 Plan view of an arrangement for the upper anterior teeth appropriate for a female patient.

Fig. 17.2 Plan view of an arrangement of the upper anterior teeth designed to produce a heightened masculine effect.

the required incisal edge level of the teeth and the centre line should have been marked. The anterior teeth should then be arranged in conformity with the information provided by the occlusal rim. Tight contacts should be developed with the posterior abutment teeth which are present.

In Chapter 11, which dealt with the principles of tooth selection, reference was made to the work of Frusch and Fisher in the development of 'Dentogenic Restorations'. Their principles can also provide a useful guide at the stage of tooth arrangement. For a female patient, an appropriate arrangement may be achieved by setting the labial surfaces of the upper anterior teeth to lie on a smooth arc (Fig. 17.1). In contrast, masculinity may be signified by developing a more angular (cuboidal) tooth arrangement. For a male patient whose personality is judged to be at the vigorous end of the spectrum, the masculine effect may be heightened by setting the two upper central incisors so that they lie a little anterior to the lateral incisors, the labial surface of all four incisors facing anteriorly (Fig. 17.2).

ARRANGEMENT OF THE POSTERIOR TEETH

In the introduction to this chapter reference was made to the role of the posterior teeth in developing masticatory efficiency in a removable partial denture. The level of masticatory efficiency which is achieved will depend mainly on the cuspal form of the posterior teeth which are used and on arranging the teeth so that optimal stability is obtained. Stability, in turn, will be influenced by three factors:

1. The positioning of the teeth relative to the underlying residual alveolar ridge.

2. The positioning of the teeth relative to the

environmental musculature (the neutral zone concept).

3. The degree to which occlusal balance is attained.

Often, these factors present opposing needs in tooth placement. The interplay of the factors and the way in which a compromise setting is decided upon to achieve optimal stability is considered in some detail in Chapter 24, which deals with the parallel situation in complete denture construction.

It should be noted that occlusal balance is often more difficult to achieve in partial dentures than in complete dentures. This is due in part to the irregular nature of the occlusal surfaces presented by many natural teeth. In addition, guidance from the contact relationship of the natural teeth often results in a steeply inclined mandibular movement path. In all instances, though, every effort should be made to develop the highest possible level of occlusal balance. This can be helped by the use of replacement teeth with a cuspal form similar to that of any natural posterior teeth which are present.

When setting the replacement posterior teeth, it is important that the role they play in developing the aesthetics of the dentition should not be overlooked. Although of less importance than the anterior teeth in terms of direct display, the first premolars at least are often visible when the patient smiles. If an unnatural appearance is to be avoided the first premolars should be set to present a balanced length relative to the adjacent canines. A sudden transition in length between the anterior and posterior teeth, especially in the maxilla, is rarely seen in the natural dentition and should be avoided when setting the replacement teeth on a partial denture.

Further features of the arrangement of posterior teeth can best be considered according to the presence or absence of posterior natural teeth.

Where some posterior teeth only are to be replaced

Where the posterior teeth are to be set in a bounded saddle situation, they should normally be set to lie in a straight line drawn through the centres of the abutment teeth. Either a normal or cross-bite arrangement may be developed, as indicated by the situation of the opposing dentition. In all instances, an adequate buccal overjet should be developed to reduce the risk that cheek-biting will occur.

It should be noted that in partial denture prosthesis, substitution of teeth relative to the natural predecessors is permissable and, indeed, is often desirable. For example, where an upper first premolar is to be replaced and the jaw relationship is such that little if any functional contact can be developed with the lower opposing teeth, a more aesthetic result will often be achieved by substituting an extra canine for the premolar. In many instances it will be found that tilting and drifting of the natural teeth leaves less space for the positioning of the replacement teeth than the space originally occupied by their natural predecessors. In such instances substitution may again be required. For example, the space originally occupied by two molars may only now present space for the placement of, say, a premolar and molar as the replacement teeth.

Where the posterior teeth are to be set on a free-end saddle, the procedures considered in the next section should be followed.

Where all the posterior teeth are to be replaced

The free-end saddle situation encountered here poses special problems in posterior teeth arrangement, especially in the case of a lower denture.

Basically, the teeth need to be arranged to achieve optimal stability and this requires that they be set in a manner similar to that used in the posterior segments in complete denture construction (considered in Chapter 24). Where opposing natural posterior teeth are present, some departure from the 'ideal' arrangement may be necessary in order to achieve a functionally acceptable occlusal relationship.

Modifications in tooth arrangement in the free-end saddle situation may also be necessary to reduce the load which is applied to the tissues underlying the saddle. The rationale for this move is considered in Chapter 21. Load reduction, where indicated, may be achieved by reducing the size of the occlusal table. This can be done by reducing the number of teeth which are set (for example, omitting the second molars) or by using smaller teeth than might otherwise have been used. Reducing the bucco-lingual width of the replacement teeth relative to that of the natural predecessors will help. It is, indeed, often advocated that such width reduction should be applied in all instances where posterior teeth are replaced and not just in the free-end saddle situation.

FURTHER READING

Frush J P and Fisher R D 1956 How dentogenic restorations interpret the sex factor. J Prosthet Dent 6: 160
Frush J P and Fisher R D 1956 How dentogenics interprets the personality factor. J Prosthet Dent 6: 441
Frush J P and Fisher R D 1957 The age factor in dentogenics. J Prosthet Dent 7: 5
Proctor H H 1953 Characterization of dentures. J Prosthet Dent 3: 339

18

The trial denture stage of treatment

INTRODUCTION

This stage of treatment may require action in two phases:

1. Trial of a cast metal framework, where one is included in the design of a partial denture.

2. Trial of the partial denture, with the replacement teeth arranged on a temporary or 'permanent' (metal) baseplate.

The examination procedure which should be carried out in each of these phases is considered in the following sections. Advice will also be given on the actions necessary where faults are detected in the course of the examination procedure.

TRIAL OF A CAST METAL FRAMEWORK

Checking fit

It is generally advisable for this to be carried out before any wax additions have been made to the metal framework. The absence of wax facilitates visual examination of the fit of the framework and also makes it easier to carry out modification of the framework where this proves to be necessary.

The framework should be positioned correctly over the standing natural teeth and gentle seating pressure applied along the path of insertion selected when the study cast was surveyed. It should be found to slide easily into the fully seated position, only moderate resistance being encountered corresponding to the retentive value of any clasps which are present. If any undue resistance to movement is encountered in the seating process, excessive force should not be applied as this may cause discomfort or make it difficult to remove the framework subsequently without over-stressing the periodontal attachment of the tooth or teeth concerned. By visual and tactile examination, an attempt should be made to determine where resistance to further movement is occurring. Location of the exact site of resistance can be assisted by the use of the a disclosing wax. An even layer of the wax, approximately 1 mm thick, should be applied to the fitting surface of the framework in the area under investigation. The framework should then be inserted up to the point where resistance to further movement is encountered. The insertion path of the framework should be carefully reversed and the fitting surface then examined. The resistance area will be revealed as the area where the wax has thinned to display the underlying metal.

Often, resistance to movement will be found to arise at interproximal metal/tooth contact areas or at the origin of clasp arms. If the thickness of metal at the resistance area is such that it is felt that the metal could be reduced without adversely affecting the strength of the framework, then grinding may be undertaken. Carborundum stones may be used for grinding a gold alloy framework but special abrasion-resistant stones, usually based on aluminium oxide, should be used to trim a cobalt-chromium alloy casting. The procedure of trial insertion of the framework, location of resistance areas and grinding of the areas should be repeated until either satisfactory insertion is obtained or it is judged that any further modification by grinding would endanger the strength of the denture. Where the latter applies, it will be necessary to take a further impression, prepare a new metal framework and repeat the examination procedure.

When satisfactory insertion of a framework has

been obtained, the fit of all the component elements should be examined with the aid of a mouth mirror. A probe may also be used to check the closeness of fit of any elements contacting the teeth. Clasp arms should be checked for non-traumatic placement relative to the gingival margins of the teeth. The various component elements should also be checked for correct positioning relative to the soft tissues. For example, gingivally-approaching clasp arms should not enter soft tissue undercuts. Palatal connectors on an upper framework should be in contact with the underlying tissues. Where a lingual bar has been used in the design of a lower framework, it should be correctly positioned relative to the gingival margins of the standing teeth and the functional level of the lingual sulcus.

The patient should be questioned as to whether or not they feel any discomfort when the framework has been inserted. Where the patient can detect a pressure area, particularly in relation to covered soft tissues, it may be necessary to relieve pressure in the area concerned by grinding the fitting surface of the framework. Disclosing wax may be used, where necessary, to locate the site of pressure. Before grinding is applied, the framework should be carefully examined to check that the intended reduction in section will not unduly prejudice its strength.

Checking retention and stability

Retention should be checked by attempting to displace the framework from its fitted position in a direction reversing the path of insertion, noting the resistance that is encountered. Due allowance needs to be made for the fact that full retention may not be present at this stage. Where the design includes the use of wrought clasps these are unlikely to be present at the stage of trial of the metal framework, but will be added later.

Stability of the framework should be checked by applying pressure on various elements — rests, saddles and palatal connectors in particular — and noting whether any rotational displacement occurs. Special attention is necessary when checking the stability of a framework carrying one or two free-end saddles. It is usual for the free-end saddle portion of a metal framework to have been relieved from tissue contact in the constructional procedure, to enable the saddle to be relined where this is subsequently required. Before testing the stability of the free-end saddle element of a metal framework which has been relieved from tissue contact, it is advisable that a wax baseplate be positioned to bridge the gap between the metalwork and the underlying tissues.

Where the design of the partial denture includes the use of a stress-breaker, especially where this is of Type 1, (Chapter 13, page 113), an appreciable degree of rotational displacement should be observable when pressure is applied to the metalwork of the free-end saddle. Where no stress-breaker has been used, and yet an appreciable degree of rotational displacement of the free-end saddle occurs when this check is applied, there is a need for subsequent action to be taken to overcome this instability. This will usually involve relining of the free-end saddle at the insertion stage of treatment.

Checking aesthetics

The framework should be inserted and its appearance noted when the patients lips are at rest and when the patient is smiling. If any elements of the metalwork are visible when the patient smiles, it is advisable to point this out to the patient and show them what is involved with the aid of a hand mirror. If proper care has been applied in the stages of treatment planning and denture design, objections to the aesthetics of a metal framework should be rarely encountered. Where objections do arise, they usually relate to an unaesthetic display of clasp arms or incisal rests. Where this is due to an unnecessary thickening having occured in the construction of the framework, it may be possible to overcome the objections by reducing the thickness of the element concerned by grinding.

Checking the occlusion

The framework should be inserted and the occlusal relationship of the teeth checked. In those cases where the natural teeth contact at the required occlusal vertical dimension, the relationship which occurs with the framework inserted should be the same as that which occurs when the framework has been removed. If the presence of the metal framework is seen to cause any disruption to the occlusal relationship of the natural teeth, articulating paper should be used to indicate where premature contact is occurring. Caution must be exercised when analysing the contact pattern produced by articulating paper, as its interpretation requires careful visual observation in order to ensure that markings arise from tooth contact. Correction may be applied by grinding either the metalwork or the natural tooth at the point of premature contact. The metal should be selected for grinding only where it is judged that this can be carried out without undue weakening of the framework. Often, a combination of grinding of both tooth and metal is used, to avoid undesirable disruption of either. The process of detection of points of premature contact and their reduction should be continued until occlusal harmony is re-established.

Where the natural dentition does not contact at the required occlusal vertical dimension and the design of the framework includes onlays, a check should be made that with the framework inserted the opposing natural teeth and the metalwork contact evenly at a vertical dimension providing an acceptable freeway space. Where necessary, articulating paper can be used to detect the site of any premature contact areas. Where interference has been shown to be present, grinding of the natural teeth and/or of the metal framework should be applied until an acceptable occlusal relationship has been established.

General observations

On completion of the above check procedures for a metal framework, it will be possible to develop an over-all appraisal of its satisfaction or otherwise. In all cases where one or more of the checks have revealed the presence of unsatisfactory features which cannot be corrected in the ways indicated, it will be necessary to take a new impression and prepare a new metal framework. This may repeat the original design or may involve modifications where indicated. The check procedures listed above should be applied to the new framework. Only when a framework has been shown to be fully satisfactory should the next stage be undertaken — that of setting the replacement teeth to develop a trial denture.

It should be noted that it is inadvisable to attempt to rectify any faults which are present in a framework (for example, inadequate retention in clasp arms) by bending the framework. It is virtually impossible to apply bending without disrupting the essential passive placement of the elements relative to the oral tissues. A bent framework may well give rise to appreciable tissue damage.

TRIAL OF THE PARTIAL DENTURE

The procedures used in checking a partial denture at the trial stage are similar to those used at the corresponding stage of complete denture construction and they should be applied in the same order. The procedures are as follows.

Checking extension, retention and stability

The extension of the baseplate on the master cast should be checked for conformity with the outline requested on the design prescription form. The denture should be inserted and the extension of any flanges which are present should be checked in relation to the levels of the functional sulci. Where appropriate, the position of the posterior border of an upper baseplate should be checked for correct relation to the vibrating line. Where extension faults are found to be present, they should be corrected by addition or subtraction to the baseplate as necessary.

The fit of the baseplate on the master cast should be noted. The denture should then be inserted and a check made that a similar fit is present on the hard or soft tissues covered by the baseplate. Where a discrepancy is evident between the fit of the baseplate on the master cast and the fit in the mouth, there is an indication that an error has occured in the previous stages of impression-taking or cast preparation. Before proceeding further, it will then be necessary to repeat these and other intermediate stages and to prepare a new partial denture for retrial.

When the fit of the baseplate has been shown to be satisfactory, the retention of the denture should be checked. This involves determination of the resistance to displacement which arises when a force is applied to the denture in a direction reversing the path of insertion. It should be noted that the retention present at this stage, except where a cast metal framework incorporating cast clasps forms the baseplate, is likely to be appreciably less than that achievable in the final (processed) denture. The presence of reasonable retention is, however, a prerequisite for being able to carry out satisfactorily subsequent check procedures and when absent consideration should again be given to the need to repeat the impression and subsequent stages before proceeding further.

Stability of the denture should be checked by applying pressure in a tissuewards direction to the replacement teeth at a series of points around the arch. If a rotatory displacement of the denture is seen to occur, the cause of this should be sought and an appropriate remedy should be applied. The most common finding will be that the replacement teeth have been positioned buccal or labial to the crest of the residual alveolar ridge to an excessive degree. Where this applies, the teeth should be reset to a position where stability is achieved.

Where a free-end saddle is present, it should be checked for the display of antero-posterior rotatory displacement when pressure is applied to the teeth on the saddle.

As previously noted in relation to the trial of a metal framework (page 146), where such displacement arises it may be an intentional feature of the design of the denture, as where a Type 1 stress-breaker type has been used. Alternatively, where no stress-breaker has been used, subsequent action will be necessary to overcome the rotation. This will usually involve relining of the saddle at the insertion stage of treatment.

Checking aesthetics

The denture should be inserted and the appearance of the patient noted with the mouth closed, with the lips slightly parted and with the patient providing a full smile. The patient should also be given a hand mirror and invited to make similar observations.

Where the visible aspect of the occlusal plane and/or the centre line of the dentition is developed by the replacement teeth, these features should be checked for compliance with the appropriate facial landmarks.

It should be borne in mind that the result will be influenced not only by the replacement teeth but also by the form of any buccal or labial flanges carried by the denture. Of particular importance will be any gingival contouring which is displayed when the patient smiles. This should harmonize with that of any natural teeth which are visible.

Where either the operator or the patient are unhappy about any of the aesthetic features of the denture, chairside modification should be carried out until a mutually acceptable result has been achieved. This may involve resetting of the replacement teeth and/or modification of the form of the flanges.

Checking the vertical component of the jaw relationship

Where the occlusal vertical dimension is defined by the contact of opposing natural teeth, the denture should be inserted and a check made that both the natural teeth and the replacement teeth on the denture meet evenly at this vertical dimension.

Where the natural standing teeth do not meet at the occlusal vertical dimension, the denture should be inserted and a check made that even contact of the artificial teeth and the natural teeth (including onlays where used) occurs at a vertical dimension which provides an acceptable value of freeway space.

The procedures that should be used to correct any errors found to be present at this check stage are considered in conjunction with those used to correct any errors found in relation to the horizontal component of jaw relationship and appear below.

Checking the horizontal component of jaw relationship

Note should be made of the inter-cuspal relationship of the natural and artificial teeth as developed on the articulator. Where the number and relative positioning of the natural teeth provide a definite inter-cuspal relationship in the horizontal plane, the denture should be inserted and the patient persuaded to close into this relationship. In all other cases the patient should be persuaded to close into the retruded jaw relationship. The intercuspal relationship which is present intra-orally should coincide with that previously observed on the articulator.

Where this requirement is not satisfied, or where an error was found to be present at the previous stage of checking the vertical component of jaw relationship, a new registration must be taken.

Where an error was found to be present in the vertical component of jaw relationship, this should be corrected first. The artificial teeth should be removed from the denture and the corresponding areas replaced by wax occlusal rims. The height of the rims should be adjusted until contact occurs between the rims and opposing natural teeth, and/ or between opposing rim surfaces, at the required occlusal vertical dimension.

A new registration should then be made of the horizontal component of jaw relationship. Where natural teeth oppose a rim surface, the registration should normally be obtained by adding softened modelling wax to the rim surface and registering the indentations of the teeth in this wax when the patient closes into retruded jaw relationship. Where the registration is to be made between opposing rim surfaces, a notch should be cut in the upper rim and about 2 mm should be removed from the surface of the lower rim in the area opposite the notch. Softened modelling wax should then be built up on the lower rim surface to an extent judged to be necessary to fill the notch in the upper rim. The previous step of reducing the depth of the lower rim provides an escape way for any excess wax which is present. The patient should then be persuaded to close into retruded jaw relationship until the rim surfaces contact. It should be noted that where a decision was made to use a low-pressure registration procedure when the original registration was made (usually because of the presence of a free-end saddle), this procedure should also be used in re-registration.

At the conclusion of re-registration of the horizontal component of jaw relationship, a check should be made that an acceptable freeway space is still present. Unless the procedures for registration of the horizontal component have been carefully

applied there is a risk that the previously-developed vertical component will be changed.

The casts should then be remounted on the articulator to the relationship given by the new registration, and new trial dentures developed by resetting of the replacement teeth. The checks listed for application at the trial denture stage should then be repeated at a subsequent visit of the patient. If necessary, the procedures for re-registration and re-development of a trial denture should be repeated until satisfaction is achieved. Authority for finishing the denture should never be given until both patient and operator are fully satisfied with the result at the trial denture stage.

When satisfaction has been achieved, two final observations should be made, where necessary, before the patient is dismissed:

1. Where an upper denture is being provided and a palatal plate in a polymeric denture-base material is to be used, if the plate is to extend to the vibrating line then the correct position for the posterior border of the denture should be clinically determined. Note should also be made of the displaceability of the tissues in this area via the use of an instrument such as a ball-ended burnisher. A post-dam preparation should then be made on the cast in the manner used in complete denture construction (Chapter 25).

2. The denture-bearing areas should be examined and a decision made as to whether any relief zones are required where the denture will not come into contact with the underlying tissues. Where relief is required, the tissue areas concerned should be mapped out on the casts.

PRESCRIPTION WRITING

When a trial denture is returned to the laboratory for finishing, the following information should be provided:

1. The colour and nature of the denture-base material to be used.

2. Details of position and depth of any peripheral seal lines required at the borders of palatal connectors in an upper denture.

3. Details of any areas which require relief. Information on the site and depth of relief areas should be given in the written prescription, sup-

plemented by the mapping out of the required extent of relief areas on the casts. Sites which frequently require relief include a torus palatinus which is to be covered by an upper denture base and the gingival areas of standing teeth, where these are to be covered by connectors.

FURTHER READING

Applegate O C 1965 Essentials of Removable Partial Denture Prosthodontics. 3rd Edn. Saunders, Philadelphia
Osborne J and Lammie G A 1974 Partial Dentures. 4th Edn. Blackwell Scientific Publications, Oxford
Swoope C C 1970 The try-in — a time for communication. Dent Clin North Amer 14: 479

19

The insertion stage of treatment

EXTRA-ORAL EXAMINATION

Before attempting to insert the finished partial denture, it should be carefully checked to ensure that no blemishes are present which could traumatise the oral tissues. Particular attention should be paid to the fitting surface of the denture. Where part, at least, of this has been constructed in a polymeric denture-base material such as acrylic resin, the surface should be checked for the presence of any blebs arising from the presence of air cavities in the corresponding area of the cast on which the denture was processed. Where blebs are found to be present they should be removed by the use of a sharp cutting instrument or by grinding, care being taken not to damage the surrounding surface of the denture.

Where metallic elements are present on the denture they should be checked to ensure that no potentially traumatic features are present. For example, the free end of clasp arms should be rounded and not tapered to a sharp point.

Where connectors or other elements cross gingival margins, a check should be made that adequate relief has been provided.

The denture should be examined for the presence of any undercuts which might interfere with its insertion. Where undercuts are present, they may need to be modified in the course of the subsequent intra-oral examination procedure.

INTRA-ORAL EXAMINATION

The check stages which are used in the intra-oral examination of a finished partial denture are similar to those used at the trial denture stage and they should be applied in the same order. If a regular routine is developed for checking dentures at both the trial and insertion stages of treatment, the risk that any individual stage will be overlooked will be reduced.

The following sections provide details of the checks that should be applied, along with advice on dealing with any problems that arise.

Checking fit

The denture should be positioned correctly in the oral cavity in relation to the standing natural teeth and gentle pressure should be applied along the path of insertion. It should glide into a fully-fitting position, the only resistance encountered corresponding to retentive features such as clasps which are present on the denture.

Where any appreciable degree of resistance to further movement is met in the course of attempted insertion of the denture, additional force should not be applied. Instead, an attempt should be made to determine the cause and site of the resistance. Providing that all unwanted undercuts on the standing teeth have been correctly blocked-out in the course of denture construction, the resistance to movement will commonly be found to be arising from the presence of undercut flanges. These should have been noted during the extra-oral examination of the denture. The site where an undercut flange is becoming impacted on the underlying tissue as denture insertion is attempted is often made apparent by blanching of the tissues in the area concerned. The patient may also be able to provide evidence of the impaction area by indicating where pressure or pain is arising in the course of attempted insertion of the denture.

Any undercut flanges which are found to be preventing denture insertion should be modified to reduce, or, where necessary, eliminate the undercut which is present. This may be achieved by reduction of flange extension or, where flange thickness permits, by the trimming of the fitting surface of the flange.

Modification of the denture should be continued until insertion into the fully-fitting position has been achieved.

Checking extension, retention and stability

The extension of the inserted denture should be checked for compliance with the level of the functional sulci. Any peripheral over-extension which is found to be present should be removed by trimming of the area or areas concerned.

Retention should be checked by inserting the denture and applying a force in a direction away from the underlying tissues and along a path reversing that of insertion. A definite resistance to displacement should be observable, the value of which must be at least equal to the displacing forces which arise during mastication if denture displacement in function is to be avoided. Because of its subjective nature, the retention check presents difficulty for the inexperienced operator.

Stability should be checked by inserting the denture and applying pressure in a tissueward direction to the replacement teeth at a series of points around the arch. No displacement of the denture should occur except, perhaps, where free-end saddles are present. The latter may show an antero-posterior rotatory displacement when pressure is applied to the teeth on the saddles. This may be an intentional feature of the design of the denture where a stress-breaker is present. In other cases, where no stress-breaker has been used, the finding implies a need for corrective procedures to be applied. These usually involve the relining of free-end saddles. The special impression procedures which are used in the relining of the saddles are considered in Chapter 15, page 134.

Checking aesthetics

The denture should be inserted and the appearance of the patient noted with the mouth closed, with the lips slightly parted and with the patient providing a full smile. The patient should also be given a hand mirror and invited to make similar observations.

The result should simulate that approved by both patient and operator at the trial denture stage. Occasionally, some modification of the depth or width of flanges may be necessary to achieve the required degree of support for the facial tissues. This need should only arise where flange form has been accidentally modified in the course of denture finishing.

Checking the vertical component of the jaw relationship

Where the occlusal vertical dimension is defined by the contact of opposing natural teeth, the denture should be inserted and a check made that both the natural teeth and the replacement teeth on the denture meet evenly at this vertical dimension.

Where the natural standing teeth do not meet at the occlusal vertical dimension, the denture should be inserted and a check made that even contact of the artificial teeth and the natural teeth (including onlays where used) occurs at a vertical dimension which provides an acceptable value of freeway space.

If either of these conditions is not satisfied, a thin grade of articulating paper should be used to determine the point or points where premature contact is occurring. Premature contacts should be ground and this process repeated until full harmony between the natural and artificial dentition has been established at the required vertical dimension.

Checking the horizontal component of the jaw relationship

Where the inter-cuspation of the natural dentition provides a definitive position in the horizontal plane, the denture should be inserted and the patient persuaded to bring the teeth into contact in this relationship. In all other instances, the patient should be persuaded to bring the teeth into contact in retruded jaw relationship. The observed inter-digitation of the natural and artificial teeth should be the same as that approved at the trial denture stage. If a minor error in the occlusal relationship of the teeth is apparent, the site of premature contact should be determined by the use of a thin grade of articulating paper. Selective grinding of premature contacts should be carried out until a harmonious relationship of the natural and artificial dentition has been established.

Where any major error in the occlusal relationship of the teeth is seen, remaking of the denture will usually be necessary.

It should be noted that procedures for remounting and selective grinding of dentures on an articulator are rarely used for partial dentures, because of the difficulties which arise from the presence of natural teeth.

INSTRUCTIONS TO THE PATIENT

When a partial denture has been found to be satisfactory by application of the check procedures detailed above, the patient should be given verbal instructions on the care and maintenance of the denture and the associated oral tissues. It is desirable that the verbal instructions should be reinforced by the provision also of written instructions. This is particularly important where the patient is either elderly or handicapped, since there is a risk that verbal instructions alone will be either misunderstood or forgotten.

The instructions should be designed to enable the patient to learn to use the denture as quickly as possible and to get the greatest possible benefit from it. The points covered both verbally and in written form should be as follows:

1. Eating may be difficult at first. Food should be cut into small pieces and adequate time allowed for chewing. Tough and sticky foods are best avoided in the initial learning period.

2. Difficulty may be experienced in removing a new partial denture. Where the denture contains thin metal parts, these should not be used to lever out the denture. Instead, only the plastic parts of the denture should be held, both when removing and replacing the denture.

3. The denture should be removed from the mouth and cleaned after each meal. A soft brush, soap and cold water are satisfactory for cleaning. Alternatively, a proprietary denture cleanser may be used, following the manufacturer's instructions. Household bleach solutions should not be used as they may damage the denture. Where metal parts are present on the denture, great care should be taken not to bend these during cleaning or the denture could be ruined.

In addition to the denture, the natural teeth must also be cleaned thoroughly after each meal. With the denture removed, a toothbrush and toothpaste should be used in the usual way. This is very important since a partial denture can lead to food being trapped around the natural teeth, with associated increased risk of tooth decay or gum disease occurring.

4. The denture should be removed at night and stored in water, to prevent drying-out and warping.

5. Pain and soreness may occur when a new denture is first worn and adjustment of the denture may be necessary to overcome this. If the pain becomes severe the denture should be left out and an appointment arranged with the dental surgeon as soon as possible. The denture should be worn on the day of the appointment so that the sore area will be visible. The patient should not attempt to adjust the denture or irreparable damage could arise.

FURTHER READING

Addy M and Bates J F 1977 The effect of partial dentures and chlorhexidine gluconate gel on plaque accumulation in the absence of oral hygiene. J Clin Period 4: 41

Bassiouny M A and Grant A A 1975 The toothbrush application of chlorhexidine. Brit Dent J 139: 323

Blatterfein L 1958 Rebasing procedures for removable partial dentures. J Prosthet Dent 8: 441

Lawson W A 1965 Information and advice for patients wearing dentures. Dent Pract Dent Rec 15: 402

Lawson W A and Bond E K 1969 Speech and its relation to dentistry. Dent Pract Dent Rec 19: 150

Smith D C 1966 The cleansing of dentures. Dent Pract Dent Rec 17: 39

Storer R 1962 Partial denture saddle correction. Brit Dent J 112: 454

20

The review stage of treatment

INTRODUCTION

Following the insertion of a partial denture, the patient should be given an appointment for review in approximately seven days time.

At the review visit, the patient should be questioned concerning any problems that have been experienced when wearing the denture. A detailed examination should then be carried out of the oral cavity and the denture, in the course of which signs of symptomless tissue damage may be noted. A diagnosis is then made of the cause of all problems revealed in the history and examination procedures. Appropriate treatment should then be applied to overcome these problems.

HISTORY OF THE PATIENT'S EXPERIENCES

The patient should be asked to give an account in his own words of any difficulties that have occurred since the denture was inserted. The commonest complaint will be that of pain. Where this applies, the patient should be asked how long the pain has been present and whether it is relieved by leaving out the denture. Note should also be made as to whether the pain is localised to one area of the oral tissues or is widespread and whether any analgesics or other medication have been used to try and alleviate the pain. The operator should also establish whether the pain is present continually when the denture is being worn or if it only arises at certain times, for example, when eating.

The second most commonly encountered complaint is that the denture seems to be loose. Where this applies, the patient should be asked if the denture is loose all the time or only when chewing food or speaking. The patient should also be asked to indicate whether displacement seems to initiate from a particular area of the denture, and, if so, where this is.

Less commonly, the patient will complain that the denture has caused problems with appearance or speech. Where the complaint relates to appearance, the patient should be asked to indicate the exact nature of the problem. For example, where anterior teeth are replaced by the denture, do the teeth seem to be too large or too small, or do they show too much or too little. Alternatively, are denture flanges producing exaggerated or deficient support for the lips and cheeks. In relation to complaints concerning speech, the patient should again be asked to indicate the exact nature of the problem. For example, does whistling or lisping arise during pronunciation of the 's' sound or is difficulty being encountered with the 'plosive' sounds, 'p' and 'b'.

A further complaint which is occasionally encountered is that of intolerance to the presence of the denture in the oral cavity. Where this problem arises, the patient should be asked how long he can wear the denture before it has to be removed. He should also be asked whether any special circumstances arise which necessitate removal of the denture. For example, does it make him feel sick or produce actual retching. Alternatively, does it produce the sensation of an unpleasant taste in the mouth or lead to a 'gripping' feeling in the mouth which could be likened to the effect which the wearing of a new pair of shoes can produce on the feet.

EXAMINATION OF THE ORAL CAVITY AND THE DENTURES

The denture should be removed from the mouth and a thorough examination made of the oral tissues with the help of a mouth mirror. Particular attention should be paid to any areas where the patient has experienced discomfort, but all the oral tissues should be examined, since symptomless changes may be observed which warrant treatment. The soft tissues should be checked for signs of injury or inflammation which may vary in intensity from mild hyperaemia to frank ulceration. Where the patient has complained of discomfort in relation to the standing natural teeth, the crowns of the tooth or teeth concerned should be re-checked to exclude the presence of any disease process. The level of oral hygiene being maintained by the patient should be noted. The periodontal status of the tooth or teeth concerned should also be re-assessed, including a test for the presence of tenderness to percussion. Radiographic examination should be carried out where thought to be necessary.

The denture should be examined extra-orally to re-check that no irregularities are present on the fitting surface which could have caused tissue irritation. The denture should then be inserted and the peripheral form examined for the presence of any areas of over-extension. Retention should be checked for adequacy and stability checked by applying pressure in a tissue-wards direction on tooth-bearing areas of the denture. The aesthetic effect of the denture should be observed, particularly in relation to any complaints of poor appearance raised by the patient. The occlusal vertical dimension should be checked to ensure than an acceptable value for freeway space is present. The dentition should also be checked to ensure that the natural and artificial teeth develop a harmonious relationship when closure occurs in retruded jaw relationship or, where appropriate, in the jaw relationship dictated by the inter-cuspal relationship of the natural dentition.

THE CAUSE AND MANAGEMENT OF PATIENTS' COMPLAINTS

The history of the patient's experiences when wearing a new partial denture and the examination of the oral cavity and the denture should enable a diagnosis to be made of the cause of the patient's complaints. A decision must then be made of the appropriate treatment, which may, for example, involve modification of the denture where this is indicated.

In this section, the common causes of patients' complaints will be considered and advice given on the necessary treatment. The subject will be discussed under a series of headings representing major patient complaints.

Pain

Where pain has arisen in a *localised* area of the soft denture-bearing tissues, the likely causes are one or more of the following:

1. Over-extension of the periphery of the denture.

2. Excessive engagement of an undercut by a denture flange.

3. Inaccuracy in the denture fitting surface, for example, the presence of an irregularity not paralleled in the corresponding area of the soft tissues.

4. The presence of a premature contact in the occlusal relationship of the dentition, arising in either a static occlusal relationship or during dynamic movements of the dentition.

5. Accidental damage to the denture, for example, a clasp arm having been bent during cleaning.

6. Attempts by the patient to remove or insert the denture along paths other than the intended paths of withdrawal and insertion.

The above causes will usually have produced clearly visible signs of inflammatory changes in the soft tissues in the areas concerned. Visual examination of the inserted denture will usually have provided an indication of the area of the denture responsible for the tissue change. Where necessary, though, disclosing wax or pressure relief cream may be used to indicate the causative area of the denture.

Treatment of causes 1, 2 and 3 will require

modification of the denture by trimming of the area concerned until painful symptoms have been relieved. Cause 4 will require adjustment of the occlusion by selective grinding until the premature contact has been obliterated. Cause 5 will require replacement of the defective clasp unit where this is feasible, otherwise remaking of the denture will be necessary. Cause 6 will necessitate the patient receiving further instruction in the correct procedures for inserting and removing the denture.

Where the complaint of pain arises from a *diffuse* area of the soft tissues covering most, if not all, of the denture-bearing zone, the likely cause will be the presence of an excessive occlusal vertical dimension. If examination of the denture revealed the absence of an acceptable value for freeway space, treatment of the condition will necessitate remaking of the denture at a reduced value of occlusal vertical dimension.

At other times, a complaint of diffuse pain may be restricted to only a part of the denture-bearing tissues. Here, the cause often relates to anatomical abnormality in the tissues concerned. For example, a sharp mylohyoid ridge may be present or, where a lower partial denture carries an anterior saddle, the pain may relate to the presence of a sharp superior margin in the residual alveolar ridge or may be due to atrophy in the overlying mucosa. In some instances, relief of pain arising from these causes may be obtained by judicious relief of the corresponding area of the fitting surface of the denture to reduce the pressure which is applied on the tissue area concerned. Where this is unsuccessful, treatment may necessitate surgical intervention. For those patients for whom surgery is contraindicated the placement of a resilient lining in the denture may be considered.

Where the complaint of pain is localised to one of the standing natural teeth, the cause is likely to be overstressing of the periodontium of the tooth. This may arise through the application of excessive vertical load to the tooth, as where an occlusal rest on the tooth is in premature contact with the opposing dentition. Where this applies, the appropriate treatment will be occlusal adjustment to remove the premature contact. Alternatively, the problem may arise through excessive force application to the tooth in the horizontal plane, as where a clasp arm has been accidentally bent by a

patient so that it engages an excessive undercut. Treatment here will require the damaged clasp unit being replaced where this is feasible, otherwise remaking of the denture will be necessary.

In some instances, a complaint of pain will relate to oral soft tissues external to the denture-bearing zone. For example, tongue irritation may arise through the presence of a sharp superior margin on a metal plate. Both the tongue and the cheeks may be injured by over-sharp ends on clasp arms. Any such traumatic features should be removed by smoothing the elements concerned.

More commonly, though, the complaint will be due to tongue or cheek biting. The usual cause of this problem is lack of buccal overjet on the posterior teeth or, in the case of tongue biting, narrowing of the arch leading to inadequate provision of space for the tongue.

Where a complaint of cheek-biting of a relatively mild degree arises in a case in which a lower denture provides replacement of the posterior teeth, resolution of the complaint can often be effected by grinding the buccal aspects of the lower molar teeth and rounding over the bucco-occlusal margins to develop an improved buccal overjet. If, in a similar type of case, the complaint is that of tongue biting of a relatively mild degree, grinding the lingual aspect of the lower posterior teeth may successfully resolve the condition by increasing the space available for the tongue. Where either tongue or cheek biting have occurred to a severe degree, it will usually prove to be necessary to reset the teeth to achieve the arch form or buccal overjet necessary to overcome the complaint.

Looseness of the denture

If the patient complains that the denture is loose when they are talking and eating and at other times when no definite function is being performed, the probable causes are:

1. Over-extension of the periphery of the denture relative to the level of the functional sulcus. If examination shows over-extension to be present, the area of the denture concerned should be reduced by peripheral trimming.

2. Incorrect shaping of the denture relative to the environmental musculature. This cause is particularly liable to affect a lower partial denture if

inadequate space has been allowed for the tongue. In some cases the problem can be overcome by grinding of the lingual aspect of the denture (including the teeth where necessary) to increase tongue space, but often remaking of the denture will prove to be necessary

3. Inadequate retention. In mucosa-supported dentures this may arise due to inaccurate fit of the denture base or inadequate development of contact points between the artificial and natural teeth. Alternatively, in a tooth-supported denture where clasps have been placed on the abutment teeth to obtain retention, the clasps may be incorrectly positioned relative to available undercuts. Where this applies, treatment will usually necessitate re-making of the denture.

If the patient complains that the denture is only loose when they are masticating foods, the likely cause is a lack of occlusal balance in the artificial dentition. Thin articulating paper and visual examination should be used to detect cuspal interferences which arise during protrusive and lateral excursions of the mandible. Selective grinding should then be carried out until the maximum possible level of occlusal balance has been achieved.

Where a partial denture carries free-end saddles, a complaint by a patient may arise that the denture moves during mastication of food (and sometimes at other times too). Examination may reveal the presence of an antero-posterior rock of the free-end saddle when pressure is applied to it. Treatment of this condition will usually involve relining of the saddle.

Problems with the appearance of the denture

A complaint of unsatisfactory appearance should rarely arise if adequate care was taken at the trial denture stage. Where complaints concerning the appearance of the denture are brought out by the patient at the review stage, questioning will often reveal that they arise from comments provided by the patient's relatives and friends. As far as possible, an attempt should be made to overcome the complaints by modification of the denture. For example, flanges may be modified in depth or thickness to increase or reduce as necessary the support of the facial tissues. Changes in

tooth colour or tooth arrangement, where called for, can usually only be effected by remaking the denture.

Speech problems

Many patients encounter a minor speech disruption when a new denture is first worn. They should be reassured that this is likely to go in a period of a month or so as the oral tissues adapt to the presence of the denture.

In some instances, though, the speech disruption may be such as to warrant denture modification. One instance of this is where pronunciation of the letter 's' is affected. The sound 's' is most commonly produced by the tip of the tongue being placed close to the palatal aspects of the upper anterior teeth and the anterior palatal tissues to develop a narrow air channel. Where an upper partial denture has been provided which replaces the anterior teeth, if the teeth have been set too far forward the air gap may be excessive and the patient may 'whistle' when pronouncing the letter 's'. Alternatively, if the anterior teeth have been placed too far back or the anterior palatal aspect of the denture is too thick, the air channel may be too narrow and the patient may lisp when pronouncing the letter 's'. Treatment of a whistling effect will require the air channel being reduced by wax additions until the correct sound is produced, the added wax subsequently being converted into the appropriate polymeric denture-base material. To correct lisping, the air channel should be increased by grinding the palatal aspects of the teeth and the denture base material in the anterior palatal area until the correct 's' sound is produced.

Another condition which will require treatment is where the patient complains of difficulty with the 'plosive' sounds 'p' and 'b'. These sounds are formed by the lips being closed to allow intra-oral build-up of air pressure. The lips are then suddenly parted to allow escape of air and development of the required sound. If the patient complains of difficulty with these sounds, the problem may arise due to the presence of an excessive occlusal vertical dimension which makes it difficult for the patient to effect the necessary lip seal. If the patient presents with this speech problem the vertical dimension of the dentures should be carefully checked. If found to be excessive, treatment will require remaking of the dentures.

Intolerance to wearing a partial denture

Although uncommon, this problem is by no means rare and can be very distressing to a patient. Usually found in association with the wearing of an upper partial denture, the main cause is enhanced sensitivity in the posterior palatal tissues producing an abnormal retching reflex action. Increased sensitivity in the dorsum of the tongue can also initiate retching if the denture contacts the tongue.

Where the problem is of a severe nature, it will almost certainly have become evident in the early stages of treatment, particularly during impression-taking. Appropriate steps should then be taken in denture design to minimise the problem. Where the sensitivity lies in the palate, the palatal connector of an upper partial denture should be shaped to avoid coverage of the posterior palatal tissues. Where the sensitive organ is the tongue, an upper partial denture should be designed to have maximum retention and a lower partial denture should provide the greatest possible space for the tongue.

Where the problem has only become evident at the review stage, the treatment required will depend upon the length of time that the patient can wear the denture before it has to be removed. With an upper denture, if the time is short — a matter of seconds or minutes only — it will usually be necessary to reduce the extension of the denture in the posterior palatal region until tolerance improves. A posterior palatal seal should then be added at the new level of connector extension. Where the onset of the problem is delayed for a longer period — perhaps six to eight hours after insertion, the cause may lie in excessive bulk in the denture. In this case the base should be thinned to the limit allowed by strength requirements. Otherwise, all that will usually be required is reassurance of the patient that with persistence the problem will be overcome.

Further aspects of the problem of intolerance to denture wearing appear in the chapter devoted to a consideration of the review stage in complete denture treatment (Chapter 27).

Other complaints

The patient may raise a number of complaints at the review stage not covered in the above list. Frequently, there will be a complaint of excessive salivation. Where the denture includes metallic elements there may be a complaint of a metallic taste in the mouth. Dentures with metallic elements which are fitted in a mouth in which metallic restorations are present in the natural teeth, may also give rise to a complaint of occasional pain in the natural teeth through galvanic action.

Complaints of this nature are usually of a short life span and the patient should be reassured that the problems will resolve in the fullness of time.

General note

In all instances where the periphery, teeth or polished surface of the denture have been modified at the review stage, the areas concerned must be carefully repolished before the denture is returned to the patient.

Where severe tissue damage was noted at the review stage, the patient should receive an appointment for further review in approximately seven days time to ensure that the treatment provided has effected resolution of the condition. Further reviews at intervals of approximately six months should be arranged in all cases so that both the denture and the standing natural teeth can be re-examined and any necessary treatment carried out.

FURTHER READING

Appleman R M 1948 Why partial dentures fail. Dent Digest 54: 490
Farrell J 1968 Partial denture tolerance. Dent Pract Dent Rec 19: 162
Kovats J J 1971 Clinical evaluation of the gagging patient. J Prosthet Dent 25: 613
Lawson W A and Bond E K 1969 Speech and its relation to dentistry. Dent Pract Dent Rec 19: 150
Miller E L 1973 Types of inflammation caused by oral prostheses. J Prosthet Dent 30: 380
Morstad A T and Peterson A D 1968 Post-insertion denture problems. J Prosthet Dent 19: 126

21

The free-end saddle partial denture

INTRODUCTION

In this chapter some of the problems faced in the design and construction of removable partial dentures carrying free-end saddles will be discussed. Dentures of this type are used to provide replacement of missing teeth in Kennedy Class I and Class II dentitions. The reader is reminded of the need to satisfy the biological requirement in partial denture prosthesis which places the preservation of the remaining tissues as the first priority.

Reports of surveys which have appeared in the literature serve to illustrate the difficulties which can arise in meeting this aim in the free-end saddle situation.

For example, where such dentures have been designed to be of a simple, mainly mucosa-supported form, Anderson and Lammie reported a widespread tendency for the periodontal tissues of the standing teeth to be traumatised, involving gingival inflammation, retraction of the gingivae and increased mobility of the abutment teeth. In another survey on dentures of that form, Koivumaa reported the occurrence of inflammatory reactions of the mucosa supporting the denture base as well as a hastening of the rate at which resorption occurred in the edentulous alveolar ridges.

Where, instead, the dentures had been designed to include support from the standing dentition, a somewhat improved picture of tissue response has been reported, although tissue damage still occurred. For example, Carlsson, Hedegård and Koivumaa found that after only twelve months wear of such dentures, many patients showed inflammatory changes in the tissues at the gingival margins of the abutment teeth, along with increased mobility of the teeth. These changes were particularly apparent where the patient had failed to maintain a high standard of oral hygiene.

Despite the difficulties which are highlighted by surveys such as those quoted above, the chance of achieving biological acceptability with a free-end saddle type of partial denture will be improved where the patient has been motivated to maintain a high standard of oral hygiene. The operator should also have an understanding of the design problems which are peculiar to this type of denture so that other steps can be taken to minimise the risk of tissue damage occurring.

DESIGN PROBLEMS

These will be considered under two main headings:
1. The provision of support for the free-end saddle partial denture.
2. The provision of retention for the free-end saddle partial denture.

The provision of support for the free-end saddle partial denture

A free-end saddle may be either mucosa-supported or tooth-and-mucosa-supported. From the biological point of view, there is much to be said in favour of the saddle being made mucosa-supported. This will ensure that when vertical masticatory forces are applied to the free-end saddle they will be spread relatively evenly over the whole of the mucosal surface underlying the saddle. The provision of mucosal support for the free-end saddle should also ensure that potentially damaging forces will not be transferred to the abutment tooth.

In the case of maxillary partial dentures, mucosal support for free-end saddles can be achieved by designing the whole denture to be mucosa-supported. As noted in Chapter 14, mucosal support is a viable proposition for maxillary dentures because of the availability of the hard palate which can be utilised to gain support. It is desirable that dentures of this type should be constructed following the principles advocated by Every in order to help the maintenance of the health of the remaining periodontal tissues.

Where only one free-end saddle is present on a maxillary denture, the Every principles can often be successfully applied, especially if two or more bounded saddles are present in addition to the free-end saddle. Where two free-end saddles are present and no additional bounded saddles exist, the prognosis for success with the Every mucosa-supported denture is much decreased due to the likely lack of the development of adequate retention and stability. To counter this problem, it will often prove to be necessary to place direct retainers on the abutment teeth. Where, as is usual, these take the form of retentive clasp arms, it will be necessary also to place rests on the abutment teeth in order to ensure correct location of the clasp arms on the teeth. The desirable principle of the free-end saddles being mucosa-supported is thereby lost, the saddles becoming tooth-and-mucosa-supported.

In the case of mandibular partial dentures carrying free-end saddles, there is an almost universal need for rests to be placed on the abutment teeth to achieve an acceptable level of support. Here, there is no hard palate available to aid the support of the denture. If rests are omitted, the whole of the vertical masticatory load applied to the saddles will fall on the relatively small area of mucosa underlying the saddles, which may respond by showing pathological change. In addition, if bilateral free-end saddles on a mandibular partial denture are to be solely mucosa-supported, it will be necessary to use a non-tooth-bearing connector such as a lingual bar. Although biologically satisfactory as far as the teeth are concerned, such a denture is likely to lack retention and stability to a level which will prove unacceptable to the majority of patients. To attempt to overcome this problem there is a temptation to replace the lingual bar with a lingual plate and to place retentive clasp arms, but no rests, on the abutment teeth. This approach, however, creates conditions which can lead to severe damage in the periodontal tissues. Over a period of time it is almost inevitable that alveolar resorption will occur in the tissues underlying the free-end saddles. Where resorption occurs, it will allow the denture to adopt a different seating position from that present at the time of insertion. As a consequence of the displacement of the denture the lingual plate may become traumatic to the gingival tissues of the covered teeth. Contact may also be lost between the lingual plate and the underlying teeth, increasing the potential for plaque retention with the accompanying risk that tissue damage will arise.

Retentive clasp arms placed on the abutment teeth may descend to a level where they become traumatic to the gingival tissues. Dentures of this type have rightly been termed 'gum strippers' and their use should be avoided. To prevent such consequences it is necessary to utilise the abutment teeth to provide support for the denture, usually achieved by the use of rests. Then, and only then, may retentive clasp arms be placed safely on the abutment teeth, the rests serving to correctly locate the clasps arms on the abutment teeth.

Thus, in a proportion of maxillary dentures carrying free-end saddles and in the majority of mandibular partial dentures carrying free-end saddles, it is necessary to place rests on the abutment teeth. This results in the free-end saddles becoming tooth-and-mucosa-supported rather than mucosa-supported as ideally desired. The creation of a condition of tooth-and-mucosa support in a free-end saddle raises the need to develop an equitable distribution of load between the two supportive tissues. If either the abutment tooth or the tissues underlying the free-end saddle are overloaded, irreparable damage may arise.

However, achieving the desired equitable distribution of load between the abutment tooth and the tissues underlying the free-end saddle can be difficult. To illustrate this point, consider the position in a mandibular partial denture with a free-end saddle providing replacement of $\overline{5\ 6\ 7}$. An occlusal rest, rigidly attached to the saddle, has been placed on the disto-occlusal fossa of the abutment tooth and clasp arms, to provide bracing, retention and reciprocation, have also been placed on the abutment tooth.

When vertical masticatory loads are applied to the free-end saddle they will be transferred both to the abutment tooth (via the rest) and to the mucosal tissues underlying the saddle. The anterior end of the saddle will be mainly tooth supported, the descent of the saddle under load being restricted by the fibres of the periodontal membrane of the abutment tooth. The posterior end of the saddle will be able to descend to a greater extent, lying as it does on the much more displaceable mucosa overlying the alveolar bone (Fig. 21.1). As a consequence, a rotatory torque will be applied to the abutment tooth in the sagittal plane.

Laterally directed forces in the horizontal plane will also be applied to the saddle when masticatory movements of the saddle occur. At the anterior end of the saddle, movement will be restricted by

Fig. 21.1 Displacement of a free-end saddle under vertical load.

Fig. 21.2 Displacement of a free-end saddle under horizontal (lateral) load.

the link between the saddle and the abutment tooth via the occlusal rest and the clasp arms. Posteriorly, the saddle is freer to move, as the underlying displaceable mucosa offers less resistance (Fig. 21.2). A rotatory torque thereby arises on the abutment tooth in the horizontal plane.

Additional torque will be applied to the abutment tooth where posterior teeth of the anatomical form have been used. This torque force arises during protrusive mandibular movements where opposing cuspal surfaces meet in a protrusive position and sliding then occurs to return the mandible into the maximal inter-cuspal contact position. By an inclined plane effect, a horizontal force component arises which is directed anteriorly in the maxilla and posteriorly in the mandible.

The combined effect of the above forces may well result in permanent damage to the periodontal tissues of the abutment tooth. If prolonged, exfoliation of the tooth can be the eventual outcome.

In addition to the effect on the abutment tooth, the effect on the supporting tissues underlying the saddle must also be considered. Here, the applied loads will be concentrated posteriorly due to the lack of posterior tooth support. This may result in an accelerated degree of alveolar resorption occurring posteriorly. Once this has occurred, the descent of the posterior aspect of the saddle under vertical load will take on a dynamic quality and a vicious circle of progressively increasing damage to both the abutment tooth and the supporting tissues underlying the saddle will be set in motion. It is clearly important that steps should be taken to reduce to a minimum the risk that such tissue damage will arise. The available procedures are considered in a subsequent section.

The provision of retention for the free-end saddle partial denture

There are two aspects of retention which need to be considered:
1. The provision of direct retention
2. The provision of indirect retention

The provision of direct retention

The potential for achieving direct retention in a free-end saddle by placement of tooth-borne direct retainers is likely to be less than that of a bounded saddle as retention can only be obtained at the mesial end of the saddle. Where it is desired to obtain direct retention by placement of a clasp unit on the single abutment tooth, the absence of useable undercuts on the tooth creates an additional problem.

Careful attention needs to be paid to the rigidity of a minor connector used to join a tooth-borne direct retainer on the abutment tooth to the free-end saddle. In general, the greater the rigidity of this connector, the greater will be the risk that potentially damaging torque forces will be applied to the abutment tooth when masticatory forces are applied to the saddle.

The provision of indirect retention

The fact that partial dentures may show rotatory displacement in function has been noted in Chapter 14, page 120. The problem is encountered most commonly in partial dentures carrying bilateral free-end saddles and no bounded saddles (Kennedy Class I dentition). When the patient is chewing sticky foodstuffs, the denture may rotate about an axis joining rests placed on the abutment teeth on each side. The free-end saddles move away from the underlying tissues whilst simultaneously the anterior portion of the denture (forward of the axis of rotation) is depressed in a tissuewards direction. If rotatory displacement of this type occurs it can be a source of embarrassment to the patient and can also give rise to appreciable tissue damage anteriorly.

POSSIBLE SOLUTIONS TO THE DESIGN PROBLEMS

These will be considered under the same headings as used in the consideration of the design problems:

1. Possible solutions to the problem of providing support for the free-end saddle denture.
2. Possible solutions to the problem of providing retention for the free-end saddle denture.

Possible solutions to the problem of providing support for the free-end saddle partial denture

Four main procedures have been suggested for use. In a given case, they may be used singly or in any possible combination. They are as follows:

1. Selective load distribution between the supporting tissues.
2. Reduction of the load applied to the saddle.
3. Optimal spreading of load.
4. Use of pressure impressions.

Selective load distribution between the supporting tissues

When load is applied to a free-end saddle which is tooth-and-mucosa-supported, part of the load will be applied to the abutment tooth (via the support/ retention unit on the tooth) and part will be applied to the mucosa underlying the free-end saddle. The distribution of the applied load between these two supporting tissues can be altered by varying the rigidity of the connector used to join the support/retention unit on the abutment tooth to the saddle. If the rigidity of this connector is high, the proportion of the load applied to the abutment tooth will be at a maximum. Where, instead, a flexible connector is used, the proportion of load applied to the abutment tooth will decrease and that applied to the mucous membrane under the saddle will increase. The more flexible the connector which is used, the greater will be the proportion of the load falling on the mucous membrane. Flexible connectors used for the purpose of achieving such selective load distribution are termed stress-breakers. The various types of stress-breakers that may be used in association with either a precision attachment or a clasp unit on the abutment tooth are considered in Chapter 13, page 113.

The decision as to whether or not a stress-breaker is to be used and, where indicated, the type of stress-breaker to be chosen for use, is based on a clinical assessment of the load-bearing potential of the two supporting tissues. Where it is judged that the abutment tooth can safely bear the brunt of the applied load, the use of rigid connection between the saddle and the support/retention unit on the abutment tooth is indicated. At the opposite end of the scale, where the periodontal status of the abutment tooth is suspect and the trabecular structure of the alveolar bone underlying the free-end saddle indicates that a favourable response to load-bearing by the bone is likely, the use of a flexible type of stress-breaker would seem to be indicated. Intermediate clinical findings may indicate the use of a stress-breaker of moderate flexibility. It should, however, be pointed out that the period for which flexible stress-breakers remain functionally active in service can be disappointingly short. Doubts have also been expressed as to whether their theoretical benefits are fully achieved in the clinical stituation.

Reduction of the load applied to the saddle

If the load which is applied to a free-end saddle during the mastication of food is reduced, the risk that the load will cause damage to the supporting tissues will be correspondingly reduced. It has been found that load reduction can be achieved by reducing the size of the occlusal table of the free-end saddle.

To explain this load reduction, it has been suggested that during the mastication of food the masticatory muscles only apply the level of force which is needed to crush the amount of food placed on the occlusal table by tongue and cheek action. If the size of the occlusal table is reduced, the volume of food placed on the table will normally be proprortionally reduced, correspondingly reducing the load applied to the free-end saddle by the masticatory muscles.

An alternative explanation for the load reduction which occurs when the size of the occlusal table is reduced is based on the fact that for a given applied load higher pressures will develop between opposing teeth. As a corollary to this, the level of pressure necessary to achieve efficient mastication can be achieved at a lower level of applied force than that necessary where a larger occlusal table is present.

There are three main ways by which reduction in the size of the occlusal table may be obtained:

1. By reducing the number of teeth set on the saddle. For example, on a saddle which would normally replace the premolars and first and second molars, the second molars may be omitted.

2. By reducing the occlusal size of the teeth which are set on the saddle, relative to the size of their natural predecessors. This is most commonly achieved by reducing the bucco-lingual dimension of the replacement teeth.

3. By substitution of the teeth. For example, a canine may replace a first premolar, or a premolar may replace a molar.

There is a limit to which this procedure can be applied, dictated by the need to maintain a reasonable level of masticatory efficiency in the replacement dentition. Some reduction in the occlusal table is, however, nearly always indicated in the free-end saddle situation, relative to the size of the occlusal table in the original natural dentition.

Optimal spreading of load

The more widely spread be the applied load, the less will be the load per unit area which the supporting tissues have to bear. Load spreading can benefit both the abutment tooth and the mucous membrane and alveolar bone underlying the free-end saddle. The support obtained by placement of a rest on the abutment tooth may be aided by positioning an additional rest on an adjacent tooth. In some cases other teeth may also be used to provide auxiliary support. For example, where the design of a lower partial denture includes the use of a lingual plate, part of the load borne by the free-end saddle will be transferred to all the teeth covered by the lingual plate. A continuous clasp, when present, will perform the same function.

Useful though it is, the principle of optimal spreading of load on the natural teeth must be applied with caution in partial denture design. The desirability of keeping the design of a partial denture as simple as possible should always be borne in mind. All coverage of tooth substance, especially when associated with coverage of the gingival margins, increases the risk that caries or periodontal problems will arise.

No such caution is necessary in the application of the principle of optimal load spreading to the tissues underlying the free-end saddle. In all cases the saddle should extend to the limit defined by a functionally trimmed impression bucally and lingually. Posteriorly, an upper free-end saddle should extend to the pterygo-maxillary fissure (hamular notch) and a lower free-end saddle should extend over the anterior third of the retromolar pad.

Use of pressure impressions

On page 160 attention was drawn to the tissue damage which can arise where tooth-and-mucosa support is used in a free-end saddle. When load is applied to the saddle, the risk that rotatory displacement of the saddle will occur will be at a maximum when the impression of the denture-bearing tissues has been recorded using a minimal pressure technique. This condition will be approached when, as is common in partial denture prosthesis, alginate has been used as the impression material.

If, instead, a pressure impression was taken, the problem of rotatory displacment of the saddle under load would be reduced. Both the teeth and the tissues underlying the free-end saddle would be recorded under pressure. Only minimal displacement of the teeth would occur to the extent permitted by the fibres of the periodontal membranes. A greater degree of displacement would occur in the tissues underlying the free-end saddle, the extent to which this occurs depending upon the value of the applied pressure. In theory, when a denture which has been made on a cast prepared from a pressure impression is inserted, it will fit in position with the tissues underlying the free-end saddle in a condition of displacement corresponding to that present when the pressure impression was taken. There is thus less scope left for displacement of the tissues to occur when masticatory or other loads are applied to the saddle, thereby lessening rotatory displacement under applied load.

As noted in Chapter 15, a pressure impression of a partially edentulous dentition may be obtained by the use of a sectional compound impression. An alternative approach is to limit pressure to the edentulous area of the impression, using alginate in the tooth-bearing portion of the impression and compound or compound plus alginate wash in the edentulous area. Unfortunately, it is difficult to control the level of pressure which will be developed by such impression prodedures. If the pressure reaches an excessive level it may give rise to highly undesirable conditions when the denture is inserted.

Since the denture when seated in position causes displacement of the tissues under the free-end saddle, the tissues will react by producing an upward force on the saddle as they endeavour to return to their resting state. If the direct retention of the denture is such that the denture stays in the fitted position, the tissues under the saddle will be under constant pressure. If this is excessive, the soft tissues may show a pathological reaction varying from hyperaemia to necrosis. Alternatively, if the direct retention of the denture is inadequate to maintain it in its fitted position, the recoil of the displaced tissues will cause the denture to move away from the tissues and except when under biting load the denture will no longer attain its correct position in the oral cavity.

Because of the problems which may arise where pressure impressions are taken at the impression stage of treatment they are rarely used. A safer alternative is considered to be that in which the denture is constructed on a cast prepared from a minimum pressure impression but a saddle relining procedure is then applied, either during or at the end of denture construction. By this means a more controlled level of displacement of the tissues underlying the free-end saddle can be achieved. This serves to reduce the level to which rotatory displacement occurs when load is applied to the free-end saddle but doesn't reach the level where the problems associated with the use of pressure impressions arise.

The procedures that may be used include the Applegate 'altered cast' technique and relining the free-end saddle of a completed denture prior to insertion. The necessary clinical and laboratory procedures are considered in Chapter 15, page 134.

Possible solutions to the problem of providing retention for the free-end saddle denture

These will be considered under the headings used in the discussion of the problems:

1. Possible solutions to the problem of providing direct retention.

2. Possible solutions to the problem of providing indirect retention.

Possible solutions to the problem of providing direct retention

Where it is desired to obtain direct retention for a free-end saddle by placement of a clasp unit on the single abutment tooth, and yet the tooth possesses no useable undercuts, it will be necessary to seek alternative means of obtaining retention. The available alternatives are considered in Chapter 13, page 99. For example, they include the placement of a crown on the tooth to artifically develop undercuts, or alteration of tooth contour by the application of acid etch composite to a suitable surface.

Where the direct retention developed by the placement of a clasp unit on the abutment tooth is judged to be inadequate to meet the retentive needs of a free-end saddle, additional retention can be obtained by positioning a second clasp unit on the contiguous tooth.

When designing a clasp unit to be used to obtain direct retention on the abutment tooth, it should be remembered that in the absence of a posterior abutment tooth the saddle will possess a wide zone of possible translatory paths (Fig. 21.3). Often, the only useable undercut area on the abutment tooth will be found to be present on the disto-buccal surface near the gingival margin. If a gingivally-approaching arm of the Roach 'L' form is used to engage this undercut (Fig. 21.4) it will not prevent posterior displacement of the saddle. If posterior displacement of the saddle arises in function, the clasp arm will correspondingly move

Fig. 21.3 Zone of translation of a free-end saddle (limits indicated by arrows).

Fig. 21.4 A gingivally-approaching clasp arm of the Roach 'L' form on the abutment tooth of a free-end saddle.

Fig. 21.5 A gingivally-approaching clasp arm on the abutment tooth of a free-end saddle, designed to resist posterior displacement of the saddle.

Fig. 21.6 An occlusally-approaching clasp arm on the abutment tooth of a free-end saddle, designed to resist posterior displacement of the saddle.

posteriorly and it will cease to have a retentive action.

To avoid the risk of this happening, if it is desired to use a gingivally-approaching retentive clasp arm, the portion of the clasp contacting the tooth should be extended to enter the interproximal embrasure on the mesial aspect of the tooth (Fig. 21.5). Alternatively, resistance to posterior displacement of the saddle can be provided by the use of an occlusally-approaching clasp arm (Fig. 21.6).

Where the survey line on the abutment tooth permits the use of either an occlusally-approaching or gingivally-approaching retentive arm, the preference is often for use of the gingivally approaching type in that its inherent greater flexibility results in less risk of damaging torque forces being applied to the abutment tooth during masticatory function. This will particularly apply where a decision has been made not to incorporate a stress-breaker in the denture design.

Where direct retention on the abutment tooth of a free-end saddle is to be obtained by use of a precision attachment, the selection of a type of attachment incorporating a stress-breaker may be preferable to avoid undue torque being applied to the abutment tooth. Suitable attachments are considered in Chapter 13, page 113.

Possible solutions to the problem of providing indirect retention

As noted previously, the need to provide indirect retainers to obtain resistance to rotatory displacment of a free-end saddle will be encountered most commonly where bilateral free-end saddles are present (Kennedy Class I dentition). The various types of indirect retainers that may be used are considered in Chapter 13, page 104.

The type most commonly selected for use because of its mechanical advantage is the continuous clasp. Alternatives include Cummer arms, anterior placement of occlusal rests and, in the case of an upper denture only, the use of anterior palatal bars, palatal arms or anterior extensions of a palatal plate.

The improved stability which can be achieved in a partial denture by placement of indirect retainers needs to be weighed against their possible disadvantages. The latter include the biological disadvantages arising from increased coverage of soft or hard tissues of the mouth and the fact that they may give rise to irritation of the tongue or other oral tissues. Their use is particularly indicated where long free-end saddles are present.

FURTHER READING

Anderson J N and Lammie G A 1952 A clinical survey of partial dentures. Brit Dent J 92: 59

Carlsson G E Hedegard B and Koivumaa K K 1961 Studies in partial denture prosthetics. II. An investigation of mandibular partial dentures with double extension saddles. Acta Odont Scand 19: 215

Hindels G W 1952 Load distribution in extension saddle partial dentures. J Prosthet Dent 2: 92

Kroll A J 1973 Clasp designs for extension base removable partial dentures. J Prosthet Dent 29: 408

Lane R P 1947 Practical stress breaking in partial dentures. Dent J Austral 19: 314

Nairn R I 1966 The problem of free-end denture bases. J Prosthet Dent 16: 522

Neill D J 1958 The problem of the lower free-end removable partial denture. J Prosthet Dent 8: 623

Osborne J and Lammie G A 1954 The bilateral free-end saddle lower denture. J Prosthet Dent 4: 640

Preiskel H W 1977 The distal extension prosthesis reappraised. J of Dent 5: 227

PART III

Special Aspects Relating to Complete Denture Treatment

22

The impression stage of treatment

INTRODUCTION

As pointed out in Chapter 8, to enable accurate impressions of the oral tissues to be obtained, it is mandatory that a two-stage impression procedure is used. Pressure impression methods can produce uncertain results, particularly when a closed mouth technique is used, and it is not recommended that they be attempted by the inexperienced operator.

It is proposed to consider minimal pressure and selective pressure impression procedures for complete dentures. The choice of impression methods and materials for a patient under treatment is dependent on the clinical conditions present. Using the procedures to be described, a wide range of clinical conditions can be satisfied.

PRIMARY IMPRESSIONS

Impression compound is a thermoplastic material which is suitable for use in obtaining primary impressions of edentulous mouths. It is incapable of reproducing undercuts, but has very useful properties which enable an impression to be modified by trimming with a sharp knife to reduce excessive bulk, or additions to be made where underextensions exist, and for the impression to be reseated in the mouth as part of the modification procedure.

Impression compound is supplied in flat sheets of some 4 mm thickness. To prepare the material for use it is placed in a water bath at 60°–65°C when it softens to form a plastic mass. Kneading of the softened compound helps to incorporate water into the mass which acts as a plasticiser and also ensures that the material is softened uniformly throughout and is free of any lumps. When fully softened and kneaded the compound is returned to the water bath to await its use.

Selection of stock trays

For the edentulous patient, stock trays having a curved form to the body of the tray are selected (see Fig. 8.1). The trays should be oversize to the extent of providing some 3 mm of space between the inner surface of the tray and the tissues to be impressed, and the flanges should not impinge on the frenal attachments.

The upper tray must extend posteriorly to cover the maxillary tuberosity and hamular notch regions while being supported in correct relationship to the residual alveolar ridge in the anterior part of the mouth. The lower stock tray is selected to ensure coverage of the retromolar pads while the tray is maintained in its correct relationship to the anterior aspect of the residual alveolar ridge.

Where the patient has existing dentures, tray selection is facilitated by observing the denture outline in relation to the stock tray. This is simply effected by resting the denture in the tray. The tray is unlikely to be of exactly the same form as the denture or the mouth to be impressed, and some form of compromise will almost certainly be required.

While generous dimensions of the trays have been recommended, gross overextension should be avoided as this will cause distortion of the peripheral regions of the impression as a result of stretching of the tissues.

The upper primary compound impression

The selected stock tray is carefully warmed and dried by passing it above the flame of a Bunsen burner. Kneaded compound is removed from the water bath and moulded into the form of a ball which is placed in the centre of the palatal region of the tray. Using the thumbs while supporting the tray with the fingers, the compound is spread across the inner aspect of the tray being careful to avoid creases or folds forming on the surface. At the same time, a shallow trough form is developed in the surface of the compound approximately corresponding to the form of the residual alveolar ridge. This form will aid in seating the loaded tray in its correct relationship to the residual alveolar ridge. During this procedure the temperature of the surface of the compound will have fallen, thus reducing its flow properties. To increase the flow properties, and thereby the ability of the material to record surface detail without the application of high pressures, it will be necessary to heat the exposed surface of the compound. This is conveniently carried out by flaming the surface of the impression material. Flaming consists of rapidly passing the exposed compound surface several times over the flame of a Bunsen burner when the surface will appear very smooth and shiny. Burning or sizzling the compound must be avoided.

The temperature of the compound surface will, at this stage, be too high to place in the mouth of a patient without the tissues being damaged and the compound must be tempered before proceeding. Tempering the compound consists of immersing the loaded tray into the water bath in which the compound was originally softened. The temperature of the compound should now be tested gently with the wet palm of the hand. When satisfied that no tissue damage will occur in the mouth, the tray is inserted into the patient's mouth in the manner described in Chapter 8. The tray is centred over the crest of the residual alveolar ridge and pressure in an upwards and backwards direction is applied to the tray. Excess material will be observed to flow into the labial and buccal sulci and onto the soft palate. The patient should be advised to breathe through the nose during the impression procedure so that the oral cavity will be sealed from the naso-pharynx, thus reducing any tendency to gag or retch on the part of the patient.

While the compound is cooling, the tray should be maintained steadily in position using one hand while the other hand is used to carry out border moulding procedures around the periphery of the labial and buccal sulci. These procedures require tissue movements with traction on the tissues in the general direction in which muscle activity would affect the form of the sulci. Particular attention should be paid to the region of labial and buccal frenae.

When the compound has hardened, the impression is removed by requesting the patient to partly close the mouth when the cheek may be reflected on one side using the forefinger of the unoccupied hand to break the peripheral seal and at the same time applying downward pressure. After removal from the mouth, the impression is washed in cold running water and examined. There should be no folds, creases or breaks in the continuity of the surface of the compound, and the anatomical landmarks of the denture bearing surface should be readily distinguishable (Fig. 22.1).

The tray flange should not be visible through the compound. Where a minor deficiency, e.g. in the region of the tuberosity, is present, the compound should be dried and some fresh material softened and added to the impression in the region of the deficiency. After flaming and tempering of the added compound the impression may be reseated into position in the mouth and border moulding

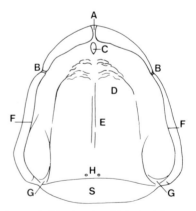

Fig. 22.1 Anatomical landmarks which should be apparent in the maxillary primary impression. A, Labial frenum; B, Buccal frenum; C, Lingual frenum; D, Groove produced by the Depression produced by the Zygomatic process; G, Hamular notch; H, Fovea palatinae; S, Soft palate.

reapplied. Where gross deficiencies are apparent, the impression must be repeated.

When a satisfactory impression has been obtained steps must be taken to reduce the possibility of cross-contamination between the surgery and the laboratory. A satisfactory method of achieve this is to immerse the impression in a suitable antiseptic solution, for example 1 : 20 aqueous solution of Savlon hospital concentrate, after which it may be transported to the laboratory for casting.

The lower primary compound impression

Following kneading, the compound is rolled into a cylindrical form approximately 1.5 cm in diameter and sufficiently long to cover the tray which is then prepared in a similar manner to that described for the upper primary compound impression.

The loaded tray is rotated into the mouth which should not be opened to the maximum extent as this restricts the oral opening in the lateral dimension, making placement of the tray in the mouth difficult. The patient should be instructed to partly close the mouth and raise the tongue when the tray is in the mouth. The tray is centred over the residual alveolar ridge and the cheeks are reflected outwards to reduce the possibility of tissue entrapment. The patient is then instructed to relax the tongue as the tray is seated firmly downwards over the ridge, while the mandible is supported by the operator's thumbs.

Border moulding is then carried out. Lingually the border is moulded by requesting the patient to protrude and elevate the tongue and move it to the left and the right sides of the mouth while the tray is held firmly in position. Labial and buccal border moulding requires the tray to be supported by one hand — the thumb under the chin and with the fingers in the premolar region of the tray — while the free hand provides the necessary traction and simulated activity of the buccal and labial tissues. After the compound has hardened the tray is removed from the mouth by reflecting the tissues in the buccal sulcus to break the seal and removing the tray by means of the handle. The patient is requested to maintain the mouth only partly open during removal to ensure that the temporoman-

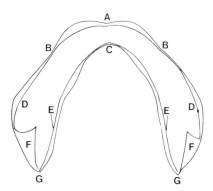

Fig. 22.2 Anatomical landmarks which should be apparent in the mandibular primary impression. A, Labial frenum; B, Buccal frenum; C, Lingual frenum; D, Groove produced by the external oblique line; E, Groove produced by the mylohyoid line; F, Retromolar pad; G, Extension into the retromylohyoid fossa.

dibular joint is protected from possible damage. The impression is washed in cold water and then examined. Landmarks which should be present on the impression are shown in Figure 22.2.

No folds, wrinkles or breaks in the continuity of the surface of the impression should be present, and the border of the tray should not be visible. Additions or repetitions of the procedure are carried out where necessary, and when satisfactory precautions against cross-contamination between the clinic and the laboratory are carried out as described for the upper impression.

Prescription writing

The instructions to the laboratory should include a request to cast the impression in dental plaster being careful to preserve all margins. The material of which the special tray is to be made and the space to be provided for the secondary impression material should be noted and also whether the tray is to be perforated (see Table 8.1). The form of the handle required should also be specified.

In respect of the extensions to be provided for the special tray, under ideal circumstances the cast produced from the primary impression should be made available and the extensions scribed thereon by the operator in accordance with the anatomical requirements of the patient. When this is not possible an alternative method is for the operator to draw an outline on the compound impression using a wax pencil and the outline will be transferred to the cast during the casting procedure.

Other primary impressions

1. Where bony undercuts exist in the mouth of the patient, alginate may be the material of choice for the primary impression. A perforated stock tray of suitable dimensions is selected and an alginate adhesive applied to the tray. The alginate is mixed in accordance with the manufacturer's instructions, the tray loaded and inserted into the mouth as described in Chapter 15 for partial denture impressions. Alginates cannot be modified where deficiencies may exist in an impression and where faults are present, the impression must be repeated. Before passing the impression to the laboratory for casting, anti cross-contamination measures should be observed as described above.

2. Alginate may also be used as a primary impression material when a selective pressure impression technique is to be used at the secondary impression stage (page 175).

3. Where the residual alveolar ridge is so readily displaceable to the extent that severe distortion of the tissue form would result from the use of compound, a fluid type of alginate may be used for the primary impression. This situation most commonly arises in the upper anterior aspect of the residual ridge. Alternatively, where these conditions exist a primary impression may be obtained using impression plaster in a stock nonperforated tray. The method of use of impression plaster is described below.

SECONDARY IMPRESSIONS

Several methods are described below in relation to their application to either the upper or lower jaw. It should be appreciated that they may be equally suitable to either jaw where dictated by the clinical conditions.

The following methods are considered:
1. Plaster impression for the upper jaw.
2. Alginate impression for the upper jaw.
3. Zinc oxide and eugenol paste impression for the lower jaw.
4. Selective pressure impression for the lower jaw.

5. Impression to define the form of the lower denture.

It has been our experience that the first three of the above methods produce satisfactory results for a wide range of patients where no special problems related to the oral conditions exist. The other lower methods to be described have been proved to be useful in dealing with less commonly occurring clinical situations.

Plaster impression for the upper jaw

Modified plaster of Paris when used in a special tray is a very accurate impression material which produces minimal tissue displacement when used in the method to be described. It is less satisfactory for use as a material for obtaining impressions of the lower jaw, being slightly soluble in water and therefore the risk of loss of surface detail from a lower impression is present because of its accessibility to saliva.

Plaster being a brittle material allows reassembly following fracture and provided this is carried out with care, the resultant impression will retain the accuracy which was present before fracture occurred. The special tray for impression plaster impressions is constructed to provide for a uniform layer of 2 mm thickness of the material and to allow 2 mm of freedom from the reflected tissues of the sulcus. The handle of the special tray must not interfere with the actions of the lip so that a simple stub handle is required, or one where a sufficiently long vertical section before it passes between the lips is provided to minimise any manipulative obstruction. Self-curing acrylic resin or shellac baseplate material may be used to construct the tray.

On delivery from the laboratory the special tray should be placed in an antiseptic solution to provide a barrier against cross-contamination. Any cast brought to the clinic from the laboratory must be clean and free of any adherent debris.

As the tray was constructed with a spacer of 2 mm thickness, stops of this dimension must be placed in the tray to enable it to be maintained in correct relationship to the tissues during its use. It is convenient to place one stop in the posterior palatal region of the tray as this will help to control the flow of the impression material and reduce

Fig. 22.3 The hatched areas indicate suitable sites for positioning stops.

discomfort to the patient. Anterior stops of small diameter may be provided in the premolar region as shown in Figure 22.3. A region of minimum displaceability of the soft tissues should be chosen for the stops so that possible distortion of the impressed surface resulting from localised pressure may be avoided. The stops may be incorporated in the material from which the tray is constructed or may be added using carding wax. With the stops in position, the tray is tried in the mouth and careful observation of the relationship of the tissues to the tray made. Posteriorly the tray should cover the vibrating line and the hamular notches and peripherally, the tray should be clear of the reflected tissues of the sulcus by 2 mm. Where over extension is present the tray should be reduced and where underextensions exist, tracing stick compound should be added to correct the extension.

When the tray is satisfactory the patient is instructed to rinse the mouth to remove adherent mucous. Impression plaster is mixed in accordance with the manufactures instructions and placed on the special tray when a creamy consistency is achieved. Sufficient plaster to cover the palatal aspect of the tray and fill that part corresponding to the ridge form is required. When the mix just fails to fall from the tray on its inversion, it is ready for insertion in the mouth. Where the palate has a high vault some of the excess material in the mixing bowl may be placed directly on the palate

of the patient before insertion of the tray. Similarly, some mixed plaster may be placed lateral to the tuberosities before the loaded tray is inserted. These are areas in which air entrapment may prevent ready flow of material during impression taking. The tray is rotated into the mouth and carried tissue-wards with a slight vibratory motion until resistance of the stops indicate that the correct tray/tissue relationship has been achieved. The tray is gently supported in position while border moulding procedures are carried out. Commercial impression plasters are formulated to prolong the initial setting stage to allow time for border moulding to take place. The setting of the plaster is tested using some of the excess material remaining in the mixing bowl. When a clean break of the plaster sample accompanied by a snapping sound can be produced, the impression is ready for removal from the mouth.

Removal is effected by requesting the patient to partially close the mouth. The lips are then parted and the forefinger of one hand passed along the side of the tray so that the pad of the finger lies between the zygomatic process and the border of the tray. Wedging the finger in this position while lifting the lip should break the seal about the impression and allow its removal. The seal posteriorly can be broken by asking the patient to cough. This causes the soft palate to elevate away from the set impression. If difficulty in breaking the seal is encountered, a few drops of water from the water syringe should be placed at the periphery of the impression and the removal procedure repeated. Immediately on removal of the impression from the mouth, it should be placed on the bracket table and the mouth inspected for any fragments which may be remaining. Common sites from which a portion of the flange of the impression has fractured are the labial border and the tuberosity region. Any broken fragments should be removed from the mouth using dressing tweezers and placed carefully on the bracket table. The patient may then be invited to rinse the mouth.

After thorough drying the broken pieces are fitted into place in the impression. As each piece is seen to fit accurately to place it is held in position using molten sticky wax which is applied to the outer aspects of the impression — not, of course, to the fitting surface. In the completed impression the surface should be intact and free of defects. The tray should not be visible through the plaster and all of the anatomical landmarks previously described for the upper denture bearing surface should be clearly visible. The impression is then ready for the cross-contamination prevention procedure to be carried out prior to casting.

Alginate impression for the upper jaw

Where bony undercuts exist and alginate material has been selected, a tray is produced of similar form to that described for use with impression plaster, except that perforations and a 3 mm spacer are required. After coating with an alginate adhesive the tray should be loaded with alginate mixed in accordance with the manufacturer's instructions. Only sufficient material to obtain the impression is required — gross excess must be avoided as this will result in distortion of the peripheral tissues. Alginate material may be placed directly in the mouth as described for the plaster impression. When set, the tray is removed from tissue contact using a rapid action following breaking of the peripheral seal by elevating the lip. After removal from the mouth the impression is washed in running water and inspected. When satisfied that the impression is acceptable, it is inserted into an antiseptic solution before removal to the laboratory for casting. No additions can be made to set alginate and where an impression is deficient, it should be removed from the tray and the impression repeated.

Zinc oxide and eugenol paste impression for the lower jaw

For this method, a close fitting acrylic resin tray is required. When tried in the mouth, the peripheral extensions should be clear of the reflection of the soft tissues by some 3 mm. A short stub handle which does not interfere with lip or tongue activity should be provided.

Zinc oxide and eugenol paste is an accurate impression material provided that it is fully supported so that it is necessary to use an impression tray which covers the whole of the usable denture supporting tissue. To achieve this, the periphery of the special tray is accurately border moulded

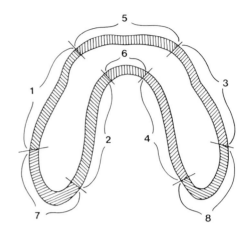

Fig. 22.4 Suggested sections about the periphery of a lower special tray which are manageable for border moulding, using tracing stick compound.

using tracing stick compound. It is not possible to border mould the entire periphery in a single operation and the procedure is carried out in conveniently manageable sections until the border is complete.

It is suggested that some eight sections might be used as shown in Figure 22.4. Having checked in the mouth that the special tray is underextended to the extent of some 3 mm around the periphery, the section to be moulded is dried. Tracing stick compound is carefully heated above a Bunsen burner flame and then attached to the margin of the impression tray in the chosen section. This should be done neatly avoiding coverage of the fitting surface of the tray. After tempering in the water bath at 65°C, the tray is inserted in the mouth and border moulding is carried out as described for the primary impression procedure. When satisfactory, the procedure is repeated for each section of the margin until border moulding is complete. There should be no visible joins between each section. The special tray is now ready for a wash impression to be taken using zinc oxide and eugenol paste. The paste is mixed in accordance with the manufacturer's instructions and a thin complete layer of the material is spread over the fitting surface of the tray. This is inserted into the mouth and seated to contact the mucoperiosteum covering the residual alveolar ridge, taking care to avoid trapping the lingual and buccal tissues during seating. Border moulding procedures are carried out and the impression is removed from the mouth after setting as indicated by the development of a firm, non-sticky surface of the excess material. After gentle washing in running cold water the impression is examined for defects. There should be a thin covering of paste over the border moulding compound and a defect-free continuous covering of paste over the whole surface of the impression. The impression is now ready for immersion in an antiseptic solution prior to its removal to the laboratory for casting in dental stone.

Selective pressure impression for the lower jaw

In some circumstances a selective pressure impression may be indicated for the mandibular residual ridge. For example, the mucoperiosteum covering the crest of the ridge may not appear to be able to tolerate the forces transmitted to it during normal mastication without the patient experiencing considerable pain and discomfort and the peripheral tissues may be considered better able to tolerate the major thrust of the forces developed during chewing. The first stage of the selective pressure impression for such a patient is to obtain a primary impression of the lower ridge and the peripheral tissues using an alginate impression material in a stock tray. It may be necessary to modify the stock tray using impression compound as described for partial denture impressions in Chapter 15. The objective of this impression is to obtain a cast of the lower ridge where the mucosa has not been subjected to the displacing forces which would be applied using a more viscous material such as compound.

The impression is cast in laboratory plaster and a perforated special tray is produced in acrylic resin using a 2 mm spacer, and with the periphery some 3 mm short of the reflection of the tissues in the sulci. Three short stub handles should be provided — one in the midline anteriorly and one on each side in the first molar region. Using impression compound an impression of the primary cast is obtained in the special tray. This compound impression purports to represent the form of the undisplaced tissues overlying the ridge. The compound lined special tray is then tried in the mouth of the patient and border moulding procedures are carried out around the entire periphery of the tray.

On completion of the border moulding, all the impression compound overlying the crest of the ridge is cut and scraped away, exposing the perforations in the special tray, but leaving the moulded border complete. The tray should then be tried back in the mouth when the patient should confirm that the tray is not in contact with the crestal mucoperiosteum. A freely flowing mix of zinc oxide eugenol paste is then loaded into the tray which is then inserted into the mouth and pressed firmly to contact the underlying tissues. The fingers should be located on the posterior stub handles to apply constant pressure while the mandible is supported by the thumbs. The perforations will allow free escape of the excess impression paste over the crestal tissues without the development of high pressures while the peripheral tissues will be displaced under the effects of the forces applied by the fingers. Border moulding procedures are required during setting of the paste to avoid overextension developing. The impression, when satisfactory, should be cast in dental stone after taking the usual cross-contamination prevention measures.

Impression to define the form of the lower denture

Because of the difficulties experienced by some patients in the management of a complete lower denture produced using conventional methods, special methods have been developed which aim to determine the form of an appliance in relation to the immediate environmental tissues during certain muscular activities. These methods delineate the space available for the lower denture within the large opposing muscle groups associated with the tongue and cheeks.

The method to be described assumes that a satisfactory upper denture can be produced or is already available. Where both upper and lower dentures are to be produced the conventional procedures for complete dentures are carried out up to the stage of registration of the retruded jaw relationship, and allowing for an increased freeway space of up to 1 mm in addition to the average value of 2–4 mm. The upper denture is then set up to meet the aesthetic requirements of the patient within the limits permitted by the available

Fig. 22.5 Denture form impression technique. Left: Coronal section through the molar region of a suitable tray for the denture form impression. Right: Lateral view of the upper denture and prepared tray. A, Upper denture; B, Perforated special tray; C, Cast of the lower residual alveolar ridge.

anatomical form of the tissues. A further special tray is then constructed. The body of this tray is of the form which would be used for an alginate impression, i.e. of acrylic resin which is spaced and perforated. The special tray carries a vertical diaphragm which is constructed to contact the occlusal surfaces of the upper posterior teeth and anteriorly to contact lightly the lingual aspects of the upper teeth near the incisal edges. The diaphragm is thin to provide minimum interference with the tissues and broadens out on the superior aspect to occlude with the upper teeth in the retruded jaw relationship (Fig. 22.5).

The diaphragm is perforated as well as the body of the special tray and stops are required to locate the tray in its correct relationship to the patient's tissues.

To obtain the impression, the patient is first instructed in the muscular activity to be used in forming the impression material. The activities include grimacing, sucking and swallowing, and the patient is required to carry these out three times with the tray and upper denture in the mouth while closed into the retruded contact position. The tray is then removed from the mouth and dried after which it is coated on all surfaces with alginate adhesive. Mixed alginate is then coated on all surfaces of the tray which is returned to the mouth and the patient requested to carry out the rehearsed activities. Because of the time required for the impression to be moulded adequately, it is necessary to select a slowly setting alginate. When set, the alginate impression is removed from the mouth and carefully inspected. While such an impression is not likely to have a conventional appearance, careful inspection will indicate any absence of surface continuity or badly formed borders. Incorrect positioning of the vertical diaphragm will be indicated by its exposure through the alginate. In such a case the impression should be repeated after relocating the diaphragm. It must be borne in mind that in addition to the conventional 'fitting' surface the denture-form impression utilises all surfaces as fitting surfaces.

The usual precautions are taken in respect of protection against cross-contamination and the impression is then forwarded to the laboratory for casting. All surfaces of the denture-form impression must be recorded in the cast so that sectional casting is required. The casting can be dismantled for removal of the impression and subsequently reassembled. The production of the various sections of such a cast requires a high degree of technical skill.

The reassembled cast will delineate the space formerly occupied by the impression and this represents the space available for, and the form which, the lower denture should take. Its location in relationship to the upper denture will also have been registered in the impression as the swallowing action used in obtaining the impression will cause the mandible to assume the retruded contact relationship.

This brief description is only one of several methods available for defining the form of the lower denture. It has been included as an illustration of a way in which the denture space may be delineated. The upper denture form can be similarly delineated and the student is referred to the literature for more comprehensive information on this aspect of complete denture treatment.

IMPRESSIONS FOR RELINING AND REBASING COMPLETE DENTURES

Dentures which have been in use for a prolonged period often become ill-fitting because of changes such as continuing bone resorption, which have taken place. In these circumstances, rather than produce new dentures, relining or rebasing the existing denture. Both procedures require an alternative. Relining consists of adding denture base material to the fitting surface of a denture to improve its adaptation to the tissues. Rebasing is the process of providing a new denture base to an existing denture. Both procedures require an impression to be obtained using the existing denture as an impression tray.

Apart from improving the fit of an existing denture a relining or rebasing impression may be required where a soft lining is to be incorporated in a denture.

Only the impression stage will be described in this section. The reader is referred to the literature for the indications and contra-indications for the procedures and for the technical aspects of the processes used.

A careful examination of the mouth and of the existing dentures is required before commencement. Where there has been a loss of vertical dimension for example, the procedure may be contra-indicated, although some increase in vertical dimension can be produced in certain cases.

In general, the impression for both procedures is similar and involves using the existing denture as a special impression tray. For an upper denture, where the tissues are traumatised, a period of use of tissue conditioning material may be required to produce a healthy tissue base for the new impression. When taking the impression, all undercuts are removed from the existing denture and the denture flanges shortened to ensure clearance from interference with the reflected tissues about the periphery of the denture seating area. As the impression will be obtained using zinc oxide and eugenol paste, accurate support of this material is required and border moulding of the denture base using tracing stick compound may be required wherever deficiencies in extensions are present. Once the denture has been prepared to the form of a special, close fitting impression tray having border moulded flanges, it is ready for use. Zinc oxide and eugenol impression paste is mixed in accordance with the manufacturer's instructions and spread over the fitting surface of the denture. Where displaceable tissue is present, the palate of the denture may be perforated, prior to loading with the mixed paste, in order to prevent the development of high pressures during the impression procedure. The denture is then carried firmly to contact with the oral tissues and the patient asked to close into the retruded contact position so that a check on the occlusal relationship with the opposing dentition can be made. If satisfactory, the patient is asked to open the mouth and the denture supported in position while border moulding is carried out. A similar procedure, but using stops of the required thickness formed with impression compound can be used where an increase in the occlusal vertical dimension is required as part of rebasing procedure. This is not a recommended procedure to be attempted by the inexperienced operator because of the difficulties likely to be encountered in respect of possible gross changes in the retruded contact position between opposing dentures.

For the lower denture the preparation for the relining impression is similar. All undercut areas are eliminated by grinding and the peripheral form of the denture is corrected wherever necessary by border moulding using tracing stick compound. A zinc oxide and eugenol impression paste impression is then taken using an open mouth method as described above for the complete lower denture impression.

FURTHER READING

Boucher C O 1973 The relining of complete dentures. J Prosthet Dent 30: 521.

Christensen F T 1971 Relining techniques for complete dentures. J Prosthet Dent 26: 373

Ellinger C W 1973 Minimising problems in making a complete lower impression. J Prosthet Dent 30: 553

Grant A A and Walsh J F 1975 Reducing cross-contamination in prosthodontics. J Prosthet Dent 34: 324

Lawson W A 1978 Current concepts and practice in complete dentures. Impressions: principles and practice. J Dent 6: 43

Matthews E, McIntyre H, Wain E A and Bates J F 1961 The full denture problem. Brit Dent J 111: 401

Osborne J 1964 Two impression methods for mobile fibrous ridges. Brit Dent J 117: 392

Storer R and McCabe J F 1981 An investigation of methods available for sterilising impressions. Brit Dent J 151: 217

Watt D M and MacGregor A R 1976 Designing Complete Dentures. Saunders, Philadelphia

23

The jaw registration stage of treatment

INTRODUCTION

To the inexperienced operator, this is likely to prove to be the longest and most difficult of the stages involved in complete denture construction. The length of the stage is due to the need to carry out in sequence a series of procedures, each of which can be quite time-consuming. The difficulty arises firstly from the fact that the stage calls for an element of judgement on the part of the operator, which, at times, can present problems to even the most experienced of operators. Secondly, the stage requires the exercise of controlled tongue and jaw movements by the patient. Some patients seem to lack the necessary neuro-physiological control to be able to produce at will the required movements.

The keystone to success at this stage is achieving a state of full relaxation in the patient. If a satisfactory rapport has been developed between patient and operator, the patient will be confident of the ability of the operator and will be more able to relax both mentally and physically.

The jaw registration stage is carried out using upper and lower occlusal rims. The sequence of procedures which is applied is as follows:

1. Checking extension, retention and stability of upper and lower occlusal rims.

2. Shaping the upper occlusal rim to provide a guide to the setting of the artificial teeth.

3. Registering the vertical component of jaw relationship.

4. Registering the horizontal component of jaw relationship (retruded jaw relationship).

5. Registering protrusive and/or lateral jaw relationships.

6. Obtaining a face-bow registration.

7. Selecting the teeth.

8. Preparing a written prescription.

All the above procedures need to be applied for all patients except for procedures 5 and 6. The latter are optional procedures which are selected for use where special needs apply.

CHECKING THE EXTENSION, RETENTION AND STABILITY OF THE UPPER AND LOWER OCCLUSAL RIMS

The upper occlusal rim should be inserted and the peripheral extension of the baseplate checked labially and buccally for conformity with the level of the functional sulcus. Adequate allowance should be present for any frenal attachments. Posteriorly, the baseplate should extend to the vibrating line of the palate.

Retention should be tested by attempting to pull the baseplate away from the underlying tissues by the application of force bilaterally at right angles to the alveolar ridge.

Stability should be tested by applying pressure in a tissueward direction to the occlusal surface of the rim on each side in the premolar area and noting whether any rocking of the baseplate occurs. A similar series of checks should then be applied to the lower occlusal rim. Here, the check on extension will include an examination of the lingual extension of the baseplate. Posteriorly, the lower baseplate should be seen to extend onto the anterior third of the retromolar pads.

If the extension, retention or stability of either rim is found to be unsatisfactory, and yet the baseplates are correctly adapted to the master casts, there is an indication that a fault has occurred in the secondary impression stage or subsequently in the preparation of the master casts. These stages should be repeated before proceeding further.

SHAPING THE UPPER OCCLUSAL RIM TO PROVIDE A GUIDE TO THE SETTING OF THE ARTIFICIAL TEETH

The upper occlusal rim should be inserted and the patient observed in front face and profile view to determine the degree of support for the facial tissues provided by the rim and baseplate. Wax should be added or trimmed from the labial and buccal aspects of the occlusal rim until it is judged that the correct level of support for the facial tissues has been achieved.

Where the patient is already wearing dentures and has indicated what aesthetic change, if any, they would like to be provided in the new dentures, useful guidance will be provided for the required form of the occlusal rim. Where the patient expresses satisfaction with the appearance of their present dentures, the labial and buccal form of the upper occlusal rim should duplicate the denture form. Alternatively, where the patient requests an increase or decrease in lip or cheek support relative to that provided by the present dentures, appropriate modifications should be made to the contour of the occlusal rim.

The occlusal plane should then be developed by modifying, as necessary, the occlusal surface of the rim. Correct placement of the occlusal plane is obtained by relating it to certain anatomical landmarks on the face. These are as follows:

1. In front face view, the occlusal plane is set parallel to a line joining the pupils of the eyes.

2. In lateral view, the occlusal plane is set parallel to the ala-tragal line.

3. The occlusal plane is set to lie approximately 2 mm below the lip at rest.

Choice of these landmarks is based on an observation that they bear a fairly constant relationship to the occlusal plane of most natural dentitions. By using them to guide the development of the occlusal plane on the upper occlusal rim there is a reasonable assurance that the artificial teeth will be set in a position that will provide

both acceptable aesthetics and satisfactory masticatory and phonetic functioning.

Setting the occlusal plane of the rim parallel to the indicated facial landmarks in front face and lateral view can be assisted by use of the Fox occlusal plane guide (Fig. 23.1A). This is made in either metal or plastic and has intra-oral and extra-

Fig. 23.1 A, The Fox occlusal plane guide. a = Intra-oral portion, b = Extra-oral portion. B, Illustrating use of the Fox occlusal plane guide to set the occlusal plane parallel to the interpupillary line. C, Illustrating use of the Fox occlusal plane guide to set the occlusal plane parallel to the ala-tragal line.

oral portions. The intra-oral portion is positioned to lie on the occlusal surface of the rim. The extra-oral portion serves to provide a magnified view of the inclination of the occlusal surface, facilitating observation of the rim inclination relative to that of the appropriate facial landmarks. Its use is illustrated in Figure 23.1, B and C.

In developing the level of the occlusal plane relative to that of the lip at rest (action 3), setting the plane approximately 2 mm below the lip at rest is normally satisfactory for patients in the young and middle-age groups. For elderly patients, setting the occlusal plane nearer to the level of the lip at rest may be indicated, to take account of the loss of lip tonus and attrition of the incisal edges of the natural teeth that would usually have resulted in decreased display of the natural dentition were it still present. Note should also be taken of the level of the occlusal plane in the present upper denture where one is being worn. If the patient expresses satisfaction with the appearance of the denture it is usually desirable to duplicate the level in the occlusal rim, even where this may differ from the 'normal' level.

Following completion of the development of the occlusal plane on the upper occlusal rim, certain guide lines should then be scribed on the labial surface of the rim. These lines can provide guidance in the later stage of selecting the size of the anterior teeth to be used on the upper denture and can also assist in achieving optimal aesthetics when the teeth are set up to develop a trial denture. The lines used are as follows:
1. Centre line
2. Canine lines
3. High lip line

Centre line

A central vertical line should be scribed on the labial surface of the upper occlusal rim to the level of the occlusal plane. When setting-up the upper anterior teeth, the centre line on the occlusal rim will be used to indicate the contact point of the central incisors. To achieve a symmetrical display of the dentition it is thus necessary for the centre line to mark the median line of the face, with special reference to the lips. The position of the philtrum of the upper lip has a major but not exclusive

role in deciding the most appropriate position for the centre line — deviations of the nose from the midline and any other asymmetry of the face must also be taken into consideration.

Canine lines

Vertical lines should be scribed on each side of the labial surface of the upper occlusal rim to the level of the occlusal plane, to indicate the position of the canines. As noted in Chapter 11, page 76, these may be developed to indicate either the cusp tips of the canines or their distal surfaces. Marking of canine lines at the distal surfaces is generally selected as it provides information which is more readily usable at the stage of selecting the overall width of the upper anterior teeth.

High lip line

A horizontal line may be marked on the labial surface of the upper occlusal rim to indicate the position of maximum elevation of the upper lip when the patient is smiling. This line can assist in selecting the length of the upper anterior teeth to be used. Teeth should be chosen whose length is equal to or exceeds that of the distance between the high lip line and the occlusal plane. This will ensure than an unaesthetic display of the labial flange of the denture does not occur when the patient is smiling.

REGISTERING THE VERTICAL COMPONENT OF JAW RELATIONSHIP

The importance of developing the correct occlusal vertical dimension in denture construction has been emphasised in Chapter 9. The serious consequences which can arise from the use of either an excessive or deficient vertical dimension are listed on page 64 of that Chapter.

A method that may be used to determine the occlusal vertical dimension is presented in some detail on page 63 of Chapter 9 and may be summarised as follows: The patient should be seated comfortably in a dental chair in an upright posture with the head erect. Every effort should be made to obtain a state of full relaxation in the patient. Markers (for example, self-adhesive paper dots) are attached to the nose and chin of the patient in the midline of the face, choosing sites which do not appear to move independently of the skeleton.

An initial measurement should be made of the distance between the markers when the mandible is in rest jaw relationship with the maxilla, using an instrument such as a Willis gauge. The lower occlusal rim only should be inserted when this measurement is made. The presence of the lower occlusal rim is desirable since, by providing support for the lower lip, it can influence the position of the chin marker. Also, the weight of the lower occlusal rim may influence the resting position adopted by the mandible. In distinction, the presence or absence of the upper occlusal rim has little effect on the nose marker because of the more remote position of the latter. Both rims must not be inserted at this stage since if their combined vertical height exceeded that necessary for the mandible to be at rest vertical dimension, measurement of the latter would be impossible.

To persuade the patient to adopt the rest jaw relationship, he or she should be asked to moisten the lips and then close the mouth until light lip contact is obtained. Alternatively, the patient should be asked to swallow and then relax the jaws, or to pronounce the letter 'm'. For the experienced operator, observation of the state of relaxation of the patient's facial tissues also provides guidance on when the position of rest jaw relationship has been achieved.

The initial measurement of the distance between the markers with the mandible in rest jaw relationship should be repeated several times. A consistent value over several readings is essential if reliance is to be placed on the measurement.

The upper occlusal rim should then be inserted and the patient persuaded to close up to bring the occlusal surfaces of the upper and lower rims into contact in retruded jaw relationship. If uneven contact of the occlusal surfaces of the rims is seen to occur, the occlusal surface of the lower rim should be adjusted until even contact over the whole surface is achieved. A reading of the distance between the markers should then be made with the rims in contact. The difference between this reading and the initial reading made at the rest vertical dimension will show whether any freeway space is present. Modifications to the occlusal surface of the lower rim should be made by trimming or addition of wax as necessary until an acceptable value of freeway space has been achieved (normally in the range of 2–4 mm). The value of the freeway space selected for use in the new dentures must, however, take into account any previous denture-wearing experience of the patient. If the patient is wearing dentures which have a deficient, absent or even negative value for freeway space, it is nearly always desirable for the new dentures to be made using a value of freeway space in the range 2–4 mm. Where, though, a patient has worn one set of dentures for many years and as a consequence of alveolar resorption and/or tooth wear, an increased value of freeway space has developed, for example to 8 mm, the use of a greater than normal freeway space in the new dentures is often indicated. A compromise value about half way between the 'normal' value and the freeway space of the old dentures may be selected, which would be of the order of 5 mm in the above example. Over the years it is likely that the patient's musculature will have gradually adapted to the change in freeway space, and a gross change in value in the new dentures may make it very difficult for the muscles to be able to re-adapt in the short term, leading to possible rejection of the dentures by the patient. This problem is particularly liable to occur in elderly patients.

Where adjustment of the depth of the lower occlusal rim is necessary to achieve the required value of freeway space, note should be made of the relative depths of the upper and lower rims as the modification proceeds. The aim should be to achieve a reasonable balance between the two rims, which serve as prototypes for the eventual upper and lower dentures. Excessive depth or deficient depth in the lower occlusal rim in particular should be avoided. The former can result in instability of the lower denture by 'walling-in' of the tongue, while the latter can produce a denture which is both prone to fracture and provides unsatisfactory aesthetics. Although the position of the occlusal plane of the upper occlusal rim has been developed to provide optimal aesthetics in the denture and hence should be unmodified if possible, instances arise where it may be necessary to change the initially selected level of the occlusal plane. Under these circumstances, it is permissible for the occlusal plane to be raised or lowered as necessary, to avoid the development of an unsatisfactory depth in the lower denture.

REGISTERING THE HORIZONTAL COMPONENT OF JAW RELATIONSHIP (RETRUDED JAW RELATIONSHIP)

The retruded jaw relationship is the jaw relationship in the horizontal plane at which the location of the occlusal rims will be registered. The reasons for acceptance of this jaw relationship in complete denture construction are presented in Chapter 9, page 65.

When the occlusal rims have been trimmed to the occlusal vertical dimension, the rims should be inserted and the patient persuaded to bring the occlusal surfaces of the rims into contact with the mandible in the retruded jaw relationship. Achieving this may be helped by asking the patient to curl the tip of the tongue upwards and backwards to touch the posterior border of the baseplate of the upper occlusal rim. Alternative methods which may be used to obtain retruded jaw relationship are usually based on tiring the muscles responsible for protrusion of the mandible. Reference should be made to a more advanced text for details of these methods.

With the mandible positioned in what is believed to be retruded jaw relationship, vertical lines should be scribed on the labial or buccal surfaces of both occlusal rims to indicate their location in the horizontal plane. This may be achieved by extending the previously-marked centre and canine lines on the upper occlusal rim downwards onto the lower occlusal rim. Alternatively or additionally, new lines may be scribed on the buccal aspects of both rims in about the second premolar position on each side.

The patient should then be persuaded to open and then close the mouth alternately to bring the rims into contact in retruded jaw relationship on four or five occasions. The relative position of the lines on the upper and lower occlusal rims should be observed each time closure occurs. If, on any occasion, the lines on the lower rim are seen to

develop a position posterior to the corresponding lines on the upper rim, new lines should be marked in this position and the check procedure should then be repeated. Only when a consistent pattern of coincidence of the lines is seen to occur on repeated closure should the developed position be accepted as that of retruded jaw relationship. When this has been achieved, registration of the rims in this position should be established.

To obtain the registration, 'V' shaped notches, approximately 5 mm deep, should be cut in the occlusal surface of the upper rim in about the second premolar position on each side. The posterior segments of the lower occlusal rim should then be reduced in height by about 2 mm. This reduction should be carried out from the first premolar area of the rim on each side to the posterior extremities of the rim. This is necessary to provide space for the wax which will be built up on the lower occlusal rim at a later stage. It also provides an escape way for any excess wax which is present. The unreduced anterior segment of the lower rim serves to preserve the previously-developed contact position of the rims in the vertical plane at the occlusal vertical dimension.

Softened modelling wax should then be added to the posterior segments of the lower rim to a height considered to be just a little in excess of that needed to restore the original height of the rim, with some heaping up of the wax in the regions opposing the notches cut in the upper rim. The occlusal rims should be inserted and the patient persuaded to close in retruded jaw relationship until the anterior segments of the rims come into contact. The lines previously scribed on the rims to denote the position of retruded jaw relationship should again be seen to coincide. If not, the registration must be repeated until this condition is satisfied. The assembled upper and lower occlusal rims should then be removed from the mouth, cooled under running cold water and the rims then separated. The upper and lower occlusal rims should then be re-inserted and tested by repeated closure to ensure that a consistent position of full mandibular retrusion has been registered. The patient should also be asked to indicate if even contact of the rims is occurring.

The rims should then be fitted on the casts and a check made that no distortion of the baseplates has occurred in the registration procedure. Via use of the registration notches, the rims should then be located in the registration position and a check made that neither the baseplates nor the land areas of the casts are interfering with rim location. Where any interference is seen to occur, the baseplates and/or the land areas of the casts should be trimmed until location of the casts is provided only by the contacting occlusal surfaces of the rims.

The casts may then be mounted on an articulator in the position registered by the occlusal rims, in preparation for the development of the trial dentures.

Registration of the horizontal component of jaw relationship using the procedure described above will prove to be successful for the majority of patients requiring the provision of complete dentures. In the treatment of a minority of patients considerable difficulty may be experienced, though, in achieving a consistent position of mandibular retrusion. These patients often give a history of having been edentulous for a number of years but of never having worn any dentures. The need to chew on edentulous ridges over a prolonged period often leads to the development of a habit of mandibular protrusion which may be difficult to break in the above registration procedure. Habitual protrusive posturing of the mandible may also occur where the patient has worn one set of dentures for a prolonged period and an excessive freeway space has developed as a consequence of alveolar resorption and/or tooth wear.

Where the problem of achieving a consistent position of mandibular retrusion is encountered, the use of an alternative method of recording the horizontal component of jaw relationship may be considered. This is by the method of gothic arch tracing. The tracing may be carried out extra-orally or intra-orally, a range of apparatus of varying design being available for use in each method. As an example of the use of gothic arch tracing, a procedure involving intra-oral tracing using one of the available range of apparatus will be considered. Reference should be made to a more advanced text for details of the alternative procedures.

The apparatus used consists of two trapezoidal-shaped metal plates, each having a maximum width of approximately 4 cm, a depth of 2 cm and a thickness of 1 mm. One of the plates has a 3 mm diameter hole at its centre, the hole being provided with a screw thread which allows a pointed screw to be raised and lowered relative to the plate. A locknut is provided to allow the screw to be set at any required position.

The apparatus is used in association with upper and lower occlusal rims, the upper occlusal rim first being shaped as described above (page 180). The lower occlusal rim should then be trimmed to provide an exaggerated freeway space of about 5 mm. The two metal plates should then be attached securely to the upper and lower occlusal rims, spanning the central region of each, the plate carrying the screw normally being attached to the upper rim. A plan view of the metal plates in position on the occlusal rims is shown in Figure 23.2

The rims should then be inserted and the vertical positioning of the screw carried on the upper metal plate adjusted until the tip of the screw contacts the lower metal plate at the occlusal vertical dimension. The locknut on the screw should then

Fig. 23.2 Plan view of the apparatus for intra-oral gothic arch tracing in position on upper and lower occlusal rims.

Fig. 23.3 Anterior view of the occlusal rims and the apparatus for intra-oral gothic arch tracing.

be tightened to maintain this position. An anterior view of the occlusal rims and tracing apparatus is shown in Figure 23.3.

The patient should be persuaded to make a range of horizontal jaw movements, during which a check should be made that the point of the screw remains in contact with the lower metal plate, and that contact does not occur between the rims or baseplates. Where contact between rims and/or baseplates is seen to occur, they should be trimmed to remove the obstruction.

A coating should then be applied to the upper surface of the lower metal plate to allow a tracing to be developed. This may be achieved by the use of engineer's marking ink, a wax pencil or carbon from a candle flame. The upper and lower rims with the attached tracing apparatus should be inserted and the patient persuaded again to make a series of mandibular movements in the horizontal plane. A tracing of the form shown in Figure 23.4 should be produced, the apex of the gothic arch form marking the position of maximum mandibular retrusion (retruded jaw relationship). To enable the rims to be sealed together in the indicated position of retruded jaw relation, a small disc with a central perforation should be fixed to the lower

Fig. 23.4 Plan view of a gothic arch tracing on the lower metal plate.

metal plate, with the perforation overlying the apex of the gothic arch tracing. The rims and tracing apparatus should be inserted and the patient persuaded to adopt the position of the mandible in which the tip of the screw enters the central perforation of the disc fixed to the lower plate. Location of upper and lower rims in this position should then be achieved by placing a mix of impression plaster between the rims in the premolar and molar areas on each side. The assemblage of occlusal rims and tracing apparatus should then be positioned on the casts in preparation for the mounting of the casts.

Certain clinical conditions contraindicate the use of gothic arch tracing for the registration of the horizontal component of jaw relationship. For example, the method is difficult to apply where gross Class II or Class III skeletal jaw relationships are present. To allow tracing to occur, the upper and lower tracing plates need to be positioned on the rims so that they lie approximately one above the other. Such a setting can be difficult to achieve where there is a gross discrepancy in the anteroposterior relationship of the upper and lower jaws. The method is also not recommended for use where the mucosa of the denture-bearing areas shows marked variation in displaceability, as this can give rise to tilting of the baseplates as tracing proceeds.

REGISTERING PROTRUSIVE AND/OR LATERAL JAW RELATIONSHIPS

These relationships are recorded where it is desired to provide individual adjustment of the condylar guidance mechanism of an articulator. Theoretical aspects of their use are considered in Chapter 9, page 65.

It is usual practice to obtain records of protrusive and/or of lateral jaw relationships by the utilisation of the occlusal rims which are also being used to obtain a record of retruded jaw relationship. Where multiple recordings of jaw relationship are to be undertaken using one set of occlusal rims, it is essential that the rims should posses a high level of resistance to distortion at oral temperatures. This can best be provided by the use of rims constructed in impression compound. Because of the greater difficulty likely to be encountered in the shaping of impression compound rims relative to those in wax, it is helpful if an initial registration is taken using wax occlusal rims following the procedures described above. The casts can then be mounted on a simple hinge articulator in the position provided by this registration. Upper and lower impression compound rims can then be constructed on the casts to duplicate the form of the wax rims. Only minimum modification of the impression compound rims should then be necessary in their subsequent clinical application.

The upper and lower impression compound rims should be inserted and the occlusal surface of the lower rim adjusted until even contact of the rim surfaces occurs when the patient closes into retruded jaw relationship. Contact should also be established at a vertical height which provides approximately 2 mm more freeway space than that required to be present in the dentures. 'V' notches, approximately 5 mm deep, should then be cut in the occlusal surfaces of both the upper and lower occlusal rims in the second premolar region on each side of the arches. A thin coating of petroleum jelly should be applied to the occlusal surfaces of both rims and in the prepared notches, to act as a separator.

A wafer of softened modelling wax, approximately 3 mm thick, should then be placed between the inserted upper and lower occlusal rims and the patient persuaded to close in retruded jaw relationship until it is judged that a vertical dimension providing the required value of freeway space has been achieved. This should then be checked by measuring the occlusal vertical dimension relative to the rest vertical dimension. Where necessary, the registration should be repeated with increase or decrease in the thickness of the wax wafer until the correct value of the occlusal vertical dimension has been established. Repeated closures should also be applied to ensure by observation of consistency of rim markings, that the retruded law relatiomship has been recorded.

The wax wafer registration should then be removed from the rims and stored in cold water to reduce the risk of distortion occurring. Labelling of the record (for example, with the letter 'R') is advisable to facilitate subsequent identification.

To obtain a record of a protrusive jaw relationship, the occlusal rims should be inserted and a wax wafer of softened modelling wax should be prepared. The wafer should be a little thicker than that used to record the retruded jaw relationship and a value of approximately 5 mm is desirable. The wafer should be placed between the upper and lower rim surfaces and the patient persuaded to close into a position providing approximately 5 mm of mandibular protrusion. It is important that the position recorded is one of true protrusion, involving an equal level of translation in both condyles. As closure on the wax wafer occurs, careful note should be made of the centre line markings on the upper and lower rims, the mandible being guided by the operator into a position of line coincidence, indicating that no lateral deviation of the mandible has occurred. The vertical dimension of the recorded relationship in protrusion is not critical, although ensuring that the wafer is at least 2 mm thick after the record has been taken will help to reduce the risk of distortion occurring subsequently. No attempt should be made to check the record by repeated closure or distortion of the wax in the notches is liable to occur. The record should be stored in cold water after suitable labelling has been carried out (for example, scribing on the letter 'P').

To obtain records of right and left lateral jaw relationships, the occlusal rims should be re-inserted and further wax wafers in softened modelling wax placed between their occlusal surfaces — one to record the right lateral relationship and a second one to record the left lateral relationship. These wafers should be of a similar form to that used to obtain the record of a protrusive jaw relationship. With one of the wafers in position between the rims, the patient should be persuaded to close into a position providing approximately 10 mm of lateral deviation of the mandible to the right side, measured in the incisor region. The degree of vertical closure that occurs in this record is not critical but it is desirable that the wafer should again not be reduced to less than 2 mm in thickness, to reduce the risk of distortion of the record occurring. Once closure to the required thickness of wafer has occurred, the mouth should be opened and the record removed from the rims. As with the record of a protrusive jaw relationship, no attempt should be made to check the position by repeated closure. The record should be stored in cold water after labelling (for example by scribing on the record the letters 'RL').

The procedure should then be repeated to obtain a corresponding wax wafer record of the left lateral jaw relationship.

Before wax wafers are used to obtain protrusive and/or lateral records of jaw relationship, it is desirable that the patient be rehearsed in the required degree of mandibular movement.

In using the records, the wax wafer registration of the retruded jaw relationship will first be used in association with the upper and lower impression compound occlusal rims to locate correctly the upper and lower casts for mounting on an adjustable articulator. Location of the wafer on the rims is provided by the wax extensions from the wafer engaging the notches in the occlusal surfaces of the rims.

The wax wafer records of the other jaw relationships may then be placed between the rims on the mounted casts and used to set the condylar inclinations of the articulator. Where right and left lateral records have been taken these are used in turn to set the contra-lateral condylar inclination (i.e. a right lateral record is used to set the left condylar inclination and vice versa). A protrusive record may be used as a sole method of setting both condylar angulations simultaneously, or may be used as a check method in association with lateral records.

OBTAINING A FACE-BOW REGISTRATION

In complete denture construction, a face-bow is used to record the relationship between the inter-condylar axis and the maxillary denture-bearing area of a patient. The relationship can then be transferred to either an average value or adjustable articulator so that the casts of the patient's jaws will assume the same relationship to the hinge axis of the articulator as that of the upper or lower jaws of the patient bear to the inter-condylar axis.

The use of a face-bow provides one link in a chain of procedures designed to ensure that an articulator will simulate as closely as possible the mandibular movements of a patient. It helps in meeting the aim that the level of occlusal balance developed when trial dentures are set up on the articulator will also be seen to be present when they are inserted in the mouth of the patient.

The registration is usually obtained using a simple face-bow.

A detailed description of the use of this instrument appears in Chapter 10, page 71. For convenience this will be summarised below:

Markers should be placed on the skin of the face of the patient overlying the condyles. The fork of the face-bow should then be securely attached to the upper occlusal rim. This should be achieved by warming the prongs of the fork in a Bunsen burner flame and then gently pressing the fork into the labial and buccal aspects of the rim, about 5 mm above the level of the occlusal plane. Care should be taken that the prongs of the fork do not perforate the fitting surface of the rim and that molten wax is not allowed to run on to the occlusal surface. The occlusal rim should then be inserted, leaving the rod of the fork protruding from the mouth. The joint on the body of the face-bow for the fork is then slipped over the rod of the fork and the condylar indicators positioned over the skin markers. The indicators are adjusted until an equal number of graduations appear on each side and the universal joint is then tightened.

Where an orbital pointer is used, the tip of the pointer should be positioned on the lowest part of the orbit and the appropriate joint tightened. After slackening off the condyle indicators, the face-bow record should then be removed from the patient.

Mounting of the maxillary cast on the articulator may then be carried out using the face-bow record.

SELECTING THE TEETH

The principles of tooth selection are presented in detail in Chapter 11. A suggested application of these principles to the selection of teeth in complete denture construction follows.

Selection of the anterior teeth

The overall width of the six upper anterior teeth is

commonly determined by reference to canine lines marked on the upper occlusal rim. Where the lines indicate the distal surfaces of the canines, a flexible ruler should be used to measure the distance between the lines around the lower border of the labial surface of the rim. A manufacturer's mould chart should then be consulted to determine the available moulds of teeth of the required width. An indication of the required length of the upper anterior teeth may be obtained by noting the distance between the occlusal plane and the upper lip line scribed on the labial surface of the upper occlusal rim. Alternatively, the length/width ratio of the patient's face may be determined and tooth length calculated by use of the formula:

$$\frac{\text{Length of face}}{\text{Width of face}} = \frac{\text{Length of teeth}}{\text{Width of teeth}}$$

In selecting the size of the lower anterior teeth, reference should be made to the manufacturer's mould chart which may indicate moulds of lower teeth which match the size of the chosen upper anterior teeth. This provides a useful basis for selection where the patient has a Class I skeletal jaw relationship. Where Class II or Class III skeletal jaw relationships are encountered, a limited change in the size of lower anterior teeth selected may be indicated. For a Class II skeletal jaw relationship, slightly narrower teeth may be selected than those indicated by the manufacturer's mould chart to take account of the decrease in area available for accommodation of the lower dentition. The opposite applies in the case of a Class III skeletal jaw relationship. Gross change in the size of the lower anterior teeth selected should be avoided as the mis-match in the relative size of the upper and lower anterior teeth will be detrimental to aesthetics. Changing the number of teeth which are set up provides a more acceptable solution than varying the width of lower anterior teeth, where gross Class II or Class III skeletal jaw relationships are present (see Chapter 24, page 193).

In the absence of more positive information, the form of the anterior teeth is generally selected by the use of Leon Williams typal theory which indicated that the shape of the crowns of the upper central incisors corresponded to the inverted outline form of the face. Where the form of the teeth is being selected by that method, note should be made of the outline form of the patient's face — square, tapering or ovoid, and teeth of a corresponding form should be selected by reference to the manufacturer's mould chart.

Alternatively, form may be selected on the basis of the sex, personality and age of the patient, following the principles developed by Frusch and Fisher.

The texture of the teeth selected should be such as to harmonise with the texture of the patient's facial tissues. Particularly where plastic teeth are to be used, the texture of the labial surfaces may be modified by grinding to develop features such as imbrication lines and surface facets where this is thought to be indicated.

Selection of the colour of the teeth is based on the patient's age and sex and the colour of the patient's facial tissues. A preliminary selection should be made from the manufacturer's shade guide after consideration of the above factors. The chosen tooth should then be tested extra-orally in relation to the colour of the patient's skin, eyes and hair and also observed intra-orally when moistened and held under the lip. Similar tests should then be applied using lighter and darker teeth until the most appropriate colour has been selected.

In relation to choice of material, either porcelain or plastic teeth may be selected. The relative merits of the two materials are presented in Table 11.1. The choice of which to use should be based on weighing up the advantages and disadvantages of each relative to the requirements of the individual patient. For example, if the patient shows a history of marked attrition of plastic anterior teeth, the use of porcelain anterior teeth may be considered to be desirable.

Selection of the posterior teeth

When choosing the size of the posterior teeth, three dimensions must be considered. These are the mesio-distal dimension, occluso-gingival dimension and bucco-lingual dimension. Guidance on appropriate values of the first two of these dimensions may be obtained by examination of the occlusal rims and casts, following the completion of the jaw registration procedures. Posterior teeth should be chosen with a mesio-distal dimension such that the lower teeth will just fill the space available between the distal surfaces of the canines and the mesial surfaces of the retromolar pads. Selection of the occluso-gingival dimension should be based on an observation of the space available between the occlusal plane and the alveolar ridges. To obtain optimal aesthetics, the length of the premolars should harmonise with that of the canines, and this point should be borne in mind when selecting the occluso-gingival dimension of the posterior teeth.

In selecting an appropriate bucco-lingual dimension for posterior teeth, the need to position the teeth in the neutral zone must be considered. This can often be helped by choosing teeth whose bucco-lingual dimension is less than that of their natural predecessors. A further benefit which may arise from a reduction of bucco-lingual width is that the load applied to the denture-bearing tissues may also be reduced.

Selection of the form of the posterior teeth requires a decision to be made on the appropriate cuspal angle. Although many different forms of posterior teeth are available, they fall into two main classes:

1. Anatomical posterior teeth, with a cuspal form approximately corresponding to that of unworn natural teeth and having a cuspal angle in the range of 20° to 30°.

2. Non-anatomical or flat-cusped posterior teeth, with a cuspal angle of 0°. Teeth of this type have grooves present below the level of the flat occlusal surface to allow food to be expressed from between the occlusal surfaces in the course of mastication.

Teeth of form 1 are commonly selected for use in complete denture construction as a means of achieving an acceptable level of masticatory efficiency. Where teeth of form 2 are used, poorer aesthetics and possibly a decrease in masticatory efficiency may arise. To compensate, teeth of form 2 will transmit less lateral stress to the denture bases and hence to the underlying supporting tissues. On that basis, they may be chosen for use where the residual alveolar ridges show substantial atrophy.

The colour selected for posterior teeth should be the same as that chosen for the anterior teeth.

Selection of the material for posterior teeth involves deciding between the use of plastic or porcelain. As in the selection of material for the anterior teeth, the basis of choice should be a consideration of the relative advantages and disadvantages of the two materials as they apply to the patient in question. Porcelain posterior teeth have the particular merit of showing a very much reduced rate of occlusal wear relative to that which can occur in plastic teeth. Porcelain teeth can be difficult to set up when the available inter-ridge space is limited. It should also be remembered that patients who are being provided with replacement dentures and who have plastic teeth on their existing dentures, may not readily tolerate replacement dentures having porcelain teeth.

PREPARING A WRITTEN PRESCRIPTION

A written prescription should be provided which will assist the technician in the development of the trial dentures. The following points should be covered:

1. Details of the anterior and posterior teeth selected for use.

2. The type of articulator to be used. Required settings of the condylar guidance angle and/or of the incisal guidance angle should be provided where appropriate.

3. A request that the maxillary (or mandibular) cast should be positioned on the articulator via use of a face-bow record, where one has been obtained.

4. A request that the maxilla/mandible relationship registered by the occlusal rims be used to provide relative location of the two casts on the articulator.

5. A request that the condylar angulation of the articulator be set by use of the protrusive and/or lateral records of jaw relationship, where these have been obtained.

6. An indication of the baseplate materials to be used in the preparation of the trial dentures.

7. Details of any special aesthetic requirements not provided by the occlusal rims. For example, the need to provide a central diastema of given dimension may be indicated.

8. Details of functional requirements should be given. For example, a requirement that the teeth

be set up in occlusal balance and where the lower teeth, in particular, should be set in relation to the alveolar ridges.

Where copying of some aspects of the existing dentures is desired for aesthetic and/or functional reasons, the provision of impressions of the exist-ing dentures obtained using alginate in stock trays of the box form will be of considerable help to the technician in achieving this aim.

9. Whether contouring and/or stippling of the labial and buccal waxwork of the polished surfaces of the dentures is required.

FURTHER READING

Frush J P and Fisher R D 1959 Dentogenics: its practical application. J Prosthet Dent 9: 914

Grasso J E and Sharry J J 1968 The duplicability of arrow-point tracings in dentulous subjects. J Prosthet Dent 20: 106

Lundquist D O and Luther W W 1970 Occlusal plane determination. J Prosthet Dent 23: 489

Payne A G L 1971 Factors influencing the position of artificial upper anterior teeth. J Prosthet Dent 26: 26

Saleski C G 1972 Color, light and shade matching. J Prosthet Dent 27: 263

Villa A H 1959 Gothic arch tracing. J Prosthet Dent 9: 624

Yurkstas A A and Kapur K K 1964 Factors influencing centric relations records in edentulous mouths. J Prosthet Dent 14: 1054

24

The principles of tooth arrangement

INTRODUCTION

The correct alignment of the teeth is essential to the production of a functionally effective and aesthetically pleasing denture. Failure to achieve occlusal balance, i.e. balanced occlusion and balanced articulation, may result in masticatory inefficiency and possible pathological change in the supporting and associated tissues because of uneven distribution of masticatory forces and instability of the appliances. Incorrect alignment of the teeth may also give rise to speech difficulties.

ARRANGING THE ANTERIOR TEETH

The contribution of the anterior teeth to appearance will possibly be regarded as their prime function by the patient and his or her close acquaintances. There are, however, other functions of the anterior teeth which are equally important to the success of the denture. These include the incision of food and their contribution to occlusal balance and to the development of articulate speech. Aspects important to the attainment of occlusal balance are considered below and the role of the teeth in speech has been referred to in Chapter 1.

Because of the individual nature of aesthetic requirements for each patient, only a general guide to arranging the anterior teeth can be given. The basis for restoration of the facial profile and lip contours has already been laid down by the contouring of the occlusal rims and the selection of the teeth as described in Chapter 23.

The labial surfaces of the upper anterior teeth will be made coincident with the labial contour of the upper occlusal rim and the incisal edges will be related to the occlusal plane developed during the jaw registration stage. These, together with the midline scribed on the upper rim and about which the upper central incisors will be orientated, provide a clear guide to the setting of the upper anterior teeth.

The lower anterior teeth contribute to lower lip support, to the development of occlusal balance, the incision of food and also assist in forming some speech sounds. They are generally arranged just anterior to the crest of the residual alveolar ridge, but must not be set further forward than the available width of the sulcus or displacement of the lower denture may result when contraction of the circumoral musculature occurs.

The inclination of the anterior teeth

The inclination of the long axis of each tooth in both the antero-posterior and mesiodistal planes, and also their relationship to the occlusal plane, is of basic importance in establishing a natural appearance and functional effectiveness in the denture. This is not to imply that all artificial teeth should be set in the same way, but rather that, as artificial teeth should simulate natural teeth in appearance, it is essential that the normal or 'classical' orientation is appreciated as a basis for positional variations to be introduced. The classical inclinations of the teeth are also the basis for descriptions of required arrangements when writing prescriptions to the dental technician for the setting of the teeth.

The classical inclinations of the upper and lower anterior teeth and their relationships to the occlusal plane are as follows (Figs 24.1, 24.2).

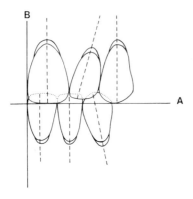

Fig. 24.1 The relationship of the anterior teeth to the occlusal plane (A), and the vertical axis (B), when viewed from the anterior aspect. The broken lines represent the vertical axes of the teeth.

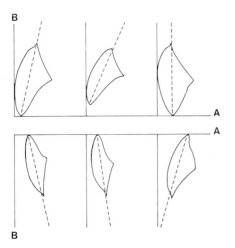

Fig. 24.2 The relationship of the anterior teeth to the horizontal plane (A) and vertical axis (B) in lateral view. The broken lines represent the vertical axes of the teeth.

Upper central incisor. The long axis of this tooth is parallel to the vertical axis when viewed from the anterior, and slopes slightly labially when viewed from the lateral aspect. The incisal edge contacts the occlusal plane.

Upper lateral incisor. The long axis inclines mesially when viewed from the anterior and the tooth has a greater degree of labial inclination than that of the central incisor. The incisal edge is approximately 1–2 mm above the level of the occlusal plane.

Upper canine. The long axes are parallel to the vertical axis. The cusp contacts the occlusal plane.

Lower central incisor. Viewed from the anterior

the long axis is parallel to the vertical axis and the crown slopes labially when viewed from the lateral aspect. The incisal edge is some 2 mm above the level of the occlusal plane.

Lower lateral incisor. The long axis is parallel to the vertical axis when viewed from the anterior and the crown has a labial inclination of lesser degree than that of the central incisor when observed from the lateral aspect. The incisal edge is some 2 mm above the level of the occlusal plane.

Lower canine. The long axis is inclined slightly mesially in anterior view and is inclined slightly lingually when viewed from the lateral aspect. The tip of the cusp is slightly more than 2 mm above the level of the occlusal plane.

In providing variation from the above inclinations for an individual patient, a clear guide to the tooth positions which existed when the natural teeth were present may be available in the form of a photograph or some other type of pre-extraction record. Where this assistance is not available the patient may volunteer particular wishes in respect of such variations as spaces between the teeth, a crowding effect or rotation of some teeth. Generally, where variation from the normal is introduced, a reasonable degree of symmetry about the midline should be incorporated, since such variation tends to be symmetrical with natural teeth. For example, the mesial incisal angles of both lateral incisors might overlap the distal surface of the contiguous central incisor; or both central incisors might be rotated about the long axis with the mesial incisal angles being rotated lingually. Subtle rather than marked irregularities may be more acceptable. Strongly rotated and tilted teeth should be avoided because of the possibility of irritation to the lips and tongue by the incisal angles.

The relationship between the anterior teeth

Where an edge-to-edge relationship is developed between the upper and lower incisors as may be used, for example, where a Class III jaw relationship exists, there is, of course, no overbite or overjet present in the anterior part of the mouth. In the case of a skeletal Class I or Class II jaw relationship the lower incisors are overlapped by the uppers. Wherever overbite is present sufficient

Fig. 24.3 Canine relationship during a left lateral excursion of the mandible.

overjet must be provided to prevent interference of the teeth in speech and mastication. Further consideration of this important aspect of setting the anterior teeth is given below. Generally, however, with the Class II relationship, in the interests of achieving occlusal balance the overbite is reduced over that which would occur with natural teeth.

In setting the canine teeth the lowers are set in relation to the upper canines such that during lateral excursions of the mandible an axial line passing through the tip of the cusp of the upper canine will contact the distal aspect of the lower canine (Fig. 24.3). This relationship is essential to the development of the correct intercuspation of the posterior teeth during lateral movements as an aspect of balanced articulation. When the lower canine teeth have been set to provide for this canine relationship in lateral movements, the mesiodistal space available for the lower incisors is defined.

Slight irregularities of the lower incisors can be helpful in providing a non-artificial appearance to the lower denture when it takes the form of slight rotation with a mildly crowded effect. Spacing of the lower incisors is only rarely necessary, and when present can sometimes be a source of tongue irritation. Where a Class III jaw relationship is present the space available for the lower incisors between the canines is often generous and to avoid the use of excessively broad lower incisors, the addition of a fifth lower incisor may be considered.

Where a large overjet is present in the anterior region, difficulty may be experienced in that the space between the lower canines may be insufficient to place four incisor teeth of the correct proportional size to that of the upper teeth. Among methods by which this problem may be overcome is included crowding lower incisors of the correct size into the available space where the discrepancy is small. Where less space is available the use of slightly narrower lower incisors might be aesthetically acceptable and in a more narrow situation the use of only three lower incisors may be resorted to.

ARRANGING THE POSTERIOR TEETH

The posterior teeth have primarily a functional purpose in aiding mastication and contributing to the development of some speech sounds, although the first premolars, being placed near the angles of the mouth, also contribute to denture aesthetics.

In order to develop functional efficiency in setting the posterior teeth, it is essential to aim for occlusal balance. While setting the posterior teeth is the province of the dental technician, it is essential that the clinician has a clear understanding of the fundamentals of developing balanced occlusion and balanced articulation in complete dentures.

Occlusal balance

The contact movements which occur between opposing complete dentures may be considered in terms of protrusive and lateral movements. Hanau identified the factors involved in obtaining balance in protrusive movements of the mandible. The factors concerned are:
1. The condylar guidance angles.
2. The incisal guidance angle.
3. The cusp angles of the posterior teeth.
4. The orientation of the occlusal plane.
5. The prominence of the compensating curve.

These five factors are interdependent and when one factor is changed alteration is required in some, or all, of the others to maintain a state of balance. The 'Laws of Articulation' as expressed by Hanau define the relationship between the factors. Some of the relationships are referred to below and reference to the literature should be made for a fuller consideration of the Laws.

Of the five factors listed above, the only one which is fixed by the edentulous patient is the con-

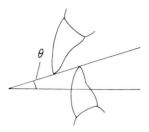

Fig. 24.4 Lateral view of upper and lower incisor teeth to illustrate the incisal angle (θ).

dylar guidance angle. Where this is steeply inclined a compensating curve of small radius, or high cusp angles on the posterior teeth, or a steeply angled occlusal plane are required to effect occlusal balance. All these factors tend to produce difficult conditions for denture management. An average value for the condylar guidance angle is some 30° and this is not regarded as a high value.

The function of the incisal guidance mechanism is to maintain the planned spacing between the casts on the articulator and to impart an opening movement to the articulator as the casts move in

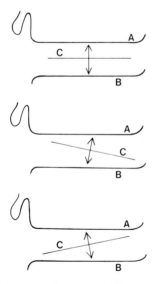

Fig. 24.5 Illustration of the effects of wide variation of the orientation of the occlusal plane on denture stability. The outlines represent the crest of the upper residual ridge (A), the crest of the lower residual ridge (B), and the occlusal plane (C). Tilting the plane down posteriorly (middle diagram) produces a tendency for the lower denture to be displaced anteriorly and the upper denture posteriorly. Tilting the plane up posteriorly (lower diagram) tends to produce the opposite effect in terms of the displacing forces developed.

imitation of the effect produced by the sliding of the lower incisors on the lingual aspects of the upper incisors in protrusive and lateral movements.

The incisal angle is usually expressed as the angle made to the horizontal by a line drawn in the sagittal plane between the incisal edges of the upper and lower incisors when the casts are mounted in the retruded jaw relationship (Fig. 24.4).

When the incisal guidance angle is steep, either high cusped teeth, or a steeply inclined occlusal plane, or a compensating curve of short radius are required to effect occlusal balance in protrusive movements. These factors should, if possible, be avoided in complete denture construction and a shallow incisal guidance angle should be chosen.

The orientation of the occlusal plane is developed during the jaw registration stage of denture production. In practical terms its angulation may be varied slightly to assist in obtaining denture stability. Wide variation from being formed parallel to the ala-tragal line should be avoided as this may result in resolved forces between the opposing dentures in occlusion, tending to displace the dentures (Fig. 24.5).

Protrusive movements

To help understand the effects of a protrusive movement of the articulator on the paths of movement of the inclined planes (i.e. the cusp angles) of the teeth, an example will be considered. Assuming that the condylar guidance angles on both sides are equal at 30°, and that the incisal guidance angle is 10°, a two-dimensional diagram can be produced as shown in Figure 24.6. Lines projected at right angles to the condylar guidance path and the incisal guidance path as shown in the diagram intersect at a point which may be termed the rotation centre. Using a compass and using the rotation centre as the central point, a series of arcs of circles has been drawn which cut the line representing the occlusal plane. The angles at which these arcs cut the occlusal plane increase in value as the condylar mechanism is approached. With the upper teeth set as shown in the diagram and the cuspal slope of the lower teeth set coincident with the paths of movement indicated by the series of arcs, balanced contact between the upper and lower teeth will be maintained when a protrusive

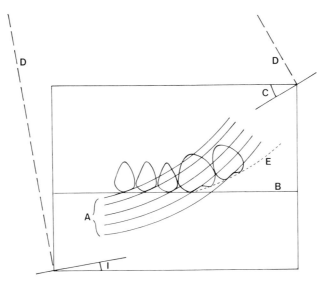

Fig. 24.6 Diagram to illustrate the way in which a compensating curve increases the effective cusp angles progressively towards the posterior. Condylar guidance angle C = 30°. Incisal guidance angle I = 10°. The dashed lines D, D, meet at the centre of rotation from which the series of arcs (A), which represent the paths of movement taken by the teeth in protrusion, have been produced. B, occlusal plane; E, compensating curve.

movement is made along the paths of movement indicated. It will be noted that this arrangement has the effect of increasing the effective cusp angle of the teeth progressively towards the posterior aspect, as the effective cusp angle is made up of the cusp angle of the tooth plus the angle of tilt provided. It will also be apparent that to achieve these circumstances, the posterior teeth are set in a curved arrangement called a compensating curve, which may be considered as analogous to the curve of 'Spee' of the natural dentition.

Lateral movements

During lateral movements, the right and left condyles are performing different actions. The side towards which the mandible moves is called the working side and the condylar movement on that side may be considered to be largely rotational about a vertical axis. The side from which the mandible moves is called the balancing side and the condyle translates downwards and forwards, and in the example given above for protrusive movement it would travel down at an angle of 30°. Consider the working side and balancing side separately.

The working side. Since only rotation has occurred, the condylar angle is effectively zero and the angles of movement are shallow, varying between 0° at the condylar guidance mechanism to 10° near the incisal guidance mechanism, and the upper posterior teeth will need to be inclined outwards (buccally) to give the required shallow working angles (Fig. 24.7).

Fig. 24.7 Example of the buccal inclinations of the first molars in the coronal plane required to maintain balance in a right lateral movement when the condylar guidance angle is 30° and the incisal guidance angle is 10°. The direction of movement of the mandible is indicated by arrows. The working side angle (θ_1) is approximately 3°, while the balancing angle (θ) is some 19°.

The balancing side. Translation down a 30° slope occurs and assuming the incisal guidance angle to be less than the condylar guidance angle, the angles of movement increase as the condylar mechanism is approached. In order to provide the necessary balancing angle to maintain contact with the opposing lower teeth, the upper teeth will need to be inclined buccally (Fig. 24.7).

In this way the buccal inclination of the teeth as described develops a lateral compensating curve (Fig. 24.8) which may be considered analagous to the curve of Monson of the natural dentition.

The factors involved in obtaining balance in lateral movements may be enumerated as:

1. The inclination of the condylar guidance angle on the balancing side.

2. The inclination of the incisal guidance angle.

3. The inclination of the plane of occlusion.

4. The compensating curves.

5. The buccal cusp height of the lower teeth and the lingual cusp height of the upper teeth on the balancing side.

6. The cusp height of the teeth on the working side.

7. Bennett movement on the working side.

Arranging the posterior teeth

Just as the starting point for the setting of the anterior teeth for optimum function and aesthetics was a consideration of the axial inclination of the teeth, so the relatively complex factors involved in the setting of the posterior teeth can also be considered in terms of the axial inclinations of the teeth and their relationship to the occlusal plane. The correct location of the teeth in relation to the residual alveolar ridge in the bucco-lingual aspect is a clinical decision and will be indicated by the position of the occlusal rim. Generally for the lower denture, the teeth will be placed with the central fossae over or slightly buccal to the ridge crest so that maximum stability to occlusal forces will result without encroachment on the tongue space. Placement of the teeth buccal to the ridge may result in displacement of the denture by interference with the action of the buccinator muscle. It is important for each patient to visualise the space available between the buccal and lingual tissues where minimal encroachment on the tissues will occur.

The axial inclinations and relationship to the occlusal plane for the posterior teeth are as follows:

Upper first premolar. The long axes of the tooth are parallel to the vertical axis. The buccal cusp contacts the occlusal plane while the lingual cusp is some 2 mm above it.

Upper second premolar. The long axes are par-

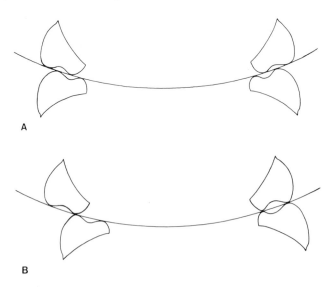

Fig. 24.8 Lateral compensating curve. A, Tooth relationship in maximal intercuspal position; B, Tooth relationship following a left lateral movement of the mandible.

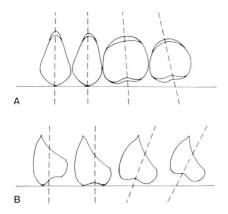

Fig. 24.9 Axial relationship of the posterior teeth to the vertical and horizontal axes. A, Lateral view; B, Anterior aspect.

allel to the vertical axis and both cusps contact the occlusal plane.

Upper first molar. The long axis slopes buccally when viewed from the anterior and distally when viewed in lateral aspect. The mesio-palatal cusp contacts the occlusal plane with the disto-palatal cusp slightly above the occlusal plane. The buccal cusps are 1–2 mm above the occlusal plane.

Upper second molar. The long axis slopes bucally more steeply than the first molar when viewed from the anterior and distally more steeply than the first molar in lateral view. All cusps are above the occlusal plane to a greater extent than those of the first molar, the buccal cusps more than the lingual and the distal cusps to a greater extent than those of the mesial.

The inclinations and relationships are illustrated in Figure 24.9, where it can be seen that these arrangements form compensating curves both anteroposteriorly and laterally.

Lower first premolar. The long axes of this tooth are parallel to the vertical axis. The lingual cusp is below the occlusal plane while the buccal cusp is some 2 mm above the plane.

Lower second premolar. The long axes are parallel to the vertical axis and both cusps are 2 mm above the occlusal plane.

Lower first molar. The long axis is inclined lingually when viewed from the front, and mesially when seen from the lateral aspect. All cusps are above the occlusal plane to a greater degree than those of the second premolar. The buccal and dis-

tal cusps are higher than the mesial and lingual cusps.

Lower second molar. The lingual and mesial inclinations of this tooth are more pronounced than those of the first molar. All the cusps are higher in relation to the occlusal plane than those of the first molar, and the buccal and distal cusps are higher than the mesial and lingual cusps.

Using the above inclinations in setting teeth having cusp angles of approximately 20° will provide a good basis for the development of occlusal balance where an average condylar angle (30°) and an incisal guidance angle of 10° are present.

Where the lower residual ridge has a broader arch form than the upper such that in the retruded jaw relationship the lower ridge lies abnormally buccal to the upper, a special arrangement of the posterior teeth may be required to provide adequate space for the tongue and stability for the dentures. This relationship may be seen where a Class III jaw relationship exists and also where resorption of the residual ridges of a patient having a Class I jaw relationship has reached an advanced stage. The arrangement of the posterior teeth which may be required is called a cross-bite arrangement. The cross-bite arrangement is such that the lingual cusp(s) of the lower teeth occlude in the central fossa of the upper teeth. In the normal arrangement, the buccal cusps of the lower posterior teeth occlude in the central fossa of the uppers. Using such an arrangement may remove the need to set the upper posterior teeth in a marked buccal relationship to the upper ridge, which would increase the risk of instability of the upper denture, while at the same time permitting the alignment of the posterior teeth in a zone of minimum conflict with the environmental tissues (Fig. 24.10).

In practice, when setting the posterior teeth, the uppers are set in relation to the occlusal plane as described above. The lower posterior teeth are then set to occlude and articulate with the uppers, balance being obtained for each tooth, in turn, during setting.

The above description applies to posterior teeth having a definite cuspal form based on the anatomy of the human teeth. Where flat cusps or other non-anatomical forms of posterior teeth are chosen, there are two commonly employed

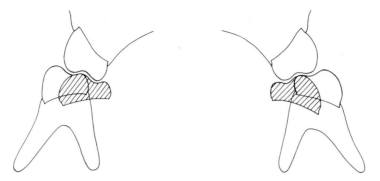

Fig. 24.10 Cross-bite relationship in the first molar region. The hatched areas indicate the normal tooth relationship.

approaches to setting the teeth. Where the biting surface has a flat form of greater mesiodistal dimensions than that of a tooth, the teeth are set to a flat plane and a 'balancing ramp' is used to provide three point balance in protrusive movements of the mandible (Fig. 24.11). Such an arrangement may be suitable for use with the Bader cutter bar or with Hardy's V.O. teeth.

Fig. 24.11 Three-point 'balance' using a balancing ramp posterior to the molar teeth in conjunction with a flat arrangement of the posterior teeth.

With flat cusp or inverted cusp type teeth, the lower teeth are set to contact a template which has the form of a portion of the surface of a sphere of some 4 inches radius. This develops antero-posterior and lateral compensating curves. When the lower teeth are set, the uppers are set to occlude and articulate with them. This arrangement allows free sliding contact in antero-posterior and lateral movements (Fig. 24.12). As might be anticipated with this method of tooth arrangement, occlusal balance in the mouth may not be exactly the same as that developed on the articulator, and some occlusal correction will be necessary to satisfy the needs of the individual patient. Because of the absence of cusps, flat cusp and inverted cusp teeth present no difficulty where the ridge relationship is unfavourable and a cross-bite arrangement is required.

In setting posterior teeth of either the anatomi-

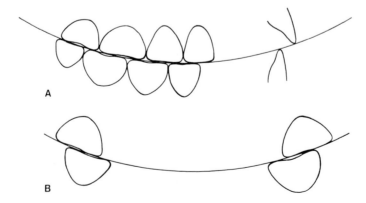

Fig. 24.12 Flat cusped teeth set in conformity with a template to develop lateral and antero-posterior compensating curves. A, Lateral view; B, Anterior view in the molar region.

cal or non anatomical type, it is important that the relationship between the upper and lower teeth in the bucco-lingual plane is such that the maximal value for buccal and lingual overjet as provided for in the tooth design is developed. Lack of adequate buccal overjet may result in cheek and tongue biting. Buccal overjet must be positively developed regardless of the cuspal form of the teeth used and whether the tooth relationship is a normal one or of a cross-bite nature.

A further important point relating to the setting of the posterior teeth is that the teeth must not be placed over the retromolar pad region as this will result in instability of the denture. Where there is a lack of space for all the posterior teeth, a premolar tooth or, where the space disproportion is greater, one of the molar teeth should be deleted from the set-up.

FURTHER READING

Beck H O 1972 Occlusion as related to complete removable prosthodontics. J Prosthet Dent 27: 246

Boucher C O, Hickey J C and Zarb G A 1975 Prosthodontic Treatment for Edentulous Patients. 7th Edn. Mosby, St Louis

Frush J P and Fisher R D 1959 Dentogenics: its practical application. J Prosthet Dent 9: 914

Hanau R L 1926 Articulation defined, analysed and formulated. J Amer Dent Assoc 13: 1694

Murrell G A 1970 Occlusal considerations in esthetic tooth positioning. J Prosthet Dent 23: 499

Nasr M F, George W A, Travalgini E A and Scott R H 1967 The relative efficiency of different types of posterior teeth. J Prosthet Dent 18: 3

Ortman H R 1977 Complete denture occlusion. Dent Clin North Amer 21: 299

Roraff A R 1977 Arranging artificial teeth according to anatomic landmarks. J Prosthet Dent 38: 120

Stephens A P 1970 Full dentures which occlude with natural teeth. Dent Pract Dent Rec 21: 37

25

The trial denture stage of treatment

INTRODUCTION

The examination procedures which should be applied to check the satisfaction of trial dentures are considered in this chapter. Advice will also be given on the actions which are necessary where faults are identified in the course of the examination procedures.

Before proceeding to intra-oral examination, the trial dentures should be examined on the articulator. The arrangement of the teeth and the form of the polished surfaces should be checked for conformity with the prescription. Note should be made of the accuracy of adaptation of the baseplates to the casts. Where the dentures have been set up on an average value or adjustable articulator, lateral and protrusive movements should be made and the state of occlusal balance present in the dentition should be noted. Where unsatisfactory features are detected in the course of the above examination, they should be corrected before proceeding further.

The trial dentures should then be removed from the casts and the fitting surfaces checked to ensure that they are clean and free from any extraneous matter. All surfaces of the dentures should be checked to ensure the absence of any sharp areas which could traumatise the patients' tissues. To reduce the risk of cross-contamination arising, the dentures should then be placed in a suitable antiseptic solution. They should then be washed in running cold water before they are inserted in the mouth at the commencement of the intra-oral check procedures.

If, in the course of intra-oral examination, the trial dentures are kept in the mouth for a period exceeding about three minutes, there is a risk that distortion will occur of any temporary base materials that have been used in their construction (for example, wax or shellac). To avoid this risk the dentures should periodically be removed from the mouth and immersed in cold water for about one minute before re-insertion.

The number and order of application of the stages used in intra-oral examination of the trial dentures should duplicate those used in the checking and subsequent development of the occlusal rims at the jaw registration stage. Adopting a consistent approach to the examination procedures helps to ensure that no stage will be overlooked. The order in which the stages should be applied is as follows:

1. Checking extension, retention and stability.
2. Checking aesthetics.
3. Checking the vertical component of jaw relationship.
4. Checking the horizontal component of jaw relationship.

CHECKING EXTENSION, RETENTION AND STABILITY

The upper trial denture should be inserted and the buccal and labial margins of the baseplate checked for conformity with the functional level of the sulcus, including the presence of adequate allowance for frenal attachments. The operator should make functional movements of the lips and cheeks of the patient and note whether any displacement of the denture occurs. Where displacement is seen to occur, the depth and/or thickness of the flange in the area concerned should be reduced until the problem has been overcome.

The posterior border of the upper baseplate should be seen to extend from one hamular notch to the other, along a line approximately 1 mm anterior to the vibrating line of the palate. Where necessary, the posterior extension of the baseplate should be adjusted until this requirement is satisfied.

Retention should be checked by applying a force at the premolar region on each side of the denture in a direction away from the tissues and at right angles to the underlying alveolar surfaces. It should be noted that the retention of the trial denture is likely to be appreciably less than that of the completed denture, due to the absence of a post-dam seal, associated with poorer adaptation of the baseplate to the tissues. As a minimum requirement, the retention of the trial denture should be such that the denture will stay in position when the mouth of the patient is opened. Otherwise, difficulty will be encountered in the subsequent stages of the intra-oral examination procedure.

Stability of the upper trial denture should then be tested by applying force in a tissueward direction in the premolar and molar regions on each side of the arch in turn and observing whether or not rotatory displacement of the denture occurs. Where displacement does occur, a likely cause is that the posterior teeth have been set in a position which lies excessively buccal to the underlying alveolar ridges. They will require to be reset into a position which provides an acceptable level of stability.

The upper trial denture should then be removed from the mouth and replaced by the lower denture. Testing of the extension of the lower denture should be carried out with the mouth in no more than the half-open position. This will ensure that the environmental musculature is in an acceptable state of relaxation. The operator should place two fingers of the left hand, into light contact with the posterior teeth on each side of the denture. The thumb of that hand should simultaneously be placed under the chin of the patient to provide mandibular support. The operator's right hand should then be used to apply functional movements to the lips and cheeks on the left

side of the patient's face, note being made of the site and extent of any displacement of the denture which arises. The test should then be repeated on the opposite side, the role played by the operator's hands being reversed.

To test the lingual extension of the denture, the operator should use both hands to apply light finger pressure to the occlusal surfaces of the posterior teeth on each side, the thumbs being used to provide mandibular support. The patient should be asked to first fully protrude the tongue, then curl it upwards and backwards so that the tip lies on the posterior palatal tissues, and finally move the tongue laterally to the right and to the left to bring the tip of the tongue into contact with the cheek on each side. Note should again be made of the site and extent of any displacement of the denture which arises.

In all cases where displacement of the denture occurs, the denture flanges should be reduced in depth and/or in thickness in the areas concerned, until displacement no longer arises.

The retention and stability of the lower denture should then be tested by applying the same procedures as described for use with the upper denture. Additionally, testing the stability of the lower denture requires observations to be made of the functional relationship of the tongue to the lower denture. The position of the tongue relative to the denture should be observed with the mouth in the half-open position. The lateral margins of the tongue should be seen to be lying over at least part of the occlusal surfaces of the posterior teeth. When this position of the tongue is adopted, it can provide an aid to retention, helping it keep the denture in position as opening and closing of the mouth occurs. Note should be made of whether the lower denture remains in position on the denture-bearing tissues when the mouth is being opened and closed. Where either or both of these requirements is not met, there is an indication that the occlusal plane of the denture may have been set at too high a level, giving rise to 'walling-in' of the tongue. Alternatively, the position of the teeth or the form of the lingual polished surfaces may be causing 'cramping' of the tongue. Where either applies, consideration should be given to the need to redevelop the denture into a form which will provide improved stability.

CHECKING AESTHETICS

The upper and lower trial dentures should be inserted and the appearance of the patient noted in front face and lateral view when the mouth is closed and also in a half-open position. The following features should be observed:

1. Whether the dentures provide adequate support for the lips and cheeks of the patient.

2. Whether the centre line of the dentition has been set in coincidence with the median line of the face.

3. Whether the occlusal plane is correctly aligned to the inter-pupillary and ala-tragal lines and to the level of the upper lip at rest.

4. Whether an acceptable display of the upper and lower anterior dentitions occurs when the mouth is in the half-open position.

5. Whether the size, form, texture, colour and arrangement of the teeth harmonize with the patient's facial features.

The patient should then be given a hand mirror and invited to comment on the appearance of the dentures. It should be pointed out to the patient that any modifications they require must be indicated at this stage. If requests for modification in tooth position are deferred to the subsequent insertion stage, they will be far more difficult to meet.

Where either the patient or the operator consider that there is a need for relatively minor modifications to be made to the dentures, they should be carried out at the chair-side. As examples of such changes, the alignment of some of the anterior teeth may be altered to provide a more personalised arrangement of the dentition, or the thickness of the flanges may be altered to provide increase or decrease as necessary in the support provided for the facial tissues.

Where major modifications are required in the dentures, for example, a change in the position of the centre line or the occlusal plane, it is advisable that the dentures be returned to the laboratory for resetting. In that case the technician should be provided with clear guidance on the modifications which are required, both by provision of a written prescription and by indicating on one of the dentures the new position of the centre line or occlusal plane. The aesthetics of the modified dentures should then be checked at a subsequent visit of the patient before finishing of the dentures is authorised.

CHECKING THE VERTICAL COMPONENT OF JAW RELATIONSHIP

Markers should be placed on the nose and chin of the patient, as used at the stage of registration of the vertical component of jaw relationship (Chapter 23, page 181). With the lower trial denture only inserted, the patient should be persuaded to adopt the position of rest jaw relationship. The distance between the markers should be determined and the measurement repeated until a consistent value has been obtained.

The upper trial denture should then be inserted and the patient persuaded to close the mouth to bring the posterior teeth into contact with the mandible in retruded jaw relationship. The distance between the markers should against be measured. The difference between this measurement and that obtained at rest jaw relationship indicates the freeway space and its value should equal that selected for use at the jaw registration stage.

Other observations may also be made to confirm the presence of a freeway space in the trial dentition. The patient can be persuaded to adopt the position of rest jaw relationship and then asked to close the mouth to bring the teeth into contact. A distinct movement of the mandible should be observable as this action is performed.

Phonetic tests may also be used. These usually involve pronunciation of the letter 's', since this sound is made with the mandible positioned relative to the maxilla at the closest speaking distance. The patient may be asked to pronounce words containing the letter 's', for example, 'Mississippi'. The teeth should be seen to come into close approximation as the 's' sound is made but neither visibly or audibly should actual tooth contact be noted, where an adequate freeway space is present. Alternatively, the patient may be asked to count slowly from one to ten and the relative positioning of the upper and lower anterior dentition observed as 'six' and 'seven' are pronounced.

Where an error is found to be present, it will be necessary to take a new registration of the vertical component of jaw relationship. The procedure for obtaining the new registration is considered below, in association with that for obtaining a new registration of the horizontal component of jaw relationship.

CHECKING THE HORIZONTAL COMPONENT OF JAW RELATIONSHIP

The upper and lower trial dentures should be inserted and the patient persuaded to close the mouth to bring the posterior teeth into contact with the mandible in retruded jaw relationship. The relationship of the posterior teeth in this position should be observed. The teeth should be in a state of maximum intercuspation, coincident with that seen when the trial dentures were examined on the articulator.

When this condition is not satisfied, a new registration of the horizontal component of jaw relationship must be obtained. Where a new registration of the vertical component of jaw relationship is also required, this should be obtained initially.

The posterior teeth should be removed from the lower trial denture and the areas previously occupied by the teeth replaced by occlusal rims constructed in modelling wax. Where a change in the vertical dimension of the dentures is required, the height of the rims on the lower trial denture should be adjusted until, when the patient closes the mouth to bring the upper posterior teeth into contact with the occlusal rims on the lower denture in retruded jaw relationship, an acceptable value of freeway space is found to be present. Where this involves a reduction in vertical height to provide an increase in freeway space, note should be taken of the relationship of the anterior dentition as reduction in height proceeds. If a point is reached in which contact of the anterior dentition arises, the anterior teeth should be removed as necessary from the lower denture and replaced by wax. To ensure the development of a correct record, it is important that the only contact between the dentures which arises when the patient closes to bring the dentures together in retruded jaw relationship is that between the upper posterior teeth and the wax rims on the lower trial denture.

In all cases a new registration of the horizontal component of jaw relationship should now be obtained. A layer of softened modelling wax, approximately 2 mm deep, should be added to the occlusal surfaces of the wax rims on the lower trial denture. The dentures should be inserted and the patient persuaded to close the mouth with the mandible in retruded jaw relationship. Closure should cease as soon as it is judged that the cusps of the upper posterior teeth have penetrated the depth of the softened modelling wax added to the lower occlusal rims. Repeated mandibular closure should be applied to ensure that the position of retruded jaw relationship has been recorded. The freeway space which is present in the newly recorded position of horizontal jaw relationship should again be checked to ensure that it still within acceptable limits.

The casts should then be remounted on the articulator in the relationship provided by the new registration and new trial dentures prepared by resetting of the lower teeth. The checks given for application at the trial denture stage should then be repeated at a subsequent visit of the patient. If necessary, the procedures for re-registration of the vertical and/or horizontal components of jaw relationship should be repeated until satisfaction is achieved.

PREPARATION OF THE CASTS FOR DENTURE FINISHING

When the trial dentures have been shown to be satisfactory, before the patient is dismissed observations must be made which will allow the casts to be prepared prior to the application of the finishing procedures. The observations which need to be made and the subsequent actions which are necessary can be considered under three headings:
1. The post-dam preparation.
2. Relief areas.
3. Undercuts and denture insertion.

The post-dam preparation

All complete upper dentures must be provided with a post-dam to ensure the development of a peripheral seal along the posterior palatal border. The border should extend from one hamular notch to the other, along a line approximately 1 mm anterior to the vibrating line. This will ensure that the maximum possible area of the posterior palatal tissues are covered, without encroaching on the moveable tissues of the soft palate.

The extension of the posterior border of the upper trial denture has been developed to the required position at an earlier stage (page 201). The denture should now be seated on the upper cast and a line drawn on the cast at the level of the posterior border of the baseplate. A groove, approximately 1 mm deep, should then be cut along the full length of the line between the hamular notches. This provides a basic preparation for the post-dam and also serves to indicate the posterior finishing line of the denture. Further preparation of the post-dam should then be based on observations of the tissue displaceability present in the post-dam region.

An instrument such as a ball-ended burnisher should be used to determine the displaceability of the tissues in this region. Often, it will be found that displaceability will be at a maximum in the mid-lateral sections of the post-dam line. This finding relates to the presence of a relatively thick sub-epithelial layer of fibrous and glandular tissue overlying the greater palatine nerves and vessels which emerge through the greater palatine foramina. In these sections, the basic post-dam groove may be deepened by an amount proportional to the observed level of tissue displacement, commonly by 1–2 mm.

Where tissue displacement permits, the post-dam preparation may also be increased anteriorly with the development of an area dam of cupid's bow form. This can be beneficial in providing a degree of maintenance of post-dam action if, for any reason, it subsequently proves to be necessary to reduce the posterior extension of the denture. This form of post-dam preparation is shown in sagittal section and in plan view in Figure 25.1. In the development of the area portion of the post-dam preparation, the cast is trimmed to provide a chamfered form tapering from zero depth at the anterior aspect of the cupid's bow to a maximum depth at the previously developed posterior groove line.

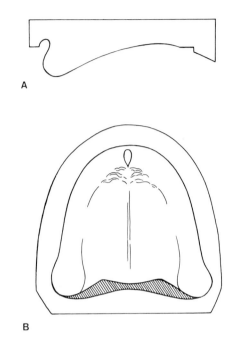

Fig. 25.1 Preparation of the maxillary cast to provide a post-dam on the upper denture. A, Prepared cast shown in sagittal section; B, Prepared cast shown in plan view.

Relief areas

Relief involves the provision of areas within the denture fitting surfaces in which the dentures, in the absence of occlusal load, are spaced from contact with the underlying tissues.

The upper and lower denture-bearing tissues should be palpated, both digitally and by use of an instrument such as a ball-ended burnisher, and note made of any anatomical features which are present which indicate a need for the provision of relief areas. These are as follows:

1. The presence of areas of varying tissue displaceability in the upper denture bearing zone, in cases where the secondary impressions have been taken using a minimum-pressure procedure. The areas of minimum tissue displaceability should be noted as those which require relief. Unless relief is applied to these areas, when the denture is subjected to occlusal loading tissue displacement will occur in some areas and the load will be concentrated on the remaining areas where the bone is thinly covered by mucosa, possibly giving rise to discomfort. The denture may also pivot about the area of high loading in function, giving an in-

creased risk that denture fracture will occur. An area of minimum tissue displaceability often occurs along the mid-palatal raphe, especially where a torus palatinus is present.

2. The presence of a torus mandibularis in the lower denture-bearing zone.

3. The presence of bony spicules which show sensitivity to pressure in either the upper of lower denture-bearing zones.

4. The presence of the mental foramina within the lower denture-bearing zone, where they show sensitivity to pressure.

5. The presence of sharp mylo-hyoid ridges which are sensitive to pressure, where the lingual flanges of the lower denture are to extend over the ridges.

All areas which are found to require relief should be mapped out on the casts. Relief will normally be obtained by cementing metal foil of an appropriate thickness to the casts in the indicated areas.

It should be noted that relief will reduce the area in which dentures are separated from the underlying tissues by a thin film of saliva. It will correspondingly reduce the retention developed by the physical forces (see Chapter 2). The provision of relief areas should thus be kept to the minimum compatable with denture comfort and stability.

Undercuts and denture insertion

The upper and lower casts should be examined for the presence of any undercuts which could prevent insertion of the denture. Where undercuts are present, the oral tissues should be examined in the areas concerned to determine if the undercuts are in soft tissues or hard (bony) tissues.

Where the undercuts are present in relation to soft tissues, a decision may often be made to extend the denture flanges into the undercut areas, as displaceability of the tissues may allow engagement of the undercuts during the insertion of the dentures. Some reduction of the undercuts may prove to be necessary when insertion of the dentures is attempted, which will necessitate reduction of the undercut engaged by trimming of the fitting surface of the dentures in the areas concerned. This possible need should be anticipated by instructing the technician to thicken the flange

in the undercut areas, so that, after trimming, a reasonable flange thickness will still be present.

Where unilateral hard tissue undercuts are present, it may be possible for them to be engaged by choosing an appropriate path of insertion for the denture. However, where bilateral or multiple undercuts are present of a depth greater than approximately 1 mm, appropriate steps must be taken in relation to the forming of the denture flanges if insertion of the denture is to be possible.

Three options are available for use:

1. One millimetre of undercut should be retained to aid denture retention, any additional undercut being blocked out in plaster on the cast and the denture flange then being extended to the full depth of the sulcus (Fig. 25.2A).

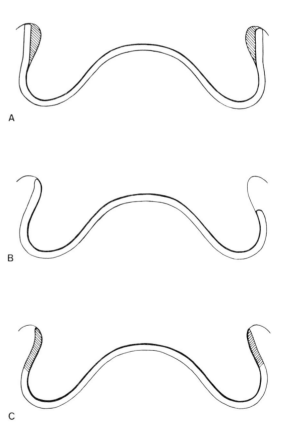

Fig. 25.2 Flange development in areas of hard tissue undercuts. A, Undercuts in excess of 1 mm have been blocked out and the flanges extended to the base of the sulci; B, Flange extended only to the level where 1 mm of undercut has been engaged on one side; C, Flange extensions developed in a resilient lining material beyond the level where 1 mm of undercut has been engaged.

2. The denture flange should extend only to the level providing 1 mm engagement of undercut on one or both sides (Fig. 25.2B).

3. The flange extensions into one or both of the undercut areas may be developed in a resilient lining material. The use of a modified acrylic type of material is preferable for this application because of its superior bond strength to an acrylic resin base, relative to that achieved by a silicone type of liner (Fig. 25.2C).

None of these options provides an ideal result. Option one may provide excessive support for the facial tissues in the undercut area and option two can provide deficient support for the facial tissues. With option three, separation of the resilient lining from the main base may occur in a disappointingly short period. The general preference is for use of option one, although option three may be chosen when the extra retention conferred by the resilient flanges is of special need.

PRESCRIPTION WRITING

When the trial dentures are returned to the laboratory for finishing, they should be accompanied by a written prescription providing the following information:

1. The colour and nature of the denture base material which is to be used.

2. Details of any modifications required in the polished surfaces of the dentures. For example, an indication for flange thickness to be increased in undercut regions, where reduction of the fitting surfaces may be required to permit denture insertion. Where contouring and/or stippling of the labial surfaces is required, this should also be stated.

3. Details of the site and depth of relief areas which are required, supplemented by the mapping-out of the areas on the casts.

FURTHER READING

Colon A, Kotwal K and Manglesdorf A D 1982 Analysis of the posterior palatal seal as related to the retention of complete dentures. J Prosthet Dent 47: 23

Kemnitzer D F 1956 Esthetics and the denture base. J Prosthet Dent 6: 603

Pound E 1954 Lost — fine arts in the fallacy of the ridges. J Prosthet Dent 4: 6

Silverman S E 1971 Dimensions and displacement problems of the posterior palatal seal. J Prosthet Dent 25: 476

Winkler S, Morris H F, Ortman H R, Staab R M and Baitz H C 1970 Characterization of denture bases for people of color. J Amer Dent Assoc 81: 1349

Wright S M 1974 Prosthetic reproduction of gingival pigmentation. Brit Dent J 136: 367

26

The insertion stage of treatment

INTRODUCTION

The insertion of dentures represents an important event for the patient and unless a careful approach is made to this stage of treatment, the success of the dentures may be prejudiced. While the preparation of the dentures following the trial stage will have been carried out by the dental technician, it must not be overlooked that the dentures are the responsibility of the dental surgeon and the laboratory work must be carefully assessed to ensure that it is of an acceptable standard. Only then can a trial of the dentures in the mouth be contemplated. Even when this step appears satisfactory and the dentures meet the required clinical criteria, the manner in which information is presented relating to the use and care of the mouth and the appliances, and of any anticipated difficulties, will play an important part in the successful outcome of the treatment.

EXTRA-ORAL EXAMINATION OF THE DENTURES

This stage is carried out after delivery of the dentures from the laboratory and before the patient arrives for the insertion appointment.

Each denture should be carefully checked for any faults which might be present. It is not uncommon for small nodules of acrylic resin to be present on the surface of the dentures. These result from the flow of acrylic resin into small surface or sub-surface air spaces present on the master cast on which the denture was processed, or the investing gypsum. Any nodules must be removed using a scraper or similar instrument or

carefully ground off using a mounted stone. The surrounding denture base must not be damaged during this process. Common sites for such nodules are the fitting surfaces and between the teeth, and while they may be difficult to see, they are readily detected by lightly moving the tip of a finger over the denture surface. Other surface imperfections which might be present include those resulting from surface damage to the master cast. These may result from accidental knife marks or small chips of gypsum lost from the cast surface. The denture surface will require careful adjustment in the regions concerned using a small mounted stone.

Where a relief area has been incorporated in the denture, the edges must be carefully examined to ensure that they are not sharp, as this could cause tissue damage when the denture is loaded in function.

The edges of any sharp relief area should be carefully smoothed using a mounted stone to merge the margin into the surrounding denture base. The denture margins should be examined to ensure that their form is continuously curved and free of any sharp angles which may traumatise the tissues.

Finally, the dentures should be fitted together with the teeth in the maximal intercuspal position as a means of detecting contact or interference between the posterior aspects of the denture bases which will affect contact relations between the dentures when placed in the mouth. Any such contact will need to be removed by reducing the thickness of the upper and/or lower denture in the area(s) concerned.

Following the extra-oral examination of the dentures and completion of any required adjustments, the dentures should then be stored in a suitable antiseptic solution to await the arrival of the patient.

INTRA-ORAL EXAMINATION OF THE DENTURES

On the arrival of the patient, any existing dentures should be removed and the mouth carefully examined for evidence of any oral damage which might be present, as this may affect the patient's reaction to the new dentures. If any tissue damage is present this should be pointed out to the patient and any necessary treatment instituted.

Extension, retention and stability of the dentures

Each denture should be assessed in turn, commencing with the upper denture. Where undercuts of an unyielding nature are present in the mouth, allowance will have been provided for these during the laboratory stages of denture production in accordance with the instructions provided in the laboratory prescription. Because of the dimensional changes which accompany the processing of acrylic resin, resistance may be met on attempting to insert the denture. Should this occur, no attempt should be made to force the denture into place. Similarly, where undercuts associated with more yielding tissues are present, it may have been decided not to eliminate these in the denture on the grounds that they may be useful as a means of providing additional retention. Such a denture may also meet resistance on attempted insertion. Where resistance is felt in the direction of the planned path of insertion, careful observation may enable the detection of tissue blanching in the region of resistance where relief of the denture is required. A low viscosity pressure relief cream is a very useful aid for the detection of undercuts. The cream is applied to the denture base and an attempted insertion of the denture is made and the denture removed when resistance occurs. Inspection of the denture base will show that the pressure relief cream has been removed from the area of contact with the tissues. The area from which the cream was removed should be carefully relieved and the whole process

repeated until the denture is fully seated into position in the mouth.

Once seated against the basal tissues, the denture should be checked for accuracy of extension and effectiveness of retention and stability. These procedures and the steps to be taken in the event of any faults being detected have been fully described in Chapter 25. Modified areas must be smoothed and polished on completion of the required adjustment.

The upper denture should then be removed and the lower denture placed in the mouth following a similar procedure to that outlined above for the upper denture.

Aesthetics

When any adjustments required to effect insertion of the dentures have been completed, both dentures are inserted into the mouth together and the appearance checked by the operator as described in the previous chapter. This is to ensure that the form of the flanges and contours, as accepted at the trial stage and requested in the laboratory prescription, have been incorporated in the denture. Only errors in relation to excessive fullness of the flanges could be corrected at this stage by grinding and subsequent repolishing.

Poor aesthetics resulting from inadequate contouring or displacement of a tooth or teeth from the position accepted at the trial stage cannot be corrected at the chairside and will require reprocessing after correcting the deficiency, or possibly remaking of the denture(s).

Occlusion

With both dentures in the mouth, the vertical and horizontal components of the jaw registration should now be verified. Because of the dimensional changes known to occur during processing between the trial denture stage and the production of the completed denture, an increase in the vertical height of the dentures is anticipated. This will result in a reduction in the freeway space of the order of 0.5–1 mm when measured as described in Chapter 9. Correction of this error will take place during the process of selective grinding of the teeth (below). It is, however, possible that an error in the jaw relationship has been incorporated in the dentures by virtue of the acceptance of an incorrect horizontal or vertical component or both, and this can generally be detected at this stage.

Occasionally the tooth movement which occurs during processing results in gross interference between opposing teeth. This will be apparent when the patient is asked to close into the retruded jaw relationship. Where gross interference of this nature is observed it is usually associated with a single premature contact and should be eliminated by grinding the offending contact(s) after first accurately locating the position using articulating paper. The vertical component of the jaw relationship can then be checked. Both the rest vertical dimension and the occlusal vertical dimension are measured to verify the presence of freeway space.

Where the freeway space is excessive or absent, one or both of the dentures may have to be remade. Only very rarely can sufficient tooth substance be removed by grinding, to provide for freeway space without gross mutilation of the tooth surfaces.

The horizontal component of the jaw registration is then checked. While the occlusion will not be perfect at this stage because of processing changes, lack of coincidence between maximum intercuspation and the retruded jaw relationship can be readily detected. Where this exceeds a distance in excess of approximately one quarter of the mesiodistal dimension of a cusp, it is unlikely to be correctable by occlusal grinding, and it will be necessary to reset the posterior teeth of one or both dentures or to remake the dentures.

Where the occlusion is substantially correct, or has only a minor error which may be corrected by occlusal modification, the next step is that of perfecting the occlusion by selective grinding following remounting on the articulator.

Remounting the processed dentures

The upper denture is mounted on an average value or adjustable articulator using a face-bow record so that the denture is correctly related to the hinge axis of the articulator. The lower denture is then mounted on the articulator in the retruded jaw relationship by means of a wax interocclusal record. This is obtained by attaching a layer of modelling wax approximately 2 mm thick to the occlusal surfaces of the lower posterior teeth, while the upper denture is seated in position in the mouth. The wax on the lower denture is thoroughly softened, the denture placed in the mouth and the patient persuaded to close into the retruded jaw relationship. Closure is stopped just before complete penetration to the opposing teeth occurs. If closure to contact of the opposing teeth is permitted, cuspal interferences may guide the mandible into an unacceptable position. Such a record may be referred to in the literature as a 'pre-centric registration'. The denture and the attached interocclusal record are removed from the mouth and placed in cold water to harden the wax thoroughly. The wax is then trimmed to remove any excess wax beyond the indentations of the cusps of the upper teeth, as the excess may form guiding planes which might influence the path of closure. The denture and the attached record is reinserted and checked for coincidence with the retruded jaw relationship. When satisfied with the accuracy of the wax record, it is used to assist attachment of the lower denture to the articulator with the dentures in the retruded jaw relationship. Selective grinding can then be carried out.

Selective grinding

The aims of selective grinding are to provide balanced contacts between the teeth in the retruded jaw relationship and in lateral and protrusive contact relations, and free sliding contact movements to eccentric positions without cuspal interferences. At the same time the occlusal vertical dimension must be maintained.

Selective grinding to the retruded jaw relationship. After remounting the dentures on the articulator, the wax interocclusal record is removed and the occlusion observed. Typically, contact between the opposing teeth will occur towards the posterior aspect of the occlusal table. Using thin articulating paper interposed between the opposing teeth the upper bow of the articulator is closed to record the points of first contact of the teeth. Those points will be marked by the articulating paper and a decision must be made as to whether the prominent cusp of the tooth or the fossa or other region which it contacts will need reduction.

In general, where a premature contact is present only in the retruded position and does not cause interfering contacts when lateral excursions of the articulator are made, fossa reduction should be undertaken. Where a cusp produces premature contacts in the retruded relationship and also in lateral relationships, cusp reduction may be required. It should be appreciated that the vertical dimension of dentures having a normal occlusal relationship of the posterior teeth, is maintained by the buccal cusps of the lower teeth and the palatal cusps of the upper teeth and their opposing fossae. Thus, once the originally planned occlusal vertical dimension of the dentures is restored, no further reduction of those parts of the teeth concerned with vertical dimension maintenance should be undertaken.

Where minor mesiodistal inaccuracy of the contact relations between the opposing teeth is present, grinding of the cuspal inclined planes may be required. This should be done in such a way that the cuspal angles are maintained. Grinding of the mesial inclined planes has the effect of producing a more distal position of the tip of the cusp and vice versa (Fig. 26.1).

Fig. 26.1 Diagram to illustrate the effect of grinding cuspal inclines (shaded) to correct a minor mesiodistal error in occlusion. Note that the cuspal angles have been maintained. Buccal aspect. A = mesial.

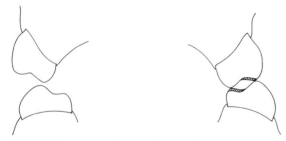

Fig. 26.2 Illustration of a coronal section through the molar region of a denture during a lateral movement with premature contact on the working side. To produce contact on the balancing side, the shaded areas will need to be reduced.

Selective grinding for lateral excursions. Once balanced contact has been achieved in the retruded relationship, balance in lateral excursions may be sought. Thin articulating paper is placed between the opposing teeth and the condylar mechanism is operated to produce a lateral excursion to the right. If, when the buccal and lingual cusps are in contact on the working side and the balancing side of the denture teeth are out of contact (Fig. 26.2), the buccal cusps of the upper teeth and/or the lingual cusps of the lower teeth should be reduced. The lower buccal and upper palatal cusps must not be ground as these are required for the maintenance of vertical dimension. Similarly, if the lower lingual cusp and the upper palatal cusps occlude prematurely in a lateral excursion, the lower lingual cusp will need to be reduced.

Grinding the buccal upper and the lingual lower cusps to obtain balanced occlusion in lateral movements is often referred to as grinding to the B.U.L.L rule.

Should the balancing side show premature occlusion between the lower buccal and the palatal upper cusps, the buccal cusp of the lower tooth may be reduced in preference to the palatal cusp of the upper tooth.

When balance has been achieved for the right lateral excursion, a similar procedure is followed to produce balance for the left lateral excursion.

Selective grinding for protrusive excursions. Following selective grinding to produce balance in the retruded jaw relationship and lateral excursions, the main premature contacts for protrusive excursions may be associated with the anterior teeth. This may require limited grinding of the incisal edges of the lower teeth which should be carried out in such a manner as to simulate attrition of the teeth.

Final milling and polishing the teeth. In order to ensure that the movements of balanced articulation in excursions of the mandible can be achieved smoothly, selective grinding may be followed by the use of a paste of fine grit carborundum and glycerine. This paste is spread on the occlusal surfaces of the teeth and up to six contact sliding movements incorporating lateral and protrusive excursions can be made without possible severe reduction of the cusps.

When selective grinding is complete, the tooth

surfaces must be carefullly polished as rough tooth surfaces can be a source of severe irritation to the patient. Grinding will have been accomplished using fine grit mounted stones in a handpiece. Where procelain teeth have been used, repolishing with rubber bonded abrasive wheels and polishing cups will be required, followed by a pumice slurry applied using a large diameter buff revolving at high speed. Where acrylic teeth are concerned, a pumice slurry applied by means of a long filament heatless bristle brush will suffice.

The dentures are now ready for reinsertion into the mouth when the vertical and horizontal components of the jaw registration are checked. If any lack of coincidence between maximum intercuspation and the retruded jaw relationship is present, the above procedure must be repeated. The vertical component of the registration should now coincide with that planned at the trial denture stage of treatment.

Following selective grinding with the dentures in the mouth, the patient should be questioned regarding evenness of posterior tooth contact, as most patients are able to detect slight pressure differences from one side to the other on closure. There should now be no pressure differences appreciated. As the patient brings the teeth into contact, there should be no movement of either denture, relative to the jaws, visible. No sliding contacts should be observable following the initial contact between the dentures when the patient closes into the retruded jaw relationship.

Once satisfied that the occlusion is fully balanced, the patient is then given a hand mirror so that the new dentures can be inspected.

INSTRUCTIONS TO THE PATIENT

Prior to dismissing the patient after insertion of the dentures, instructions in the use and care of the dentures and the oral tissues must be given. Any anticipated difficulties which might arise should be discussed at this stage and a further appointment must be given so that the progress of the patient can be reviewed.

Experienced denture wearers having oral tissues in good condition will already have views on denture management, whereas those receiving dentures for the first time will look to the dentist for advice in this new experience. It is advisable to give full information to both groups of patients and verbal instructions in the use and care of the dentures should be reinforced by the provision of written instructions. The advice given should be designed to enable the patient to adjust to the dentures as quickly as possible and to understand the limitations of complete dentures.

The patient should be instructed in the insertion and removal of the dentures and should be asked to demonstrate this so that the dentist is certain that the patient has mastered the procedure. The points covered in verbal and written form should include:

1. Eating may be difficult at first. Food should be cut into small pieces and chewed slowly and carefully. Tough and sticky foods should be avoided in the initial learning period.

2. The dentures should be removed and cleaned after each meal. Cleansing of the dentures can be carried out using a soft brush with soap and cold water. A proprietary denture cleaner may be used, following the manufacturer's instructions.

3. The dentures should be removed at night and stored in water to prevent drying of the appliances and possible consequent warping.

4. A warning that pain and soreness may occur with new dentures should be given and that adjustment to the denture(s) may be required. The patient should be advised that in the event of severe pain, the dentures should be removed from the mouth and placed in water. An appointment with the dentist to review the situation should be sought as soon as possible. It is helpful from the diagnostic point of view, if the patient will return the dentures to the mouth on the day of the appointment as painful areas are not always easily detectable.

5. The patient must be warned against attempting to adjust the dentures as such a procedure can cause permanent damage to them.

Finally, an appointment is given to return for review of the mouth and dentures in seven days time. The patient should be urged to keep the review appointment even if it is felt by him or her to be unnecessary, as incipient tissue damage might be evident to the dentist and corrective measures could then be taken which will prevent possible discomfort.

FURTHER READING

Atkinson H F and Grant A A 1962 An investigation into tooth movement during the packing and polymerizing of acrylic denture base materials. Austral Dent J 7: 101

Collett H A 1967 Motivation: a factor in dental treatment. J Prosthet Dent 17: 5

Hickey J C, Boucher C O and Woelfel J B 1962 Responsibility of the dentist in complete dentures. J Prosthet Dent 12: 637

Jankelson B 1962 Adjustment of dentures at time of insertion and alterations to compensate for tissue change. J Amer Dent Assoc 64: 521

Lawson W A 1965 Information and advice for patients wearing dentures. Dent Pract Dent Rec 15: 402

MacCallum M, Stafford G D, MacCulloch W T and Combe E C 1968 Which cleanser? Dent Pract Dent Rec 19: 83

Mack A 1964 Complete dentures Part IV The finished denture. Brit Dent J 117: 52

Neill D J 1968 A study of materials and methods used in cleaning dentures. Brit Dent J 124: 107

27

The review stage of treatment

INTRODUCTION

Following the insertion of complete dentures, the patient should be given an appointment to attend for review in approximately seven days time.

At the review visit, the patient should be questioned concerning any difficulties which have arisen during the wearing of the dentures. A thorough examination should then be carried out of the oral tissues and the dentures. In the course of this examination signs of tissue damage may be noted which link to the difficulties reported by the patient. In addition, signs of symptomless tissue damage may be noted.

A diagnosis should then be made of the cause of all problems revealed by the history and examination procedures. Appropriate treatment should be carried out to resolve these problems.

HISTORY OF THE PATIENT'S EXPERIENCES

Initially, the patient should be asked to give an account of any difficulties encountered when wearing the dentures or which have occurred during insertion and removal of the dentures. Where specific complaints arise, secondary questioning should then be directed at obtaining information which will assist in diagnosis of the cause of the complaints. The complaints which commonly arise and the appropriate questioning which should be applied are as follows.

Pain

This is the commonest complaint made by patients following the insertion of complete dentures. The patient should be asked to describe as fully as possible the nature of the pain. To assist categorisation, the patient may be asked, for example, if the pain is of a sharp and stabbing nature which is brought on by the application of biting pressure to the dentures. Alternatively, is the pain of a neuralgic type which may be likened to toothache or is it better described as a burning sensation in one or both of the denture-bearing areas?

Subsequent questions asked should include the following:

1. How long has the pain been present and is it relieved by leaving out the dentures?

2. Is the pain present continually when the denture is being worn, or does it arise only at certain times, for example, at mealtimes or when the denture is being inserted or removed?

3. Is the pain localised to a small area of the oral tissues or is it widespread? The exact area affected by the pain should be established as far as is possible.

4. Have any analgesics or other medication been taken to try and relieve the pain?

Looseness of the dentures

The questions asked should include:

1. Do both dentures or only one seem to be loose, and, where the latter applies, which one is affected?

2. Does the looseness arise indiscriminately throughout the period when the denture is worn, or does it only arise when specific functions are being undertaken, for example, eating or speaking?

3. Does displacement of the denture(s) seem to

initiate in a particular area, for example, does the back part of the lower denture rise when the tongue is moved?

Unsatisfactory aesthetics

Many patients are reticent about complaining of the appearance of dentures, fearing that they may be considered to be unduly vain. Careful and sympathetic questioning is necessary if the exact nature of the problem is to be established.

Initial questioning should be directed at finding out whether the patient's complaint relates to the display of the teeth or to the support which the dentures provide for the cheeks and lips.

Where the complaint concerns the display of the teeth, secondary questioning should aim at determining the feature or features which concern the patient. For example, do the anterior teeth seem to be too large or too small? Has the occlusal plane been set at too high a level providing deficient display of the upper anterior teeth? Does the patient consider that the centre line has been misplaced or is the arrangement of the teeth unsatisfactory?

Where the problem relates to the support of the lips and cheeks provided by the dentures, the patient should be asked to indicate whether it is considered to be excessive or deficient, and whether it applies to a specific area or to the whole denture.

Speech problems

Questioning should be directed at determining the exact nature of the patient's complaint, for example, does whistling or lisping arise during the pronunciation of the 's' sound?

Intolerance to denture wearing

Where the patient complains of an inability to wear the dentures continuously because of the development of nausea, the following questions should be asked:

1. For how long can the dentures be worn before they have to be removed?

2. Does taking out only one of the dentures remove the problem and, if so, which denture is concerned?

3. Has a similar problem occurred with any previous dentures worn by the patient?

Inefficient mastication

Where this complaint arises, the patient should be asked to indicate:

1. Does the problem arise when attempting to chew all types of food, or is it restricted to the chewing of certain types only, for example, fibrous foods such as meat?

2. Are the masticatory problems accompanied by other difficulties such as pain or looseness of the dentures?

3. Does adequate room seem to be present for the placement of food in the mouth, as chewing proceeds?

EXAMINATION OF THE ORAL CAVITY AND THE DENTURES

The dentures should be removed from the mouth and a detailed examination should be made of the oral tissues with the help of a mouth mirror. Although particular attention should be paid to any areas where the patient has experienced pain, all the oral tissues should be examined since symptomless tissue changes may be noted which require treatment. The site of all the observed tissue changes should be recorded, along with an indication of their intensity, which may vary from mild hyperaemia up to frank ulceration. In all cases where it is thought that a tissue change may be associated with underlying pathology, a radiographic examination should be carried out of the area concerned.

The dentures should then be examined, first extra-orally and then intra-orally. In the extra-oral examination, the state of cleanliness of the dentures should be noted. The denture surfaces should then be examined for the presence of any irregularities which may have caused tissue irritation. For example, nodules may be found on the fitting surfaces, or sharp margins may be noted on one or more of the teeth.

Intra-oral examination of the dentures should be carried out by the application of the procedures used to check the satisfaction of the trial dentures and which are described in detail in Chapter 25. Each denture should first be checked for extension, retention and stability. The aesthetic effect of the dentures should then be observed with particular reference to any complaints relating to appearance raised by the patient. The occlusal vertical dimension of the dentures should be checked to ensure that an acceptable value of freeway space is present. The intercuspal relationship of the posterior teeth should be noted when the teeth are brought into occlusion with the mandible in retruded jaw relationship. Finally, the patient should be requested to make protrusive and lateral movement of the mandible with the teeth in contact and note made of the state of occlusal balance which is present.

Throughout the period of examination of the dentures an attempt should be made to relate the observation of any faults which are found to be present with the complaints raised by the patient. For example, a finding of overextension in a denture may relate to complaints by the patient of pain and/or of looseness of the denture.

THE CAUSE AND MANAGEMENT OF PATIENTS' COMPLAINTS

Normally, diagnosis of the cause of a patient's complaints will be possible when the history of the experiences of the patient during denture-wearing is considered in association with the findings of the examination of the oral tissues and the dentures. Occasionally, atypical conditions may be present which will require the patient being referred to an appropriate specialist before diagnosis is possible. A consideration of these conditions is considered to be beyond the scope of this text.

Once a diagnosis has been made, a decision must be made of the appropriate treatment which is necessary, for example, modification of the dentures where this is indicated.

In this section, the common causes of patients' complaints will be considered and advice given on the treatment which should be provided. The subject will be discussed under the headings previously used in the presentation of the patient's complaints.

Pain

For convenience, the complaint of pain may be considered under three sub-headings which correspond to the area of the oral tissues in which the complaint arises:

1. Cases in which the complaint of pain arises in a localised area of the oral tissues.

2. Cases in which the complaint of pain arises over a diffuse area which is restricted to part only of the denture-bearing tissues underlying one or both of the dentures.

3. Cases in which the complaint of pain arises in a diffuse area extending over most, if not all, of the denture-bearing tissues underlying one or both of the dentures.

However, it should be noted that no clear division exists between the areas involved in the first two of the following sections. Cases will be encountered in which the presenting signs and symptoms overlap the boundaries of the areas of pain concerned in these two sections. Where this arises, the treatment provided must take account of the possible causes of pain and the appropriate treatment prescribed in the consideration of each of these sections.

Cases in which the complaint of pain arises in a localised area of the oral tissues

Where the complaint arises in the denture-bearing tissues, the likely causes are one or more of the following:

1. Over-extension of the periphery of the dentures.

2. The presence of too deep or too sharp a post-dam on the upper denture.

3. Irregularites present on the fitting surfaces of the dentures, not paralleled by the form of the corresponding areas of the underlying soft tissues.

4. Localised irregularities in the inter-cuspal relationship of the dentition, either in the position of maximum intercuspation or during lateral or protrusive excursions of the mandible.

5. Excessive engagement of undercuts by the denture in a localised area.

6. Localised irregularities in the residual alveolar ridges, thinly covered with soft tissues, which have either not been relieved, or inad-

equately relieved, in the course of denture construction.

7. The presence of pathology, for example, superficially placed buried roots, in the tissues supporting the dentures.

8. The presence of the mental foramina within the lower denture-bearing area, for which either no relief or inadequate relief has been provided in the course of denture construction.

Causes one to five inclusive will usually have produced clearly visible signs of inflammatory changes in the soft tissues in the areas concerned. Visual examination of the inserted dentures will usually indicate the area of the denture responsible for the tissue damage. Where necessary, pressure relief cream may be used to indicate the causative area(s) of the denture. Where causes one to four apply, the patient will usually complain of some discomfort being present whenever the dentures are worn and that a more acute pain arises whenever biting pressure is applied. Where cause five applies, the patient may only experience severe pain when the dentures are being inserted or removed.

Visible signs of tissue damage will be seen in a proportion of cases where causes six and seven apply, but only rarely where cause eight applies. Where these causes are responsible for pain, the tissue areas concerned will be found to show increased sensitivity to pressure. Cause seven will be identified by radiographic examination of the area. For cause eight the mental foramina will be palpable within the lower denture-bearing zone. Again, pressure relief cream may be used to aid location of the portion of the denture associated with the area of the tissues where pain is arising.

Treatment of all the above causes except four and seven will require modification of the dentures by trimming of the area(s) concerned, until the painful symptoms have been relieved. Treatment of cause four will require adjustment of the occlusion by selective grinding, until full occlusal harmony of the dentition has been established. Treatment of cause seven will usually require surgery to effect resolution of the condition.

Where the complaint of pain arises in the mucosal surfaces of the lips, cheeks or tongue, the likely causes are as follows:

1. Irritation of the tissues arising from the presence of a sharp margin on one or more of the teeth.

2. Cheek biting, due to an inadequate buccal overjet having been developed in the posterior dentition.

3. Tongue biting, due to an inadequate lingual overjet having been developed in the posterior dentition, and/or the presence of too narrow an arch form, causing 'cramping' of the tongue.

Where cause one applies, treatment will involve smoothing and polishing of the sharp area of the tooth or teeth responsible for the condition.

For cause two, where the cheek biting which has occurred is of a relatively mild nature, usually associated with the development of only hyperaemia in the tissues concerned, the resolution may be achieved by the grinding of appropriate areas of the teeth to develop an improved buccal overjet. Where the posterior teeth have been set in a normal relationship, this will involve reduction of the buccal surfaces of the lower posterior teeth. Where a cross-bite arrangement of the posterior dentition has been adopted, the buccal surfaces of the upper posterior teeth should be reduced instead. In both cases the bucco-occlusal margins of the ground teeth should be rounded-over and polished, to reduce the risk of further tissue trauma arising.

For cause three where tongue biting has occurred as a consequence of the presence of an inadequate lingual overjet being present in the posterior dentition and the condition is of a relatively mild nature, treatment may be applied as described above for the condition of cheek biting. Where the posterior teeth have been set in a normal relationship, the palatal surfaces of the upper posterior teeth should be reduced and for a cross-bite relationship the lingual surfaces of the lower posterior teeth should be reduced until an adequate lingual overjet has been achieved. Rounding-over and polishing of the palato-occlusal or linguo-occlusal margins of the ground teeth should follow the above treatment.

Where tongue biting has occurred as a consequence of the arch form 'cramping' the tongue, and the condition is again of a relatively mild nature, grinding the lingual surfaces of the lower posterior teeth to increase the available tongue space may serve to resolve the condition. Where this treatment is applied, the linguo-occlusal margins of the posterior teeth should be rounded-over and polished to reduce the risk of further tissue trauma arising.

Where causes two or three have resulted in severe tissue damage arising, especially where frank ulceration of the tissues has developed, treatment of the condition will usually require the posterior teeth being reset or one at least of the dentures being remade, to provide adequate buccal or lingual overjet and/or adequate tongue space, as required.

Cases in which the complaint of pain arises over a diffuse area restricted to part only of the denture-bearing tissues underlying one or both of the dentures

The cause of this condition will most commonly found to be the presence of anatomical abnormality in the tissue area concerned. A region where this condition is often encountered is the lower anterior alveolar region.

Here, digital and radiographic examination may reveal the presence of a sharp or irregular margin in the residual alveolar ridge which may be associated with atrophy in the overlying mucosa. Pressure from a denture on such a tissue base may well stimulate a painful response. Other bony abnormalities in the lower denture-bearing tissues which may cause pain when pressure is applied by a denture include sharp mylo-hyoid ridges and the development of the genial tubercles to form a bony shelf.

In the upper denture-bearing area, pressure from the denture may give rise to pain in the area of a torus palatinus, where the area has been either unrelieved or inadequately relieved in the course of denture construction. Also in some cases, pain may arise where pressure from the denture is applied to the bone at the root of the zygomatic arch.

For all these conditions, relief of pain may be obtained by reduction of the fitting surface of the denture in the areas concerned, to reduce the pressure applied by the denture in the corresponding area. Where this is unsuccessful, treatment may necessitate surgical intervention. Alternatively, especially where surgery is contraindicated, the placement of a resilient lining in the denture may be considered.

Cases in which the complaint of pain arises in a diffuse area extending over most, if not all, of the denture-bearing tissues underlying one or both of the dentures

Two main causes may be responsible for this condition:

1. The presence of an excessive occlusal vertical dimension in the dentition.
2. Allergy or sensitivity to the denture base material which has been used.

Where cause one applies, the patient may complain of widespread pain arising in both the upper and lower denture-bearing areas. In the course of the examination of the oral tissues, inflammation of the denture-bearing tissues may be observed.

When an excessive vertical dimension is present in the dentures, the force applied by the masticatory muscles may be greater than that arising at the correct occlusal vertical dimension. Where an increase in force arises, the denture-bearing tissues may show an inflammatory response with associated pain production in the tissues. The lower denture-bearing area is particularly liable to be affected because the applied pressure is concentrated on a smaller area than that of the upper denture-bearing area. The space present between the teeth in speech will also be reduced so that the patient may complain that a clicking sound occurs in the pronunciation of some sounds as a consequence of tooth contact occurring. Difficulty may also be experienced in the production of sounds which involve contact being developed between the upper and lower lips, such as 'p', 'b' and 'm'. Where examination of the dentures shows the absence of an acceptable value for freeway space, treatment will require the remaking of one denture at least at a reduced value of occlusal vertical dimension.

Where cause two applies, the patient usually complains of a burning sensation in the denture-bearing tissues, especially in the upper jaw. On examination of the oral tissues, those in contact with the dentures may show oedema and hyperaemia.

Acrylic resin is the denture-base material which most commonly gives rise to this condition. Where allergy or sensitivity is suspected as being the responsible agent for a patient's complaint of pain, a patch test should be carried out. Details of the procedure involved in carrying out patch testing may be found in the literature relating to this topic and are considered to be outside the scope of the present text.

Where a positive diagnosis of allergy or sensitivity to a denture-base material has been made, treatment will require the dentures being remade using an alternative material (for example, vulcanite, where the allergy or sensitivity is to acrylic resin).

Looseness of the dentures

Where the patient complains that one or both of the dentures is loose throughout the period they are being worn, the cause is likely to be one or more of the following:

1. Over-extension of the periphery of the dentures relative to the level of the functional sulcus. Where intra-oral examination of the dentures shows one or more areas of over-extension to be present, the areas concerned should be reduced to the correct level by marginal trimming. A complaint of looseness of the dentures due to this cause will often be accompanied by a complaint of pain arising in the tissues in the area where over-extension is present.

2. Incorrect shaping of the denture relative to the environmental musculature. This cause is particularly liable to produce a complaint of looseness of the lower denture. The teeth may not have been set in the neutral zone (zone of minimum conflict) causing, perhaps, cramping of the tongue. Alternatively, the polished surfaces of the dentures may have been incorrectly shaped so that conflict arises between the dentures and the environmental musculature in the performance of functions such as speech. Where this cause applies, treatment will usually necessitate remaking of the dentures in a more acceptable form.

3. Inadequate retention may arise where the dentures are under-extended relative to the level of the functional sulcus. Where the upper denture is affected, a deficient post-dam may have been provided. Alternatively, the condition may arise where faults have occurred in impression-taking or in the subsequent stage of preparing the master casts. Where features of the dentures other than inadequate retention are found to be satisfactory,

relining or rebasing of the dentures may resolve the condition, (see Chapter 22, page 177 for details of the necessary impression procedures). In all other cases, treatment will involve remaking of the dentures.

Where the patient complains that the dentures are only loose when masticating food, the likely causes are one or more of the following:

1. Newness of the dentures, particularly where the patient has no previous experience of denture-wearing. Where this cause is suspected, the patient should be encouraged to persevere. It may be helpful to reiterate previous advice that the dentures are 'foreign bodies' in their mouth and that it takes time for the tissues to adjust to their presence. It may take several weeks or even months for a patient who is new to denture wearing to learn the art of denture control. The patient should be reassured that with perseverance the position will improve and that food and dentures will no longer seem to be inexorably mixed at mealtimes!

2. Unilateral instability of the dentures arising in the course of mastication, as a consequence of the teeth having been set excessively buccal to the crest of the alveolar ridges. The lower denture is particularly liable to be affected, tilting from side to side as masticatory pressure is applied. Treatment will require resetting of the teeth into a more acceptable position relative to the alveolar ridges, or remaking of the dentures.

3. Bilateral instability occurring as a consequence of a lack of occlusal balance being present in the dentition. Where this cause applies, a face-bow record and wax pre-centric record should be obtained. The dentures should then be remounted on an average value or adjustable articulator and selectively ground to develop occlusal balance. The procedures for obtaining the necessary records and carrying out selective grinding are considered in Chapter 26, pages 209–211.

Unsatisfactory aesthetics

This complaint should arise only rarely if adequate care was taken in checking aesthetics at the trial denture stage. Where the patient does raise objections to the aesthetics of the dentures at the review stage, questioning will often indicate that the objections arise from comments made by the patient's relatives or friends.

Whenever possible, an attempt should be made to overcome the complaints by modification of the dentures. For example, where the complaint is that the dentures provide excessive support for the lips and/or cheeks, the denture flanges may be reduced in thickness until the required reduced level of support for the facial tissues has been obtained. Where the complaint is that the dentures provide inadequate support for the facial tissues, wax may be added to increase the thickness of the flanges until the required level of support has been achieved. Increasing flange thickness to provide greater support for the facial tissues is often referred to as 'plumping' of the dentures. The added wax is converted into the appropriate denture base material in the laboratory, before the dentures are returned to the patient.

Where the complaint of unsatisfactory aesthetics relates to the teeth, it may concern features such as the size or colour of the teeth, the position of the centre line and the degree to which the upper and/or lower anterior teeth show when the patient is smiling or talking.

Where modification of tooth arrangements is necessary to meet such complaints, remaking of the dentures will usually be necessary.

Speech problems

Where a patient is provided with complete dentures for the first time, a period of adaptation of a month or so may be necessary before the quality of speech approches that which occurred when the natural dentition was present. In this period, the lips, cheeks and tongue will be adapting to the presence of the dentures, with gradual improvement in the quality of the sounds which are produced. The patient may be warned that this period of adaptation may be necessary when the dentures are inserted.

Some minor disruption of speech may also occur where replacement complete dentures are provided. The patient should be reassured that such a problem is likely to disappear in a month or so as the tissues adapt to the presence of the new dentures.

Where speech problems persist beyond this time, modification of the dentures may be necessary. The sounds most likely to be affected are those associated with the pronunciation of the letters 's', 'p' and 'b'. This subject is considered in some detail in the parallel section relating to the review stage of partial denture treatment (Chapter 20, page 157). That section should be consulted for details of the speech defects and of the denture modifications which are necessary to overcome them.

Intolerance to denture wearing

Where the patient complains of the development of nausea on or shortly after the insertion of complete dentures and indicates that the upper denture seems to initiate nausea, the likely causes causes are one or more of the following:

1. Over-extension of the posterior aspect of the upper denture. Where the denture extends on to the movable tissues of the soft palate, the retching reflex may be stimulated.

2. The posterior extension of the upper denture is correct by 'normal' standards, but the denture covers areas of the posterior region of the hard palate which show abnormal sensitivity. This condition may relate to the presence of an enhanced amount or abnormal distribution of nerves in the tissues overlying the hard palate.

3. Incorrect development of denture form at the posterior palatal termination. Where a ledge is present at the junction of the posterior border of the denture with the palatal tissues posterior to the denture, irritation of the dorsum of the tongue may occcur during deglutition and speech, giving rise to nausea. Enhanced sensitivity of the posterior region of the dorsum of the tongue has been said to occur in some patients as a consequence of the presence of an abnormal distribution of the glossopharyngeal nerves.

4. Inadequate retention being present in the upper denture. Nausea may arise when displacement of the denture occurs in function, bringing it into contact with the dorsum of the tongue, particularly where the latter shows enhanced sensitivity.

Where the patient indicates that the lower denture seems to initiate nausea, the likely causes are:

5. 'Cramping' of the tongue as a consequence of the provision of inadequate tongue space.

6. Over-extension of the denture postero-lingually so that contact occurs in function between the denture and the tissues of the palato-glossal arch.

Where cause one applies, the treatment required will be reduction of the posterior extension of the upper denture to a level where it lies just anterior to the vibrating line. Where necessary, a new post-dam should be provided.

For cause two, treatment will depend upon the severity of the condition. Where only mild nausea arises, not extending to actual retching, the patient may be asked to persevere with the wearing of the denture for a further trial period. With time, the tissues may adapt to the presence of the denture and the nausea will disappear without further treatment being necessary. Where this is tried but resolution of the nausea does not occur, or where the condition is found to be of a more severe nature at the initial review visit, it will usually be necessary to reduce the posterior palatal extension of the upper denture. Examination of the posterior palatal tissues should be carried out with an instrument such as a ball-ended burnisher and the area of enhanced sensitivity noted. The extension of the denture should then be reduced to avoid coverage of the corresponding tissue area. Minimum reduction of palatal coverage compatible with overcoming the complaint of nausea should be aimed at so that optimal denture retention will be achieved. A posterior palatal seal, approximately 1 mm deep, should be developed around the new posterior palatal border of the denture.

It should be noted that a complaint of severe nausea due to enhanced sensitivity in the posterior palatal tissues is unlikely to be noted at the review stage without prior warning of the condition having arisen during earlier treatment stages. Often, it will have been necessary to reduce the palatal extension of the upper special tray, upper occlusal rim and upper trial denture baseplate to overcome nausea experienced in these stages. Where this applies, the palatal extension of the finished denture should be developed to a similar level. A denture of the so-called 'horseshoe' form may be necessary where an extensive area of the palatal tissues show enhanced sensitivity.

Treatment of cause three will require trimming of the polished surface of the upper denture in the region of the posterior palatal border until the ledge has been removed.

Treatment of cause four will require action to improve the retention of the upper denture. This may be achieved by relining of the denture in appropriate cases, otherwise remaking of the denture may be necessary, as noted on page 218.

The treatment necessary to overcome cause five will depend upon the severity of the condition. Where the condition is of a mild nature, trimming of the lingual surfaces of the lower posterior teeth and/or thinning of the lingual flanges of the lower denture may provide sufficient increase in tongue space to overcome the complaint. Where the condition is more severe, treatment will usually necessitate remaking of the dentures to provide adequate tongue space.

Treatment of cause six involves reduction of the postero-lingual extension of the lower denture until contact of the denture with the palato-glossal arch no longer occurs in function.

Where the patient complains of nausea, but this only develops several hours after the insertion of the dentures, the probable cause will be a reaction of the tissues to the bulk of the dentures. Where this problem arises, the patient may again be asked to persevere with the wearing of the dentures in the hope that adaptation will develop in time and nausea will no longer be a problem. Where this is unsuccessful, the bulk of the dentures should be reduced by trimming of the polished surfaces. The palate of the upper denture should receive particular attention. Care should be taken that the reduction which is applied does not exceed the level at which the strength of the denture will be impaired.

In some instances, it may prove to be necessary to provide a denture with a metal palate (for example, in cast cobalt-chromium alloy) to achieve a tolerable thickness in the palate. Singers in particular may present this special need.

Inefficient mastication

Where a patient complains of a difficulty in chewing all types of food, the cause is likely to be one or more of the following:

1. Inexperience in the wearing of complete dentures. When a patient wears complete dentures for the first time, an induction period is usually necessary in which the patient learns the art of muscular control of the dentures. This period may extend from one week to six months or even more, being dependent upon the ability of the patient's tissues to adapt to the presence of the dentures. In general, the older the patient at the time complete dentures are first fitted, the longer is the induction period likely to be. During the induction period, the patient is likely to experience difficulty in the mastication of food.

2. The presence of an excessive vertical dimension in the dentition. This may result in the patient experiencing difficulty in placing food on the occlusal table and will require a conscious effort to increase mouth-opening beyond the normal level each time food has to be placed in the mouth.

3. The occlusal plane of the dentures having been set at too high a level. Where this applies, the tongue and cheeks may experience difficulty in re-positioning food on the occlusal table as mastication proceeds.

4. The presence of an inadequate vertical dimension in the dentition. One of the possible consequences of an excessive freeway space is that the power applied by the masticatory muscles may be reduced. This can give rise to inefficient mastication.

5. Lack of occlusal balance in the dentition. Where cuspal interferences arise in the course of mandibular movements, a reduction in masticatory efficiency is also likely to occur. This problem is particularly liable to occur where the patient has a ruminatory type of masticatory mechanism.

6. As an accompaniment of a complaint of looseness of the denture. Where the dentures are loose in the course of mastication of food, the efficiency of chewing is likely to be reduced.

7. As an accompaniment of a complaint of pain in the denture-bearing area. Where the patient is experiencing pain in the denture-bearing areas, the pain-protection reflex may limit the force applied by the masticatory muscles in the course of the mastication of food. Decrease in applied pressure may result in decreased masticatory efficiency.

Where the patient complains of masticatory inefficiency, restricted mainly to the chewing of fibrous foods such as meat, the likely causes are one or more of the following:

8. The presence of anatomical-type posterior teeth whose cuspal form has been excessively reduced, usually in the course of selective grinding.

9. The use of flat-cusped or non-anatomical form of posterior teeth. Teeth of this type may provide poorer masticatory efficiency than that provided by teeth of an anatomical form.

10. The use of acrylic posterior teeth. This problem is particulary liable to be encountered where the patient has previously worn dentures provided with porcelain posterior teeth.

Treatment of cause one will require the patient being reassured that as muscular control of the dentures is developed, masticatory efficiency should improve. Where causes two or four apply, treatment will require remaking of the dentures to provide an adequate and yet not excessive value of freeway space. Treatment of cause three will require the dentures being remade to provide a more appropriate level of the occlusal plane. This need will have to be considered in association with the need to set the occlusal plane at a level at which acceptable aesthetics will be achieved, and some compromise in the level selected for use may be necessary. Guidance on the optimal position of the occlusal plane for achieving masticatory efficiency may be obtained by observing the level of the dorsum of the tongue when the tongue is at rest. The plane should be set at the observed level of the dorsum of the tongue. Treatment of cause five will require the dentures being remounted on an average value or adjustable articulator via the use of a face-bow and wax pre-centric records and selectively ground into a state of occlusal balance. The procedures for obtaining the necessary records and for carrying out selective grinding are considered in Chapter 26, pages 209–211.

Treatment of causes six and seven will require resolution of the complaints of looseness of the dentures or pain in the denture bearing areas, following the procedures considered on pages 218 and 215 respectively.

Treatment of cause eight will require replacement of the posterior teeth by a new set, or remaking of the dentures.

Where causes nine or ten apply, the patient may be asked to persevere with use of the dentures for a further trial period. If no improvement in masticatory efficiency arises, it may be advisable to provide replacement posterior teeth, using anatomical type posterior teeth where cause nine applies and porcelain posterior teeth for cause ten.

Other complaints

The patient may raise one or more complaints at the review stage which have not been covered in the above list. For each of these, a diagnosis of the cause of the complaint should be made. This will be based on the history of the patient's experiences when wearing the dentures, considered in association with the findings of the examination of the oral tissues and the dentures. Appropriate treatment to overcome the cause of each complaint should then be provided.

One complaint that may be frequently encountered is that of excessive salivation, particularly where the patient has been provided with complete dentures for the first time. The only treatment normally required for this complaint is reassurance of the patient that the condition is likely to resolve in the fullness of time.

General note

In all instances where the peripheries, teeth or polished surfaces of the dentures have been modified at the review stage, the areas concerned must be carefully repolished before the dentures are returned to the patient.

Where severe tissue damage was noted at the review stage, the patient should receive an appointment for further review in approximately seven days time to see if the treatment provided has effected resolution of the condition. Where necess-

ary, further treatment should be applied and the patient re-examined after the same interval. This procedure should be repeated until full resolution of the condition has occurred. Where extra-oral examination of the dentures showed a poor level of cleanliness to be present, the advice given to the patient at the insertion stage concerning care of the dentures should be repeated at the review stage.

At the conclusion of the review stage, the patient should be provided with information on the likely life of complete dentures and of the need to return for further reviews.

It may be pointed out to the patient that as a consequence of the changes which occur in the denture bearing tissues and in the dentures, the average life of complete dentures is of the order of five years. However, considerable variation in this period may occur in individual cases. It is desirable that the patient should return for review at approximately two-yearly intervals. The oral tissues and the dentures can then be examined to determine if their condition is still satisfactory or if further treatment is required. Of particular importance is the fact that symptomless changes can occur in the oral tissues which require treatment. For example, hyperplasia may develop in the tissues related to the peripheries of the dentures without the patient being aware of this occurrence.

The patient should also be encouraged to seek a further appointment for review whenever circumstances arise with the dentures which give cause for concern. For example, pain may develop in the oral tissues or the dentures may become loose or provide less efficient mastication of food than that present when the dentures were first fitted.

FURTHER READING

Kovats, J J 1971 Clinical evaluation of the gagging patient. J Prosthet, Dent 25: 613
McCabe, J F and Basker, R M 1976 Tissue sensitivity to acrylic resin. Brit Dent J 140: 347
Makila, E 1974 Adjustment visits following provision of complete dentures. J Oral Rehab 1: 373
Miller, E L 1973 Types of inflammation caused by oral prostheses. J Prosthet Dent 30: 380
Morstad, A R and Peterson, A D 1968 Post-insertion denture

problems. J Prosthet Dent 19: 126
Murphy, W M 1971 The effect of complete dentures on taste perception. Brit Dent J 130: 210
Nagle, R J 1958 Post-insertion problems in complete denture prosthesis. J Amer Dent Assoc 57: 183
Yemm, R 1972 Stress-induced muscle activity: a possible etiological factor in denture soreness. J Prosthet Dent 28: 133

28

The overdenture

INTRODUCTION

An overdenture is a removable complete or partial denture which is supported by mucoperiosteum and prepared teeth or roots. The more commonly used overdentures are of the complete denture form and this chapter will be confined to a consideration of principles related to complete overdentures. For further information relating to the application of overdentures to partial denture treatment or the treatment of such defects as partial anodontia, the literature should be consulted.

ADVANTAGES OF OVERDENTURES

These largely relate to advantages which accrue from the retention of tooth substance:

1. Retained roots provide a stimulus for the retention of alveolar bone. The loss of a tooth is invariably followed by alveolar bone loss and, to date, all attempts to prevent this have failed.

2. Periodontal proprioception is retained. This is equally true for endodontically treated teeth as for vital teeth.

3. Enhanced retention over that obtainable by conventional complete dentures is possible.

4. Denture stability and support is enhanced over that of complete dentures.

5. Overdenture treatment does not preclude the provision of conventional complete dentures at a later stage should this prove necessary. In addition, as the form of an overdenture is similar to that of a complete denture, the potential of the patient for effective management of complete dentures may be enhanced.

DISADVANTAGES OF OVERDENTURES

1. The susceptibility of the overlaid teeth to caries is high and meticulous home care together with the need for frequent recall for examination of the patient is required.

2. Periodontal disease of the retained teeth may continue or even be stimulated by the presence of an overdenture. Normal stimulation of the gingival tissues by the tongue and cheeks is absent and plaque accumulation is enhanced.

3. Bony undercuts of the alveolar ridge are often found adjacent to retained teeth, especially where isolated teeth are present. Such undercuts are usually situated on the buccal and labial aspects of the arch. The possibility of varying the path of insertion of an overdenture is limited and consequently where an undercut is present, the cast must be blocked out during the processing of the denture or the flange must be foreshortened. See page 205 for further consideration of these approaches. When either blocking out or foreshortening of the flange is used, aesthetic implications exist, as the former may result in excessive bulkiness of the flange, and the latter may cause uneven lip support.

4. Encroachment beyond the denture space. The presence of a prepared tooth, particularly where a precision attachment is to be used to aid retention, may produce excessively bulky contours. These may encroach on the tongue space and cause possible speech difficulties, or in some cases may even encroach on the available freeway space.

PRINCIPLES OF OVERDENTURE TREATMENT

All unusable teeth are extracted leaving the teeth or roots which can be used for overdenture support. These teeth are then reduced in length in order to improve the crown-root ratio so that the potential for the effects of high laterally directed forces is substantially reduced. In most instances, reduction of the crown length to the extent required — some 2 mm above the gingival crest — will mean that endodontic treatment must be carried out.

Support and retention for overdentures

The choice of supporting elements for overdentures is usually very limited. Whenever possible, support which is symmetrically distributed about the jaw should be sought. For example, a canine and molar on each side of the arch will be satisfactory. However, only two teeth, especially when present in the anterior part of the lower arch, may be usefully applied. Unilateral retention of teeth is less satisfactory, although such a situation still offers advantages over the conditions which may result from total tooth loss. Even teeth which exhibit clinically demonstrable mobility may be considered for use as such movement will be found to diminish after decoronation of the tooth. The important point is that there must be at least 5–7 mm of bony support with intact gingival tissues which can be brought to a healthy state.

Endodontic treatment is carried out and the crown of the tooth removed. For the simple type of overdenture, no additional retaining device is used beyond the normal forces utilised in the retention of complete dentures, and any additional frictional forces generated by contact with the retained teeth. Where a cast coping is to be placed over the remaining root face(s) it is of a shallow dome form retained in the root canal by means of a short post, and having margins slightly supragingivally placed (Fig. 28.1). If no casting is to be used, the exposed part of the root canal is sealed with amalgam and the amalgam and dentine smoothed and polished to a rounded form. Such a form is easy to clean and maintain by the patient.

Where an attachment device is to be used to

Fig. 28.1 Section through a tooth having a shallow dome form of casting cemented in position. A, Casting; B, Gingival margin; C, Alveolar bone.

provide positive retention and/or additional support, it may be of a type requiring cementation of a threaded post into the root canal, or one requiring the soldering of the patrix portion to the root face coping. Magnetic forces using cobalt-samarium magnets have also been successfully applied to assist overdenture retention. The splinting of roots together can also be undertaken using bar devices such as the Dolder bar, which will also provide positive retention.

Fabrication of the overdenture

In the case of the simple overdenture where no precision attachment devices are included in the denture design, conventional methods are used to construct the overdenture. The overdenture is mucosa supported at rest and becomes tooth and mucosa supported when loaded. A small space is present between the root face or coping and the denture under resting conditions (Fig. 28.2). This

Fig. 28.2 Section through a simple overdenture resting in position over a prepared root. A, Overdenture; B, Space between root facing and the denture; C, Amalgam plug in the root facing.

may be provided by relieving the denture as a stage in denture processing as described on page 204 for the provision of a relief area in a conventional denture. The gingival margin region must be relieved to prevent damage to these tissues as movement of the denture occurs during function. Excessive relief must be avoided as hypertrophy of the tissues into the space created may occur.

Where precision attachments are to be used, the procedures to be followed for the impression stage and the location and incorporation of the attachments varies between the different devices and no attempt will be made to consider details of these. The major problem in the fabrication of such an overdenture is the incorporation of the retention device within the normal outline form of a complete denture. This may be found to be an impossible ideal and bulging of the denture in the region of the device is often necessary.

CARE OF OVERDENTURES

Whether the root facing is covered by a cast coping or not, the dangers of caries and periodontal disease are ever present. While the care of the gingival tissues is simplified by the loss of the crown of the tooth, the potential for plaque retention is considerably enhanced by the presence of the overdenture. Thus meticulous oral hygiene procedures and denture cleansing must be impressed on the patient. Recall of the patient every four months is recommended so that any caries or deterioration of the gingival condition can be detected early and any necessary treatment and reinforcement of oral hygiene instruction undertaken.

FURTHER READING

Brewer A A and Morrow R M 1975 Overdentures. Mosby, St Louis
Loiselle R J, Crum R J, Rooney G E and Stuever C H 1972 The physiologic basis for the overlay denture. J Prosthet Dent 28: 4
Toulson L B, Smith D E and Phillips C 1978 A 2-year longitudinal study of overdenture patients. Part I. Incidence and control of caries on overdenture abutments. J Prosthet, Dent 40: 486
Toulson L B, Smith D E and Phillips C 1982 A 2-year longitudinal study of overdenture patients. Part II. Assessment of the periodental health of overdenture abutments. J Prosthet Dent 47: 4

Further reading

Removable denture treatment cannot be undertaken successfully without acquaintance with related fields, and to this end the following list of textbooks is suggested as companions to the introductory study of clinical prosthetic dentistry:

CONSERVATIVE DENTISTRY:
Pickard H M 1976 A Manual of Operative Dentistry. 4th Edn. Oxford University Press, London

CROWN AND BRIDGEWORK:
Tylman S D and Malone W F P 1978 Theory and Practice of Crown and Bridgework. 7th Edn. Mosby, St Louis

DENTAL MATERIALS SCIENCE:
Combe E C 1981 Notes on Dental Materials. 4th Edn. Churchill Livingstone, Edinburgh

DENTAL TECHNOLOGY:
Osborne J, Wilson H J and Mansfield M A 1979 Dental Technology and Materials for Students. 7th Edn. Blackwell Oxford

ORAL MEDICINE:
Chisholm D M, Ferguson M M, Jones J H and Mason D K 1978 Introduction to Oral Medicine. Saunders London

ORAL SURGERY:
Moore J R and Gillbe G V 1981 Principles of Oral Surgery. 3rd Edn. Manchester University Press Manchester

ORTHODONTICS:
White T C, Gardiner J H and Leighton B C 1976 Orthodontics for Dental Students. 3rd Edn. Macmillan London

PERIODONTICS:
Pawlaak E A and Hoag A M 1981 Essentials of Periodontics. Mosby, St Louis

Many excellent books on removable prostheses are referred to in the text.

Index

Adhesion, role in denture retention, 19
Aesthetics
    of dentures
        checking of, 146, 148, 152, 157, 202, 208
        unsatisfactory, 157, 214, 218
    effect of tooth loss on, 87
Age of patient, and treatment planning, 46, 47
Ala, 3
Alginate, 128, 131
    primary impressions, 172
    secondary impressions, 172, 174
Allergy, 34
    to denture base material, 217
Altered cast technique, 134, 164
Alveolar ridge
    residual, 4, 5
    resorption of, 4, 5
Alveoplasty, 54
Analysing rod, 40
Anatomy
    extra-oral surface, 3
    intra-oral surface, 4
    structures influencing periphery of dentures, 6
Angle
    of mouth, 3
    naso-labial, 3
Anxiety, 30, 32
Aphthous ulceration, 53
Appearance see aesthetics
Articulation
    balanced, 24, 193
    definition, 24
    laws of, 193
Articulators, 68
    adjustable, 69, 73
    average value, 69, 73
    classification, 68
    development, 68
    selection, 73
    simple hinge, 68, 73

Bennett movement, 13
Bimeter, 63
Body image, 30
Bone loss after extractions, 5
Bracing in clasp unit, 100

Bridges, fixed, 46
Bruxism, 25
Buccal bars, 112, 124, 126
Buccinator muscle, 7, 8, 9, 22

Candida infection, 26, 52, 53
Caninus muscle, 9
Canthus, outer, 3
Carbon marker, 40
Cast, altered, technique of, 134, 164
Cast surveyor, 28, 40
Casts
    study
        dentate mouths, 39
        edentulous mouths, 43
        preparation of, 130
        surveying, 39, 42, 43
    working
        material for, 131
        preparation for denture finishing, 203
        production, 131
Cementum, 7
Cheek biting
    complete dentures, 199, 216
    partial dentures, 156
Cheilitis, angular, 52
Clasps, 96
    arms, classification of, 96
        Blatterfein system, 98
        Ney system, 97
    back-action, 97
        reverse, 98
    continuous, 105, 123, 166
        modified, 112, 124, 126
    and denture retention, 22, 120
        direct, 165
        indirect, 105
    design, 100
    functions, 100
    lateral stresses conveyed by, 25
    materials for, 43
    nervous control mechanism and, 25
    ring, 98
Cohesion, role in denture retention, 18
Columella, 3
Communication with patient, 30, 31, 32
Condylar guidance angle, 194

Connectors, 124
    as indirect retainers, 106, 108, 109, 123
    major, 107, 124
        material for, 125
        types of, 124, 125
    minor, 124
    partial division of, 114
Constrictor muscle, superior, 9
Contact, premature, 25
    partial dentures, 147, 153
Contour, maximum, location of, 39
Craddock classification of partial dentures, 89
Cross-bite arrangement of teeth, 197
Cummer arms, 106, 123, 166
Cysts, 54

Dentist-patient relationship, 29, 30, 32
Denture space, 27
    delineation, 176
Dentures
    care of, 211
    design principles, 24–28
    form, impression to define, 175
    immediate, 46
    partial see partial dentures
    periphery, anatomical structures influencing, 6
    remounting of, 209
    retention see retention
    sectional, 103
    stability see stability
    tolerance of, 26
        see also intolerance
    trial see trial dentures
    weight, 20
Depressor anguli oris muscle, 8, 9
Depressor labii inferioris muscle, 8
Design
    partial dentures, 116–126
    principles, 24–28
Diabetes, 34
Diagnosis 45
    dentate mouths, 45
    differential, 45
    edentulous mouths, 48
Digastric muscle, 13
Disabled patients, 46, 48

Drug therapy
  effects on denture treatment, 36
  identification of, 34, 35

Elastomers, 128, 131
Embrasure hooks, 94
Epilepsy, 34, 46
Equilibrium, zone of see neutral zone
Examination, 32–44
  clinical, 36
  at insertion, 151, 207
  review, 155, 214
Exostoses, 54
Exteroception, influence of dentures on,
    25

Face-bow, 71
  hinge axis, 72
  simple, use of, 71
  use in construction
    complete dentures, 187
    partial dentures, 139
Fovea palatinae, 4, 6
Freeway space, 11
Frenectomy, 54
Frenula
  buccal, 5
  labial, 5
  lingual, 5
Frenum
  buccal, 4, 5, 8
  labial, 4, 7, 8
  lingual, 5
Friction and denture retention, 21

Galvanism, oral, 15, 158
Genial tubercles, surgical removal, 55
Genioglossus muscle, 9
Geniohyoid muscle, 9, 13
Gingivae, 4, 7
Gingival crevice, 7
Gingival groove, 7
Gingival remnant, lingual, 4
Glands, mucous, 14
Gothic arch tracing, 184
Granuloma, denture, 53
Grinding, selective, 209
Guiding planes, 42
  tooth preparation, 53

Hamular notch, 8
Handicapped patients, 46, 48
Health status of patient, 34
  contraindicating dentures, 46, 48
History taking, 32
Hydrocolloids, 128, 131
Hygiene, oral, 26, 45
Hyperkeratosis, 53
Hyperplasia
  denture, 53
  papillary, 52
  surgical removal, 54

Immediate dentures, 46
Implants, 49
Impression compound, 169
Impression paste, zinc oxide-eugenol see
    zinc oxide-eugenol
Impression plaster
  for complete dentures, 172
  for jaw registration, 138
Impression trays, 56
  complete dentures
    insertion and removal, 170
    for plaster, 172
    primary impressions, 169
    secondary impressions, 172
    for zinc oxide-eugenol paste, 174
  partial dentures
    insertion and removal, 59
    primary impressions, 127
    secondary impressions, 130
Impressions
  minimal pressure, 59
  pressure, 58, 133
    free-end saddle partial dentures, 164
  primary
    complete dentures, 169
    partial dentures, 127
      choice of material, 128
      procedure, 128
  procedures, 56–60
    altered cast, 134, 164
    complete dentures, 172
    partial dentures, 128, 131
    for relining
      complete dentures, 177
      partial dentures, 134
    special, 133
  secondary
    complete dentures, 172
    partial dentures, 130
      choice of material, 131
  selective pressure, 58, 175
Incisal guidance angle, 194
Incisive papilla, 4
Incisivus labii inferioris muscle, 8, 9
Incisivus labii superioris muscle, 7, 9
Insertion
  checking prior to, 151, 207
  complete dentures, 207–212
    undercuts and, 205
  partial dentures, 151–153
  path of, 40
Instructions to patients, 153, 211
Intercuspal position, maximal, 12
Interocclusal distance, 11, 61
  measurement of, 11
Intolerance
  complete dentures, 214, 219
  partial dentures, 154, 158
  see also tolerance

Jaw
  positions, terminology describing, 11
  upper, examination of, 37
Jaw relation(s), 11
  errors in, 25

horizontal, 11
  checking, with dentures, 148, 152,
      203, 209
  establishment of, 64
    complete dentures, 183
    partial dentures, 137
    at position of mandibular retrusion,
        139
  registration, 65, 138, 183
lateral, 65, 66, 140, 185
protrusive, 65, 66, 140, 185
registration
  complete dentures, 179–190
  partial dentures, 136–141
  principles of, 61–67
rest, 11, 61
  factors influencing, 61
retruded (centric), 11, 183
vertical, 61
  checking, with dentures, 148, 152,
      202, 208
  establishment of, 62
    complete dentures, 181
    partial dentures, 136
  registration, 65, 136, 182

Kennedy classification of partial
    dentures, 89

Labial bars, 112, 124, 126
Labio-mental groove, 3
Laboratory see technician
Leukoplakia, 53
Levator anguli oris muscle, 7, 9
Lichen planus, 53
Lingual bars, 110, 124, 126
Lingual plates, 112, 124, 126
  partial division of, 114
Lining materials, soft, 49
Lisping, correction of, 157
Looseness
  complete dentures, 213, 218
  partial dentures, 154, 156

Magnetic forces to aid denture retention,
    21
Mandible
  examination of, 38
  movements of, 11
    Bennett, 13
    border, 12
    lateral, 195
    muscles producing, 13
    neuromuscular control, 24
    protrusive, 193, 194
  position of, terminology describing, 11
  support during impression taking, 59
Masseter muscle, 9, 13
Mastication
  effect of tooth loss on, 87, 89
  inefficient, with dentures, 214, 218,
      220
  muscles of, 13

Maxillary ridge, resorption of, 4
Maximal intercuspal position, 12
Mentalis muscle, 8
Metal framework, cast, 145
Modiolus, 9
Mouth
 angle of, 3
 preparation for prosthetic treatment,
  51–55
Mucous glands, palatine, 14
Mucous membrane, oral
 classification, 6
 examination, 37
 functions, 6
Muscles
 influencing denture base design, 6–9
 of mastication, 13
 role in denture retention, 22
 see also specific muscles
Mylohyoid muscle, 9, 13, 23
Mylohyoid ridge, resection of, 55

Naso-labial angle, 3
Naso-labial groove, 3
Nausea, dentures and, 154, 214, 219
Neutral zone, 27
 effect of tooth loss on, 88

Occlusal plane
 guide, 180
 placement of, 180
Occlusal rims
 prescription for, 133
 use in jaw registration, 138, 139, 140,
  179, 182, 183, 184
Occlusion
 balanced, 24
  complete dentures, 191, 193
  partial dentures, 143
 checking, with dentures, 146, 208
 definition, 11
 disrupted, restoration of, 24
 functional, 24
 modification of, 53
 vertical dimension, 61, 62
  errors in, 64
  estimation of, 64
Onlays, 95
Oral galvanism, 15
Oral hygiene, 26, 45
Oral sphincter, 9
Orbicularis oris muscle, 7, 8, 9, 22
Overclosure, 64
 tooth loss and, 88
Overdentures, 223–225
Overjet, provision of, 193, 199, 216

Pain
 from complete dentures, 213, 215
 from partial dentures, 154
  causes, 155, 156
  treatment, 156

Palatal arms, 107, 166
Palatal bars, 108, 124, 166
Palatal plates, 110, 125, 166
Palate, 5
Palatoglossal arch, 4, 9
Papillae
 incisive, 4
 sublingual, 5
Parkinson's disease, 34
Partial dentures, 87–166
 care of, 153
 classification, 89
 component elements, 92–115
  see also individual components
 definition, 87
 design, 116–126
 free-end saddle, 159–166
  design problems, 159
 impressions for see impressions
 insertion, 151–153, 207
 intolerance, 154, 158
 looseness, 154, 156
 mandibular, provision of support, 119,
  159
 masticatory efficiency, 143
 maxillary, provision of support, 119,
  160
 reasons for providing, 87
 relining see relining
 retention see retention
 review of, 154–158
 stability see stability
 support for, provision of, 118
  free-end saddle dentures, 119, 159,
   162
 as treatment choice, 47
 treatment planning for, 48
 trial stage, 145–150
Patients
 attitudes of, 29
 disabled, 46
 health status of, 34, 46
 history taking, 32
 instructions to, 153, 211
 relationship with dentist, 29, 30
Periodontal ligament, 7
 proprioceptors in, 25
Periodontal treatment of denture
  patients, 51
Periodontium, 6
Philtrum, 3
Phonetics, 15, 157
Plaque
 accumulation, 26
 control, 26, 45, 51
Plaster see impression plaster
Platysma muscle, 13
Polishing, 211
Polysulphides, 128, 131
Posterior palatal seal (post-dam), 23
 preparation, 203
Precision attachments, 22, 101, 120
 as direct retainers, 165
 as indirect retainers, 105
Prescription writing for technician see
  technician

Proprioception, influence of dentures on,
  25
Psychological factors in denture
  treatment, 29–31
Pterygoid
 hamulus, 8
 muscle, lateral, 13
 muscle, medial, 9, 13
 plates, 8
Pterygomandibular raphe, 7, 8, 9

Radiography, use in clinical assessment,
  38
Raphe
 median, 4
 pterygomandibular, 7, 8
Rebasing, impressions for, 177
Records, history taking for, 32
Relief areas, 204, 207
Relining, impressions for
 complete dentures, 177
 partial dentures, 134
  free-end saddle, 164
Rest seats
 forms of, 95
 tooth preparation, 53
Rests, 92
 cingulum, 93
 functions, 94
 incisal, 93
 as indirect retainers, 104, 122, 123
 occlusal, 92
  mesial placement, 114
 support for saddles, 118, 119
Retainers
 direct, 96, 119
 indirect, 104, 120
  choice of, 123
  placement of, 123
Retching, 154, 158, 219
Retention, 18–23
 checking, 146, 147, 152, 201, 208
 direct,
  provision of, 119
   free-end saddle dentures, 161, 165
 factors affecting, 18
  mechanical, 21
  physical, 18
  physiological, 22
 indirect, provision of, 120
  free-end saddle dentures, 162, 165
 saliva and, 14, 15, 18, 19
 trial dentures, 146, 147, 201
Retromolar pad, 4, 6
Review of finished dentures
 complete, 213–222
 partial, 154–158
Ridges, flabby, surgery of, 54
Roots, retained, 54
Rugae, 4
 palatal, 6

Saddles, 92
 bounded, support for, 116, 118

Saddles (contd)
  classification, 92, 116
  design, 116
  free-end
    relining of, 134
    support for, 116, 118
  provision of support for, 118
Saliva, 13
  and denture retention, 14, 15, 18, 19
  excessive, 15, 158, 222
  functions, 13
  state of, and denture design, 38
  variations in flow, 15
  viscosity, 19
Salivary glands, sublingual, ducts, 5
Sensitivity to denture base material, 217
Sialorrhoea, 15
Silicones, 128
Soft tissue
  disorders, treatment of, 51
  distortion of, 51
  surgery, 54
Speech
  dentures and, 15
    complete, problems of, 214, 217, 219
    partial, problems of, 154, 157
  effect of tooth loss on, 87
  production, 15, 157
Springs to aid denture retention, 21
Stability, 18
  complete dentures, checking, 201, 208
  partial dentures, 143
    checking, 146, 148, 152
Stomatitis, denture, 52
Stress-breakers, 113, 124, 146, 148, 162
Study casts see casts, study
Sublingual folds, 5
Sublingual papillae, 5
Sulci, 4
  extension, 54
Surface tension, role in denture
            retention, 18
Surveying, 39
  procedure, 42
Surveyor, cast, 28, 40

Technician, provision of information to
  with first impressions, 130, 171
  jaw registration stage, 140, 189
  with second impressions, 133
  with trial dentures
    complete, 206
    partial, 149

Teeth
  anterior
    inclination of, 191
    relationship between, 192
    see also under teeth, artificial
  artificial
    arrangement
      anterior teeth, 142, 191
      cross-bite, 197
      posterior teeth, 143, 193, 196
    colour
      anterior teeth, 79, 142, 188
      posterior teeth, 84, 189
    form
      anterior teeth, 77, 188
      posterior teeth, 81, 189
    material for
      anterior teeth, 80, 188
      posterior teeth, 84, 140, 189
    selection principles, 75–84, 140
      anterior teeth, 75–80
      posterior teeth, 80–84, 189
    size
      anterior teeth, 75, 187
      posterior teeth, 80, 188
    texture, 78, 188
  examination of, 37
  extraction as treatment choice, 47
  modification of, in denture patients, 53
  opposing complete denture, 47
  overeruption of, 88
  partial loss of, effects, 87
  premature contact between, 25
    partial dentures, 147, 153
  setting up, 180
  unerupted, 54
Temporalis muscles, 13
Temporomandibular joint, 10
  dysfunction syndrome, 64
  effect of tooth loss on, 88, 89
  pain, premature contact and, 25
  proprioception, 25
Thrush, 53
Tolerance of dentures, 26
  see also intolerance
Tongue
  biting
    complete dentures and, 199, 216
    partial dentures and, 156
  cramping of, 156, 216, 220
  and denture retention, 22, 201
  examination of, 38
  position relative to denture, 201
Torsion bars, 114
Torus mandibularis, 6, 38
  surgical removal, 54

Torus palatinus, 6, 38
  surgical removal, 54
Tracing, gothic arch, 184
Tragus, 3
Trauma caused by dentures, 26, 52
Treatment planning, 45
  dentate mouths, 45
  edentulous mouths, 48
Trial dentures
  complete, 200–206
  partial, 145–150
    cast metal framework, 145
Tuberosity, 4
Tumours
  hard tissue, 54
  soft tissue, 53, 54

Undercut areas, 39
  enclosed by denture, 42
Undercut gauge, 40, 41, 43
Undercuts
  elimination of unwanted, 41, 43
  engagement
    by clasps, 100
    and denture retention, 21
  insertion and, 205
  production of, 53, 99
  retention, 42
  surveying of, 40, 41, 43

Vacuum devices to aid denture retention,
            20
Vestibule, 4
Vibrating line, 5, 8

Wax wafer jaw registration, 136, 138,
            139, 140, 186
Whistling, correction of, 157
Willis Bite Gauge, 62, 63

X-rays, use in clinical assessment, 38
Xerostomia, 15

Zinc oxide-eugenol impression paste
  for complete dentures, 174
  use in jaw registration, 138
  for relines, 134, 177
Zone of equilibrium (minimum conflict)
            see neutral zone
Zygomatic process of maxilla, 7, 8
Zygomaticus muscle, 9